CW01506776

PHYSICAL LITERACY
THE WORLD

Physical Literacy across the World records the progress of the concept of physical literacy over the last decade. It examines developments, issues and controversies in physical literacy studies, and looks at how the concept has been implemented around the world.

Contributions from practitioners and researchers across the world tell unique stories of the way physical literacy is changing perceptions of physical activity through research and the generation of scholarly writing, the creation of new national and local policies, and the development of partnerships with a range of professions. The book argues that physical literacy has value beyond formal education, such as in occupational and recreational settings, as well as for early years children and older people, and shows how life story methods can explain our physical literacy journeys. At root, it sets out a case for the significance and value of physical literacy as making a notable contribution to human flourishing.

This is important reading for anyone with an interest in physical activity, health and well-being, sport studies, physical education, or the philosophy related to physical activity.

Margaret Whitehead is Visiting Professor at the University of Bedfordshire, UK.

Routledge Studies in Physical Education and Youth Sport
Series Editor: David Kirk, University of Strathclyde, UK

The *Routledge Studies in Physical Education and Youth Sport* series is a forum for the discussion of the latest and most important ideas and issues in physical education, sport, and active leisure for young people across school, club and recreational settings. The series presents the work of the best well-established and emerging scholars from around the world, offering a truly international perspective on policy and practice. It aims to enhance our understanding of key challenges, to inform academic debate, and to have a high impact on both policy and practice, and is thus an essential resource for all serious students of physical education and youth sport.

Also available in this series

Digital Technology in Physical Education
Global Perspectives
Edited by Jeroen Koekoek and Ivo van Hilvoorde

Redesigning Physical Education
An Equity Agenda in Which Every Child Matters
Edited by Hal A. Lawson

Play, Physical Activity and Public Health
The Reframing of Children's Leisure Lives
Stephanie A. Alexander, Katherine L. Frohlich and Caroline Fusco

Young People, Social Media and Health
Victoria A. Goodyear and Kathleen M. Armour

Physical Literacy across the World
Edited by Margaret Whitehead

www.routledge.com/sport/series/RSPEYS

PHYSICAL LITERACY ACROSS THE WORLD

Edited by Margaret Whitehead

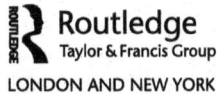

Routledge
Taylor & Francis Group

LONDON AND NEW YORK

First published 2019
by Routledge
2 Park Square, Milton Park, Abingdon, Oxon OX14 4RN

and by Routledge
52 Vanderbilt Avenue, New York, NY 10017

Routledge is an imprint of the Taylor & Francis Group, an informa business

British Library Cataloguing-in-Publication Data
A catalogue record for this book is available from the British Library

Library of Congress Cataloging-in-Publication Data
A catalog record has been requested for this book

ISBN: 978-1-138-57154-9 (hbk)
ISBN: 978-1-138-57155-6 (pbk)
ISBN: 978-0-203-70269-7 (ebk)

Typeset in Bembo
by Swales & Willis Ltd, Exeter, Devon, UK

MIX
Paper from
responsible sources
FSC
www.fsc.org
FSC™ C013985

Printed in the United Kingdom
by Henry Ling Limited

CONTENTS

Notes on contributors   *viii*

Acknowledgements   *x*

PART I

Physical literacy moving forward   **1**

1 Overview and recent developments in physical literacy   3
   Margaret Whitehead

2 Definition of physical literacy: developments and issues   8
   Margaret Whitehead

3 Aspects of physical literacy: clarification and discussion
   with particular reference to the physical domain   19
   Margaret Whitehead

4 In support of physical literacy throughout life   32
   Margaret Whitehead

5 What does physical literacy look like? Overarching
   principles and specific descriptions   45
   Margaret Whitehead

6 Charting the physical literacy journey   74
   Margaret Whitehead

PART II
International perspectives on physical literacy   **97**

7   Introduction to international perspectives on physical
literacy   99
Margaret Whitehead

8   A brief history of physical literacy in Australia   105
Richard Keegan, Dean Dudley and Lisa Barnett

9   Physical literacy in Canada   125
Dwayne Sheehan, Daniel Robinson and Lynn Randall

10   Perspectives on physical literacy in continental Europe   143
*Jeroen Koekoek, Niek Pot, Wytse Walinga and
Ivo van Hilvoorde*

11   Physical literacy in India   156
Pankaj Markandey and Nigel Green

12   Aotearoa/New Zealand's physical literacy journey   167
Karen Laurie

13   Physical and food literacy: a holistic approach to public
health in Scotland   181
Chris Topping, Jo Kopela, Isla Gibson and Sandy Whitelaw

14   Physical literacy in the United States   200
E. Paul Roetert

15   Physical literacy development in Wales   215
Helen Hughes

16   Reflection on international perspectives   230
Margaret Whitehead

PART III
Physical literacy: establishing significance and looking ahead   **237**

17   Physical literacy as a journey   239
Liz Taplin

18 Human flourishing and physical literacy 255
   Elizabeth Durden-Myers and Margaret Whitehead

19 Human flourishing, human nature and physical literacy 265
   Elizabeth Durden-Myers and Margaret Whitehead

20 The significance of physical literacy in human life,
   conclusions and the way ahead 272
   Margaret Whitehead

Explanatory glossary 278
Author Index 283
Subject Index 285

CONTRIBUTORS

Lisa Barnett is Associate Professor at Deakin University, Australia.

Dean Dudley is Senior Lecturer in Health & Physical Education in the Faculty of Human Sciences at Macquarie University, Australia.

Elizabeth Durden-Myers is Senior Lecturer in Physical Education in the Faculty of Education at the University of Gloucestershire, UK.

Isla Gibson is Research Assistant at the University of Glasgow, UK.

Nigel Green is Senior Lecturer at Liverpool John Moores University, UK.

Helen Hughes is Senior Officer at Sport Wales, Cardiff, UK.

Ivo van Hilvoorde is Professor at Windesheim University of Applied Sciences, Zwolle, and Assistant Professor at Vrije Universiteit, Amsterdam, the Netherlands.

Richard Keegan is Associate Professor of Sport and Exercise Psychology at the University of Canberra, Australia.

Jeroen Koekoek is Senior Lecturer of Physical Education and Sport Pedagogy at Windesheim University of Applied Sciences, Zwolle, the Netherlands.

Jo Kopela is Health and Wellbeing Specialist at NHS Dumfries and Galloway, UK.

Karen Laurie is Young People Consultant – Early Years and Primary age: Community Sport Team at Sport New Zealand, NZ.

Pankaj Markandey is Member of The Gopichand Academy Physical Literacy Team, India.

Niek Pot is Policy Adviser in Sports at the Municipality of The Hague/Windesheim University of Applied Sciences, the Netherlands.

Lynn Randall is Professor at the University of New Brunswick, Faculty of Education, Canada.

Daniel Robinson is Associate Professor and Chair in the Department of Teacher Education at St. Francis Xavier University, Canada.

E. Paul Roetert is Sports and Physical Activity Consultant/Researcher at Broadlands, Virginia, United States.

Dwayne Sheehan is Associate Professor of Health and Physical Education in the Faculty of Health, Community and Education at Mount Royal University, Calgary, Canada.

Liz Taplin is Associate Professor/Senior Lecturer in Primary Physical Education at Plymouth Institute of Education, Plymouth University, UK.

Chris Topping is Health and Wellbeing Specialist and Director General in Health and Wellbeing at Dumfries and Galloway Council, Dumfries, UK.

Wytse Walinga is Teacher/Researcher at Windesheim University of Applied Sciences, the Netherlands.

Margaret Whitehead is Visiting Professor at the University of Bedfordshire, UK.

Sandy Whitelaw is Senior Lecturer in Health and Social Policy at the School of Interdisciplinary Studies, University of Glasgow, UK.

ACKNOWLEDGEMENTS

There are two groups of people who I would like to thank. First, those colleagues who have played a part in the establishment and running of the International Physical Literacy Association. This includes our Trustees, Len Gooblar (rtd), Niek Pot (rtd), Jeanne Keay, Susan Capel, Chris Topping and E. Paul Roetert. Also included are the Officers of the Association, Liz Taplin, Elizabeth Durden-Myers, Nigel Green and Fiona Diffey. Their generosity in giving their support and time has been exceptional. Second, I am very grateful to all those who have played a part in the writing of this book. Most significant are the authors of the chapters in the international perspectives part of the book. Thanks are also due to those who have worked with me in relation to applying general principles to groups of participants other than those in school. Many of these people have been named in particular chapters of the book. I am also grateful for the support of colleagues from Canada, the United States and Australia who have written briefly about their different schemes to chart progress in respect of physical literacy journeys. I would also like to pay tribute to Len Almond. While he is no longer with us, he was instrumental in our work, challenging our thinking in very many areas, most notably with reference to the primacy of movement and the relationship between physical literacy and human flourishing.

In relation both to the running of the Association and writing this book, there are numerous people who have given invaluable service to the cause of promoting physical literacy. It is on account of all these people, named and not named, that physical literacy is recognised and advocated across the world. Indeed, without this dedicated, tireless and enthusiastic team of people, this book could not have been written. Alongside me for very many years was my late husband, John. I will always be grateful for his love and untiring support. Without him, I doubt my journey would have been so productive. In this book, we are sharing and celebrating a success story. A story that is only just beginning but a story that is making a difference. Together, we can be even more successful. We can reach more people and encourage more people to 'choose physical activity for life'.

PART I
Physical literacy moving forward

1

OVERVIEW AND RECENT DEVELOPMENTS IN PHYSICAL LITERACY

Margaret Whitehead

It is a privilege to edit a second book on physical literacy. It is also a very welcome opportunity to bring readers up to date with the development of the concept and to clarify a range of issues. It also allows readers to learn about the spread of the concept worldwide.

Physical Literacy throughout the Lifecourse was published in 2010, and was the outcome of over 10 years of study, presentations across the world and extended dialogue with many in the field of physical activity. The goals of this publication were threefold. First, to explain the nature and background to the concept, particularly from a philosophical point of view. Second, to enable a distinguished group of writers to share their views on the credibility of the concept from their perspective in different fields. And finally, the publication outlined the implications of adopting physical literacy as a goal of physical education. While *Physical Literacy throughout the Lifecourse* was predominantly UK-focused and school-based, the book stimulated debate both internationally and from those involved in promoting physical activity throughout the lifecourse. The book has played a key role in challenging colleagues to re-evaluate the place of physical activity in life and to debate how best to engage participants in such a way that the wide-ranging potential benefits of participation can be realised. Such has been the interest in the concept that this publication is needed not only to share developments, but also to review the fundamental nature of physical literacy.

Building on the philosophy of the 2010 publication, this new book aims to argue that the concept of physical literacy is well founded philosophically and in tune with the nature of human being, thus making it pertinent to everyone – of whatever age and wherever they live. However, at the same time, it will be suggested that it is robust enough to accommodate interpretations that reflect different cultures across the world. These aims have influenced the content of *Physical Literacy across the World*. Broadly, Part I reviews developments and issues in respect of physical literacy, and considers the value and implications of committing to work within the parameters of this concept. Part II comprises chapters from eight different countries, each of which tells a particular story of how the concept has been taken up and developed. Part III builds from the background of Parts I and II, and proposes both that physical literacy can play a significant role in an individual's life and that it can make an important contribution to human flourishing.

While the intent and the content of the two books are distinctive, they also differ from each other in their overall nature. The 2010 publication was an introduction to and explanation of the concept of physical literacy, while the 2019 publication can be seen as a resource. There are three sources of information to be found via this publication: first, the text itself; second, the material referred to on the Web; and finally, the wide range of post 2010 publications identified.

One of the major developments in physical literacy has been the founding of the International Physical Literacy Association. This was created as a result of colleague pressure and became a recognised charity in 2014. The mission of the Association is: 'To enable everyone everywhere to understand and embrace physical activity as an integral part of life by developing a culture that values and promotes physical literacy' (IPLA, 2019). Expressed briefly, the Association advocates 'choosing physical activity for life'. The Association identifies eight objectives (see www.physical-literacy.org.uk), which include: promoting the value of physical literacy worldwide; preserving the integrity of physical literacy; providing a forum to discuss and disseminate research, policy and practice relating to all aspects of physical literacy; and coordinating a global community committed to physical literacy.

Since its foundation, the Association has run a number of conferences, workshops, forums and seminars in the UK, and now has plans to organise gatherings further afield in the future. All these afore mentioned events have been attended by colleagues from across the world, and one conference was jointly organised with colleagues from the field of medicine. These events, as well as the IPLA website, have generated interest across the world. Key international players have contributed the chapters in Part II. Recently, new contacts have been made with South Korea, Japan, China, Taiwan, Malta, Singapore and Iran. In addition, over the last two years, members have presented at conferences and courses in many countries, including Luxembourg (UNESCO), Vienna (International Schools), Canada (Sport for Life), India, Greece, Jersey, Brazil, the Isle of Man, Ireland and Scotland. In addition, in 2013, the International Council of Sport Science and Physical Education (ICSSPE) asked colleagues to draw up an edition of their Bulletin. The Bulletin comprises 48 short papers covering a wide range of aspects of physical literacy, including a number written by colleagues from across the world. More recently, the IPLA has produced a short video, 'Active for Life', created a range of draft guidance material, and in 2018 worked with the editor of the *Journal of Teaching in Physical Education* to produce a special issue on physical literacy (IPLA, 2018). It is also good to report that Sport England has included reference to physical literacy in a recent paper (2019) and that *Physical Literacy throughout the Lifecourse* has been translated into Persian and Portuguese.

Content of *Physical Literacy across the World*

Space does not allow material from the first publication to be repeated; however, much of Part I in this new publication will refer back to the previous book, and readers are advised to be familiar with the earlier text to understand and position new thinking and developments. The intention is to move on from earlier work, highlighting specific key areas of discussion that have arisen through initiatives led by the IPLA and extensive worldwide consideration and debate. Such is the growing number of publications pertinent to PL that readers are advised to follow up the recommended texts as there is not room in this book to look in depth at many of these.

Physical Literacy across the World is divided into three parts. Part I is entitled 'Physical literacy moving forward'. Part II has a worldwide focus, and is entitled 'International perspectives on physical literacy'. Part III looks broadly at physical literacy in the context of human life, and is entitled 'Physical literacy: establishing significance and looking ahead'.

Part I has six chapters. Chapter 1, 'Overview and recent developments in physical literacy', updates readers on developments since the publication in 2010 of *Physical Literacy throughout the Lifecourse* (Whitehead, 2010) and outlines the content of physical literacy across the world. Chapter 2, 'Definition of physical literacy: developments and issues', sets out the subtle changes in the definition and the attributes. Alternative definitions used around the world are considered briefly. The chapter also addresses a concern that philosophy is not mentioned in the definition, and the wisdom of using the notion of 'literacy' alongside the term 'physical'. Chapter 3, 'Aspects of physical literacy: clarification and discussion with particular reference to the physical domain', covers the assumptions that have arisen around some of the domains referred to in the definition. Significant here is the place of fundamental movement skills within the physical domain. Other contentious areas are also addressed, such as the relevance of physical literacy to all and the relationship between physical literacy and physical education. Chapter 4, 'In support of physical literacy throughout life', outlines the value of physical literacy from a philosophical perspective and from a social justice standpoint. This is followed by a debate on physical literacy as an end in itself and as a means to achieve extrinsic ends. The chapter closes with a brief survey of the value of physical literacy to different groups of people. Chapter 5, 'What does physical literacy look like? Overarching principles and specific descriptions', surveys the implications of adopting physical literacy as an aspiration in promoting and participating in physical activity. Central here to maintain authentic practice is a commitment to the philosophy underpinning the concept. General principles of this adherence are set out, and these are followed by more detailed recommendations for practitioners working with different groups of participants across the lifespan. Chapter 6, 'Charting the physical literacy journey', sets out the current IPLA recommendations and then includes short pieces from Canada, the United States and Australia where instruments have been or are being devised.

Part II comprises eight chapters written by colleagues who have played a central role in developing physical literacy in their country. These are presented in alphabetical order of the countries included. The spread of constituencies in which these colleagues are based demonstrates the breadth of relevance of the concept. For example, initial interest in Canada came from an independent body, Canada Sport 4 All (CS4A), while the initial drive in Australia was created by a partnership between the national government and the university sector. Adoption of the concept of physical literacy in both New Zealand and Wales came through work in sports organisations, and adoption in a region of Scotland developed from interest shown by a local government authority. Each of the key individuals in continental Europe, the United States and India have a particular background, and thus a unique starting point in spreading the concept. In continental Europe, academics in the university sector have been particularly active, with research taking a high profile. Work in the United States burgeoned from investigations by the National Physical Education Association, and in India a national sports star was instrumental in alerting his country to the value of the concept of physical literacy for all. Each chapter tells a unique story of the debate surrounding the introduction and operationalisation of the notion of physical literacy. All have met both enthusiastic acceptance and scepticism. All have worked, and are working, tirelessly to spread the concept to a wide range of constituencies, such as those involved in working with children in the early years, participants with disabilities, the medical profession, and those caring for the elderly. Their reflections are revealing and their ambitions impressive.

Part III focuses on the value of physical literacy both from the perspective of the life patterns of individuals and in respect of enhancing human flourishing. Chapter 17, 'Physical literacy as a journey', discusses the value of seeing physical literacy as a journey. Using some examples of journeys from across the world, the chapter considers what can be learnt from looking at physical literacy as a journey. Chapters 18 and 19 discuss the place of physical literacy in respect of its contribution to human flourishing. The former, 'Human flourishing and physical literacy', considers the philosophical background to human flourishing and physical literacy, and then compares the two dispositions in respect of their constituents and characteristics. The latter, 'Human flourishing, human nature and physical literacy', looks at human flourishing and human needs. The question is raised as to how far physical literacy can be seen as an essential feature of human nature. Key considerations here relate to human needs and human potential and resources. Chapter 20, 'The significance of physical literacy in human life, conclusions and the way ahead', looks back on what has been learnt from looking widely and deeply at the notion of physical literacy across the world and speculates on the opportunities ahead. Importantly, it considers how IPLA members and other committed colleagues can best work together to realise the aspiration of developing a worldwide population committed to 'choosing physical activity for life'.

Readers should note that the material in this book was accurate at time of writing. Please follow up website references to find further developments. The IPLA is always pleased to hear from those with an interest in physical literacy. Please contact us via our website (www.physical-literacy.org.uk).

A short explanatory glossary is to be found at the end of the book.

References

Bulletin on Physical Literacy (2013) ICSSPE Bulletin no. 65. (See also on IPLA Website: www.physical-literacy.org.uk.)

International Physical Literacy Association (IPLA) (2019) *Physical Literacy across the World: Resources and References.* Available at: www.physical-literacy.org.uk/plaw-resources-and-references/ (accessed 14 March 2019).

IPLA (2018) Special issue on Operationalising Physical Literacy, *Journal of Teaching in Physical Education*, 37(3).

Sport England (2019) Active Lives. Children and Young People Survey 2019. Available at: www.sportengland.org/research/active_people_survey.aspx.

Whitehead, M.E. (ed.) (2010) *Physical Literacy throughout the Lifecourse.* London: Routledge.

2

DEFINITION OF PHYSICAL LITERACY

Developments and issues

Margaret Whitehead

Introduction

This chapter is designed to remind readers of the essential tenets of physical literacy and to present significant developments since the publication of *Physical Literacy throughout the Lifecourse* (Whitehead, 2010). Areas of discussion cover the definition of the attributes, and the legitimacy of aligning 'literacy' with 'physical'.

The definition of physical literacy

The concept of physical literacy was developed as a result of a concern for the lack of respect shown for the human embodied dimension and from the philosophical study undertaken to investigate the role of the embodiment throughout life. The concept was created as a rallying call to underline the essential contribution of this dimension to human life. The definition (see Table 2.1) should be read as having two messages. The final section identifies the fundamental *raison d'être* of physical literacy – this being the aspiration that all should 'value and take responsibility for participation in physical activity for life'. The first section proposes the means by which this aspiration may be met, being the 'motivation, confidence, physical competence, and knowledge and understanding' in respect of participation in physical activity.

Taken together, the aspiration and the means generate the definition.

TABLE 2.1 Definition of physical literacy

As appropriate to each individual, physical literacy can be described as the *motivation, confidence, physical competence, knowledge and understanding to value and take responsibility for engaging in physical activities for life.*

Since the publication of *Physical Literacy throughout the Lifecourse* (Whitehead, 2010), and influenced by the creation of the International Physical Literacy Association, there has been a modest rewording of the definition of physical literacy.

The final phrase of the definition has been changed from 'to maintain physical activity throughout the lifecourse' to 'to value and take responsibility for engaging in physical activities for life'. This change highlights that the individual should value physical activity and be self-motivated to maintain an active lifestyle.

Thus, the notion of 'physical literacy' can be seen as arising from a belief in the long-term value of engagement in physical activity, and addresses the means by which this may be realised. It is argued that working with this commitment in mind, in all organised or managed physical activity settings, can have far-reaching effects on participation. In addition, the sound philosophical base (Whitehead, 2010, 2016–2018) on which the concept is built can provide a secure foundation from which to make a case for the value of promoting physical activity.

The concept has generated a great deal of debate, which will be reflected in this text. One criticism centres on the fact that while advocating a strongly monist approach, the definition sets out a range of domains – the affective, the physical and the cognitive – that need consideration if lifelong participation is to be fostered. This can be read to indicate that there are, in fact, somewhat separate aspects of human being. As a result, the question is asked, 'Is physical literacy a truly monist concept?' The answer is in the affirmative. Monism champions the situation that while humans are comprised of a number of domains, these are inextricably related to each other. The definition cites the affective, the physical and the cognitive domains, and in most cases any human endeavour is the outcome of a close-knit relationship between these domains. In fact, it is almost impossible to isolate any of these human potentialities. That having been said, each domain carries its own specific characteristics and is studied using particular approaches. Monism reveals both the complexity of the human condition and the intra-relationship between all human domains. This can be exemplified in the philosophical assertion that there are not two things, such as the feeling of fear and the retreat from the situation. The retreat *is* the fear.

There has also been scepticism about the use of 'physical' in the definition. For example, Standal (2015) questions the appropriateness of using the notion of 'physical', on account of its all-too-ready association with the body as an object, and thus dualism. As discussed in Whitehead (2010), terms such as 'movement literacy' and 'embodied literacy' were not judged acceptable. The former was seen as having very many connotations with movement beyond that of humans, while the latter was viewed as too far from language in common use.

Notwithstanding debate surrounding the nature of physical literacy, since the publication of *Physical Literacy throughout the Lifecourse* (Whitehead, 2010), the concept has spread worldwide. This evidences a growing respect for the notion of physical literacy and substantial support for the value of physical activity through the lifespan. However, as will be seen in Part II, which is comprised of chapters written by colleagues from across the world, a number of alternative definitions have been created. For example, the United States includes the concept of desire,

Australia refers to the social domain, and New Zealand makes reference to the spiritual aspect of human being. While modified definitions can cause confusion in a number of ways, particularly in relation to implications for practice and charting progress, a survey of most current definitions shows that, broadly, two essential aspects of the concept are retained. These are: a determination to promote a commitment to physical activity for life; and the appreciation of the holistic nature of human beings that must be recognised and addressed if this first commitment is to be realised. These aspects of the definition clearly identify the value of lifelong participation and the fact that practitioners need to appreciate that those participants with whom they work are complex feeling, moving, thinking individuals. This last observation is in line with the monist principles on which the concept is based. As these two aspects are central tenets of physical literacy, it is suggested that many of the modified definitions are perspectives on the definition rather than challenges to the concept as a whole. In one sense, a particular definition could be seen as contextually functional, and should be judged on its effectiveness to generate practices that are effective in promoting lifelong participation in a particular culture.

The absence of reference to philosophy in the definition

The omission of reference to philosophy in the definition has been questioned. Given that physical literacy has evolved from philosophical writings, and that this has been explained on many occasions, it is unfortunate that some people are concerned that this grounding is not represented in the definition. It would seem that the role of philosophy in respect of the nature of physical literacy needs to be clarified further. In the case of physical literacy, philosophy provides a rationale, not a description. It is the definition that provides a description and answers the question, 'What is physical literacy?' Philosophy does not answer this question. Rather, it answers the question, 'What is the value of physical literacy?' The answer to the second question provides a reasoned case to justify the value of the concept. These two questions are of a different order. Below are two pairs of questions. In each case, the first is factual and descriptive while the second is evaluative: 'How would you describe your house?'/'What is the value of having a house?' Similarly: 'Where are you going today?'/'Why are you going to the gallery?' The questions and answers are of a different nature. Returning to physical literacy, the definition sets out the aspiration of fostering physical literacy and the means by which it might be nurtured. Philosophy has a different task; it looks behind the definition to reveal the beliefs and values that underpin the concept. Monism supports the crucial role of the embodied dimension in human life, while existentialism underwrites the value of being involved in a range of experiences. In addition, phenomenology reminds us that each participant is a unique individual and that this should be considered in the promotion of physical literacy. There is a view that to include detailed reference to the philosophical underpinning in the definition would result in a somewhat unwieldy explanation. That having been said, for those advocating physical literacy, knowledge of the philosophical justifications that underpin the definition is critical, as these provide answers to the questions of purpose and value. It is the authoritative nature of these scholarly philosophical views that give the twenty-first-century presentation of physical literacy validity. In many cases, these views have helped to initiate worldwide interest in the concept.

Attributes of physical literacy

The attributes of physical literacy are intended to clarify the nature of the concept. They are not part of the definition. When the twenty-first-century concept of physical literacy was introduced, the question was posed regarding what characteristics would be evident if an individual is making progress on their physical literacy journey. To this end, a list of attributes was drawn up to expand on the domains cited in the definition: affective, physical and cognitive. While the definition describes a human disposition, the attributes describe behaviours that are symptomatic of progress being made in respect of fostering physical literacy. Following discussion in the IPLA, the attributes listed in Whitehead (2010) have been modified. The rationale for these changes was to ensure that all the domains were adequately covered and that these descriptors could be readily understood by all practitioners. Table 2.2 sets out the current attributes in full and in simplified form.

The attributes highlight each of the domains in the IPLA definition. Motivation and confidence arise from the affective domain, and are referred to in attributes A and B. Physical competence is a manifestation of the physical domain, and is the background to attributes C, D and E. Knowledge and understanding are features of the cognitive domain, and are addressed in attributes F and G. Attribute H addresses both affective and cognitive domains.

While the attributes are designed to describe an individual who is making progress on a physical literacy journey, they can be used to guide practice in a number of ways. They can inform goal-setting, pedagogy and identifying progress. It is valuable to consider each attribute and reflect on how each can inform practice. One example is set out below with reference to attribute A. Later chapters will go into more detail of the pointers to practice signalled by the attributes. The IPLA video 'Active for Life' (see IPLA, 2019) is valuable in depicting the attributes 'in action'.

Attribute A (affective domain) refers to symptomatic behaviours that evidence 'the motivation to be proactive in taking part in physical activity, applying self to physical activity tasks with interest and enthusiasm, and persevering though challenging situations in physical activity environments'. This attribute can influence practice in that it:

- signals the need to provide realistic and achievable goals or challenges appropriate to the individual;
- points to the importance of giving positive and constructive feedback to individuals; and
- provides a focus for monitoring progress (e.g. in judging how far an individual remains on task and evidences perseverance).

TABLE 2.2 Attributes of physical literacy

Attributes	Simplified attributes
Individuals who are making progress on their unique physical literacy journey will demonstrate the following attributes:	*An individual who is making progress in respect of physical literacy will have the following characteristics:*
A. Motivation to be proactive in taking part in physical activity, applying self to physical activity tasks with interest and enthusiasm, and persevering through challenging situations in physical activity environments (affective domain)	Wants to take part in physical activity (affective domain)
B. Confidence in relation to the ability to make progress in learning new tasks and activities, and assurance that these experiences will be rewarding (affective domain)	Has confidence when taking part in different physical activities (affective domain)
C. Movement with poise, economy and effectiveness in a wide variety of challenging situations (physical domain)	Moves efficiently and effectively in different physical activities (physical domain)
D. Thoughtful and sensitive perception in appreciating all aspects of the physical environment, responding as appropriate with imagination and creativity (physical domain)	Has an awareness of movement needs and possibilities in different physical activities (physical domain)
E. The ability to work independently and with others, in physical activities in both cooperative and competitive situations (physical domain)	Can work independently and with others in different physical activities (physical domain)
F. The ability to identify and articulate the essential qualities that influence the effectiveness of movement performance (cognitive domain)	Knows how to improve performance in different physical activities (cognitive domain)
G. An understanding of the principles of holistic embodied health, in respect of a rich and balanced lifestyle (cognitive domain)	Knows how physical activity can improve well-being (cognitive domain)
H. The self-assurance and self-esteem to take responsibility for choosing physical activity for life (affective and cognitive domains)	Has the self-confidence to plan and effect a physically active lifestyle (affective and cognitive domains)

Taken together, the definition and the attributes of physical literacy represent a comprehensive springboard for the development of practitioner work that is true to the concept. As will be seen in Chapter 4, the definition and the attributes provide clear guidance in identifying the answer to the question, 'What does physical literacy look like in practice?'

Issues relating to use of the term 'literacy' in the definition

The use of the term 'literacy' alongside 'physical' has proved controversial. The next section of this chapter will look at the rationale behind this use, reminding readers of the philosophical underpinning of the concept, and thus the aptness of the notion of physical literacy. In addition, it will be acknowledged that the current use of physical literacy is not the first use of the term. Finally, a range of literacies now in use in other areas of human development will be considered alongside physical literacy.

As set out in Whitehead (2010), the notion of 'literacy' was selected on account of its alignment with the existential notion of 'interaction'. In a philosophical context, 'interaction' describes the way that human beings realise their unique nature in a two-way relationship with the world. As individuals perceive the world and act upon it, so they learn about the world and simultaneously learn about themselves. Broadly speaking, literacy can be understood as an ability to interact or engage effectively with the world in which we are situated. Effective interaction or literacy depends on the application of perceptual and actional abilities. In other words, meaningful interaction is a two-way communication process that relies on sensitive and informed perception coupled with versatile and apposite response. All those domains that enable the human to interact with the world are of potential significance in their unique contribution to self-realisation. It is argued that the human embodied dimension is one such avenue of interaction, and therefore has value in its own right (Whitehead, 2010, 2016–2018).

In adopting the concept of physical literacy, there have been a number of misunderstandings. Principal among these has been a perception that physical literacy is purely concerned with cognitive development. Early involvement with the concept in some countries, such as Canada and the United States, focused on cognitive aspects of the concept; however, this has not persisted. There is general agreement that while aspects of knowledge and understanding feature in physical literacy, this is only one domain of the concept, and by no means takes precedence over other domains. It needs to be reiterated that the notion of literacy was not selected to align specifically with, for example, linguistic literacy and mathematical literacy, as a ploy to give the concept 'academic' credibility. 'Literacy' in respect of physical literacy refers to meaningful holistic interaction, and is not to be considered as solely intellectual nor to identify a particular aspect of linguistic acuity.

It has to be said that a basic grasp of the philosophical principles underpinning the concept of physical literacy is essential for a sound understanding of the legitimacy of 'literacy' alongside 'physical'. These cover not only literacy as interaction, but also the holistic nature of humans encompassing a wide range of domains, including the physical domain (Whitehead, 2010, 2016–2018; ILPA, 2019).

It is acknowledged that the current use of the term 'physical literacy', referred to initially in 1993 (Whitehead, 1993), was not the first time that this descriptor had been used. Kiez and Kriellaars (2015) identify 16 references to physical literacy from 1927 to 1979. It is interesting to consider what was understood by 'literacy' in these earlier uses. Approximately eight focused on fitness and health, five identified mastery of physical skills, and five anticipated a variety of benefits in relation to developing communication through movement, providing an opportunity to play or furthering personal development. It is thought-provoking to note that while most uses had a somewhat dualist approach, seeing the embodiment as an object to be honed, there are some that embrace a more holistic outlook. These indicate the benefits physical activity can accrue to individuals. However, there is little evidence that any of these previous uses were founded on philosophical principles, and none generated a sustained interest in the value of capitalising on the human embodied dimension as a feature of a multidimensional individual. It is perhaps the secure grounding in philosophy, as well as support from other disciplines (see later chapters), that has enabled the 1993 concept of physical literacy to engage interest and sustain support across the world for more than 20 years.

The spread of the notion of 'literacy' in the twenty-first century

It is thought-provoking to reflect that alongside the creation and development of physical literacy, there has been considerable interest in the notion of literacy and a mushrooming of appending 'literacy' to other areas of knowledge and understanding.

For example, UNESCO has produced a range of statements on literacy. A 2004 document was written to encourage worldwide linguistic literacy. This reads:

> The United Nations Educational, Scientific and Cultural Organization (UNESCO) defines literacy as the 'ability to identify, understand, interpret, create, communicate and compute, using printed and written materials associated with varying contexts. Literacy involves a continuum of learning in enabling individuals to achieve their goals, to develop their knowledge and potential, and to participate fully in their community and wider society'.
>
> *(UNESCO, 2004)*

While this is specifically aligned with linguistic literacy, the statement is useful in the way it describes literacy as developing a form of interaction. The statement refers to individual abilities, such as understanding, the way the individuals can benefit from a variety of resources, and the potential of these features to enrich communication skills and enable individuals to reach personal goals. It is not difficult to apply this statement to other literacies. For example, with reference to physical literacy the statement could be re-presented as below. Modifications to the UNESCO statement are italicised:

Physical literacy is defined as a human capability that can be described as the ability to identify, understand, interpret, create, respond effectively and communicate, *using the human embodied dimension, within a wide range of situations and* contexts. Physical literacy involves a continuum of *meaningful experiences* enabling individuals to achieve their goals, to develop their knowledge and potential, and to participate fully in their community and wider society.

Notwithstanding the current close association of literacy with linguistics and the UNESCO (2004) statement above, a much more liberal use of the notion of literacy has developed in the last 20 years. The physical domain is certainly not unique in associating literacy with a specific area of concern other than linguistic literacy. A thorough but not exhaustive search on the Web reveals that there are over 30 current uses of 'literacy'. This is not the place to analyse, in detail, all these uses; however, it is of interest to note, as set out in Table 2.3, how far physical literacy aligns with other literacies.

Characteristics A and B show that the majority of literacies are focused on knowledge, skills, abilities, competencies and understanding that enable individuals to function effectively in a particular culture, as well as to be able to participate in practices adopted in a parent society. While physical literacy incorporates embodied techniques/movement patterns in its development, and is sensitive to the context in which these aspects of physicality are developed, it is argued that there is more to physical literacy than an instrumental means to acquire embodied techniques to accommodate cultural practices. Characteristics C, D, E and F reflect a somewhat different focus. Those literacies listed would seem to signal the value of developing the 'literacy' in the interests of the individual's quality of life. Physical literacy aligns strongly with characteristic C in its reference to lifespan value and reasoned commitment throughout life. This characteristic

TABLE 2.3 Characteristics of some literacies

Characteristics cited within description and purpose of literacies	*Literacy area*
A. Focused on developing the knowledge, skill, understanding and competencies needed to function effectively in a particular culture	Nutrition, economic, Internet/digital, climate, political, geo, aesthetic, health, emotional, computer, media, mathematics, science, historical (physical)
B. Concerned to enable effective participation in practices adopted in a parent society	Nutrition, economic, Internet/digital, climate, political, geo, aesthetic, health, emotional, computer, media, mathematics, science, historical (physical)
C. Concerned with being of value throughout life	Nutrition, economic, Internet/digital, health, leisure, computer, mathematics, food (physical)
D. Role played in developing personal responsibility	Climate/nutrition, political, geo, health, leisure, emotional, food, historical (physical)
E. Role played in furthering personal fulfilment	Artistic, geo, leisure, emotional, musical (physical)
F. Concerned with benefit to the development of the individual	Dance, emotional, leisure (physical)

is not always mentioned specifically in respect of other literacies; however, it would seem to be inferred from assertions concerning long-term benefits. Characteristics D, E and F refer specifically to the individual, and cover breadth of development, furthering personal fulfilment and taking personal responsibility. It is interesting to note that a number of literacies preface their presentations with the clear assertion that their concept goes beyond linguistic literacy and that others continue to debate the nature of literacy in their area of work.

The legitimacy of physical literacy would seem to be endorsed by its similarity to other literacies. Physical literacy is most closely aligned to emotional literacy, leisure literacy and musical literacy, particularly on account of a shared concern for the development of the individual. The principal focus of these literacies is on the individual's realisation of potential.

The motivation behind the expansion of literacies is unclear. One reason could be that the notion of a literacy can provide the opportunity to answer the questions, 'What is the purpose of a particular area?' 'What is its value?' In this context, the notion of literacy can perhaps provide a clear intention and a justification for striving to reach an aspiration. This was the case with respect to physical literacy. Philosophical study led to an appreciation of the value of capitalising on human embodied potential and suggested that lifelong participation in physical activity could contribute significantly to quality of life. The definition and attributes of physical literacy set out a defensible and valued end, interwoven with a well-grounded justification. It is interesting to note that as physical literacy has been adopted around the world, the concept has been addressed alongside other literacies. For example, the United States, New Zealand, Wales and Australia see physical literacy as closely linked to health literacy, while an area of Scotland has drawn up programmes in which physical literacy and food literacy are combined. Similarly, in the United States, there is interest to link physical literacy with nutritional concerns.

UNESCO has continued to show an interest in literacy. In their document entitled *Education for All: Literacy for Life* (UNESCO, 2006), there is a chapter entitled 'Understandings of Literacy'. The range of literacies now in existence is briefly referred to, and four categories of understandings of literacy are set out. These are:

- As a discrete set of skills, independent of context.
- As applied, practised and situated. This literacy is seen as a given set of social practices that need to be developed to gain access to a particular cultural context.
- As a learning process. Literacy here is seen as the ability to make sense of experiences, as an active and broad-based learning process. Those advocating this understanding cite experiential learning, in which learners need to engage in meaningful personal experiences that enable them to make sense of the world around as they interact with 'sociocultural realities'.
- As text. This refers to the textual nature of the discourse of a literacy. This seems to be a development of the second understanding, which was concerned with social practices, but adds to this the repository of wisdom that in some sense 'belongs to the parent culture'.

The four UNESCO 'understandings' would seem to resonate with aspects of the earlier presentation of the characteristics of other literacies; however, they do not provide an obvious home for physical literacy. Physical literacy does not aim solely to develop a set of skills independent of context, nor, it is argued, is its paramount aim to develop skills that are valued and significant to the parent culture. Physical literacy is not a process, as set out later in Chapter 3, nor is it primarily an initiation into a specific discourse. However, there are aspects of each 'understanding' that could be seen to resonate, to some extent, with physical literacy. Movement competency or development of movement patterns is an important element in the definition of physical literacy, and provides the opportunity to be involved in valued social practices is not overlooked. A well-designed learning process is essential to physical literacy as the route to fostering lifelong participation. Finally, there are philosophical discourses that underpin the concept. On these grounds, as well as on account of the characteristics that we share with other literacies, there seems to be support to argue that there is justification to use the word 'literacy' alongside 'physical'.

Physical literacy, as arising from monism, existentialism and phenomenology, has at its heart the notion of providing opportunities for the individual to realise human potential through holistic interaction with the world. It is of note that the UNESCO (2004) definition of linguistic literacy does evidence an interest in the individual. For example, mention is made of the learner and the context, and the relationship between these two features. Reference is made to 'enabling individuals to achieve their goals, to develop their knowledge and potential', to participating 'fully in their community and wider society', and to an 'ability to identify, understand, interpret, create, communicate'. In contrast, the 2006 'understandings' do not endorse this perspective, focusing rather on the 'content' in considering literacies. This is disappointing as the earlier statement describes literacy as a relationship between an individual and the world. Physical literacy is essentially person-centred and only realises its full potential when embraced by an individual. The 2006 UNESCO 'understandings' present a somewhat technical and instrumental perspective on literacies, and seem to leave aside the individual who is at the heart of the enterprise. One might ask why concern for human potential, individuality, freedom and personal responsibility have seemingly been overlooked.

However, there is a small but promising section at the end of the UNESCO (2006) paper. This makes reference to the work of Freire (1985), who writes about literacies as contributing to the 'liberation of man' and to realising his full potential, and to Bataille (1976), who proposes that literacies stimulate initiative and 'participation in the creation of projects capable of acting upon the world, of transforming it and of defining the aims of an authentic human development'. He concludes by asserting that 'literacy is a fundamental human right' (UNESCO, 2006: 154). There is clearly room for debate in relation to the nature and role of 'literacies' as human potentialities. The notion of physical literacy as a human right is picked up in Chapter 4 in relation to discussions concerning value.

Conclusion

This chapter has briefly addressed some of the issues surrounding the definition of physical literacy. The principal focus has been on the legitimacy of using the notion of 'literacy' alongside 'physical'. It has been argued that from a foundation of monism and existentialism, which together respect each human being as a composite of irretrievably interconnected characteristics that play an essential role in interacting with the world, the contemporary use of 'literacy' can readily sit alongside 'physical'. As proponents of musical literacy and artistic literacy champion the value of their area as providing unique fulfilment of human potential unrelated to linguistic literacy, so physical literacy identifies a specific characteristic of human being. It will be argued later in Part III that nurturing this human potential can make a significant contribution to human flourishing.

These discussions reflect considerations by the International Physical Literacy Association, as well as debate in the seminars, fora and conferences that the Association has mounted. The following chapter will consider a range of misunderstandings that have been evident as the concept has begun to be used more widely.

References

Bataille, L. (ed.) (1976) *A Turning Point for Literacy: Adult Education for Development. The Spirit and Declaration of Persepolis.* Oxford: Pergamon.

Freire, P. (1985) *The Politics of Education: Culture, Power, and Liberation.* South Hadley, MA: Bergin & Garvey.

International Physical Literacy Association (IPLA) (2019) *Physical Literacy across the World: Resources and References.* Available at: www.physical-literacy.org.uk/plaw-resources-and-references/ (accessed 14 March 2019).

Kiez, T. and Kriellaars, D. (2015) *Origins of Physical Literacy.* Unpublished paper, University of Manitoba.

Standal, O.F. (2015) *Phenomenology and Pedagogy in Physical Education.* London: Routledge.

United Nations Educational, Scientific and Cultural Organization (UNESCO) (2004) *The Plurality of Literacy and Its Implications for Policies and Programs.* Available at: http://unesdoc.unesco.org/images/0013/001362/136246e.pdf (accessed 6 September 2012).

United Nations Educational, Scientific and Cultural Organization (UNESCO) (2006) *Education for All: Literacy for Life.* Paris: UNESCO.

Whitehead, M.E. (1993) Unpublished conference paper, IAPESGW Congress, Melbourne, Australia.

Whitehead, M.E. (ed.) (2010) *Physical Literacy throughout the Lifecoure.* London: Routledge.

Whitehead, M.E. (2016–2018) *Physical Literacy: Philosophical Roots, Definition, Value and Implications.* Available at: www.physical-literacy.org.uk/resources/library/download-info/physical-literacy-philosophical-roots-definition-value-and-implications/ (accessed 6 December 2018).

3

ASPECTS OF PHYSICAL LITERACY

Clarification and discussion with particular reference to the physical domain

Margaret Whitehead

Introduction

This chapter addresses some of the areas of misunderstanding concerning the nature of physical literacy. As the concept has spread across the world, some confusion has been generated. In some cases, this has been caused by translation challenges, while elsewhere the definition has been interpreted to align with current practice and priorities. In respect of these last cases, the outcome has sometimes moved away from the IPLA definition and a loss of concern for some of the central tenets of the concept. Space does not permit a comprehensive consideration of the range of alternative interpretations; however, some of these will be discussed again in Part II, where colleagues from eight different countries describe the adoption of the concept in their settings. This chapter considers the relationship between physical literacy, physical competence and fundamental movement skills, and looks briefly at a range of other issues that have caused some misunderstanding.

Physical literacy and the physical domain

As the concept of physical literacy has developed across the world, there have been two common misinterpretations. The first misinterpretation has arisen from the presumption that physical literacy has a single focus on effective body management. The second misinterpretation is related to this view, but goes a step further and identifies fundamental movement skills as the sole concern, and indeed the essence, of fostering physical literacy.

Looking at physical literacy as purely concerned with the human physical domain carries dualist undertones, giving the impression that it is possible to isolate one aspect of human nature without any consideration of other features. As has been explained on many occasions (see Whitehead, 2010, 2016–2018; IPLA,

2019), the concept of physical literacy embraces the nature of the individual as an interrelated composite of a number of domains – the affective, the physical and the cognitive. This is reinforced in the reference to these domains in the definition. It can be conjectured that one reason for the current disappointing levels of commitment to physical activity for life could be the outcome of a focus solely on the physical, with the embodiment considered principally as an instrument (see explanatory glossary). It is suggested that what is needed is a more holistic, empathetic and individualised approach. This is supported by the philosophy underpinning the concept. There is no dispute over human physicality being at the heart of physical literacy, and thus providing opportunities for development that are unique to this area of human potential; however, involvement in this enterprise needs to avoid a body-as-instrument, dualistic focus. Promoting physical literacy should be a route into the holistic well-being of the individual (see Chapters 18 and 19).

Physical literacy and fundamental movement skills

While a focus on the physical is overly narrow, more concerning is the way that this perception has been reduced to the promotion of fundamental movement skills. Indeed, there is a perception that fundamental movement skills per se constitute fostering physical literacy. This is far from the case, and is corroborated by a number of writers (e.g. Barnett et al., 2016: 223). There are at least three areas to discuss here. These relate to the relationship between physical competency and fundamental movement skills, the interpretation of the notion of 'fundamental', and the implications of a focus on fundamental movement skills on practitioner pedagogical practices.

The presumption that physical competency can be interpreted solely as fundamental movement skills

Whitehead (2010) describes physical competency as the sufficiency of movement abilities to interact with a wide variety of physical activity settings. This is further clarified in attributes C, D and E, as set out in Table 2.2. Attribute C refers to the development of 'poise, economy and effectiveness in a wide variety of challenging situations'. Attribute D spells out the seminal feature of physical competence being the effective interaction with the world. This is described as 'thoughtful and sensitive perception in appreciating all aspects of the physical environment, responding as appropriate with imagination and creativity'. Attribute E identifies 'the ability to work independently and with others in physical activities in both cooperative and competitive situations'. As can be seen, within physical literacy, there is far more to physical competence than fundamental movement skills. Physical competence refers to movement patterns in context, to movement that affords effective interaction with environments and situations in the world. Pot et al. (2018) discuss this area in some detail and make a strong case for a focus on meaningful movement patterns in context, rather than isolated skills.

The legitimacy of the notion of 'fundamental' in fundamental movement skills

This can be considered from a number of perspectives, viz.:

- the definition of a skill;
- the breadth of application;
- the notion of innate movements versus learnt movements;
- the concept of 'fundamental' as being an 'ideal' model; and
- the cultural context.

On all counts, it is suggested that there are issues that need to be discussed and clarified.

With reference to definition, as used in a physical activity setting, 'skill' is usually understood as an applied technique. To have 'skill' usually describes a mover who can apply techniques perceptively, in a wide variety of settings. Fundamental movement techniques would, on this definition, be a more appropriate label. Kirk (2010) would seem to agree with this nomenclature in his description of physical education as the promotion of 'sport techniques'.

Murdoch and Whitehead (2010) proposed that the notion of movement patterns more readily describes the movement configurations that should be fostered. These are also set out by Durden-Myers et al. (2018), where a developmental model is described. This involves foundation movement patterns, general movement patterns, refined movement patterns and specific movement patterns. Throughout this progressive developmental process, movement patterns are honed both by the demands of different activity contexts and by the application of movement capacities such as coordination, control and balance. There is a view that it is these capacities that are the fundamental constituents of human movement. These capacities are described in Whitehead (2010), where it is suggested that the development of these movement abilities can facilitate the acquisition of a wide range of movement patterns (p. 177). Barnett et al. (2016) suggest that mastery of capacities within any fundamental movement 'skill', such as 'functional coordination and control', can be transferred to 'skills' across different activity contexts (p. 221). This is a proposal that has long been debated and warrants detailed investigation and research.

With regard to the breadth of application, being how far commonly used clusters of fundamental movement 'skills' represent 'skills' that are the forerunners of all types of physical activities, there are issues that need to be considered. It would appear that far from addressing the needs of a wide variety of physical activities, most programmes of fundamental movement 'skills' seem to be selectively focused on constituents of particular physical activities, namely competitive team games. For a set of 'skills' to be truly fundamental in a movement activity context, a wide range of 'skills' need to be included. For example, 'skills' that are involved in swimming, sailing, windsurfing, outdoor adventure and genres of dance – to name but a few additional activities. The creation of a programme that is relevant to a wide range of activities and addresses the spectrum of movement capacities could be valuable; however, as intimated later in this chapter, it is suggested that time may be better spent in exploring the use of techniques in context rather than in isolation.

The relationship between physical development and the progressive mastery of a cluster of foundation movement patterns is contentious in respect of how far these patterns are innate and how far they need to be taught. Barnett et al. (2016) and Pot et al. (2018) disagree on this point. Barnett et al. (2016) propose that all fundamental techniques or movement patterns need to be taught, while Pot et al. (2018) are of the view that some of the techniques are innate. This is particularly pertinent in the early years, where ontogenetic development and phylogenetic development seem to go hand in hand (see explanatory glossary). Observation of the young child would indicate that, characteristically, these young people acquire movement acuity through exploration and trial and error. The young child does not have to be taught to walk, run, jump and climb. These are all surely fundamental aspects of movement that are drawn on in very many physical activity settings. Young children readily kick and scramble up obstacles without instruction as they interact with their world. While young children may well be emulating the movement of others, there seems little doubt that these aspects of innate embodied acuity need further investigation. If the child is born with innate movement patterns, how do the batteries of 'fundamental' movement 'skills' relate to these? Notwithstanding the outcome of any research in this area, this debate begs the question: What exactly does 'fundamental' refer to?

Another concern that arises in respect of the notion of 'fundamental' movement 'skills' is the suggestion that there is one 'ideal' way to perform these movements. In many cases, they are presented as 'closed skills', 'skills' that can be learnt and applied without adaptation in a setting. This is very far from reality, and there is a great deal of writing that indicates that a named 'skill' is very seldom replicated. Pot et al. (2018) ask if, in fact, there is a 'fundamental' way to execute a particular technique (e.g. a throw). Any throw will occur in a specific context and will have particular purpose. No two throws will be the same; each will answer a particular need. Standal and Moe (2011) describe many actions in a sporting context to be 'the intertwining of a moving body-subject and the immediate environment where the movement takes place'. They suggest that 'skills' will need to be adapted to the particular environment, to the actions of other participants involved in the activity, as well as to the purpose of the action (pp. 261, 262, 265). Furthermore, it is suggested that individuals may well have a personal throwing pattern. Standal and Aggerholm (2016) cite the work of Sellinger and Crease (2002), who argue that performances differ from person to person, and therefore 'cannot be reduced to rules of thumb' (p. 271).

From the cultural perspective, there is an issue about how far any cluster of fundamental movement 'skills' can have relevance throughout the world. This is yet another dimension of the question: What is meant by 'fundamental'?

Pot et al. (2018) go to some length in arguing that there is a significant cultural influence of what could be identified as fundamental 'skills' in the context of physical activity. With respect to activities, fundamental movement 'skills' may well need to be specific to the particular physical activities that are prevalent in a country, and indeed the way that a particular activity is practised. For example, a country or culture is likely to have its own cluster of most prevalent physical activities. 'Skills' underpinning skiing and skating will be highly relevant in some countries, while 'skills' involved in baseball and basketball or 'skills' involved in a particular dance genre will be relevant elsewhere. In addition, where an activity is practised in more than one country, it could be that significant aspects of the activity or game are different. For example, soccer is played in many countries, but may have rules, procedures and 'skills' particular to the host country. This issue is picked up by Pot et al. (2018), where they refer to Mauss (1934), who argues that movement actions are shaped by culture. There remain questions to be considered about if and how far any cluster of fundamental movement 'skills' can be common across the world.

As can be seen above, there is a great deal of clarification needed to legitimise fundamental movement 'skills' within the context of physical literacy. It has been suggested, first, that it may be best to focus on movement capacities such as balance and coordination to create a sound foundation for more effective participation; and second, that the notion of movement patterns more readily describes the way that humans interact with the world. A bank of movement patterns can be seen as a resource from which an individual can draw to effect interaction with the environment. Research is needed to ascertain aspects of movement development, the nature of the movement abilities that can cater for participation in all forms of physical activity, and the best way to foster these abilities so that they are readily drawn on in activity situations. The recommendation that movement patterns are best established in a context is the subject of the following section on pedagogy.

Fundamental movement skills and pedagogy

An additional area of concern is the procedures used to promote fundamental movement 'skills' in a managed physical activity setting. On account of the suggestion that there *is* one ideal way to perform each of these 'skills', it is all too easy for practitioners to use pedagogical practices that, it could be conjectured, are less likely to promote enthusiasm for participation. For example, the specific focus on a particular 'skill' can result in teaching being didactic and drill-like, with learning all but replication and repetition. As argued by Pot et al. (2018), in the teaching of fundamental 'skills', the focus tends to be solely on how a 'skill' is to be performed. Where, when, with whom, and why are not considered. Not only can practices of copying and repeating of skills be demotivating, but where skills are worked on in isolation from meaningful contexts, experiences can lack purpose and be less than satisfying (see explanatory glossary).

A commitment to long-term aspirations needs to be borne in mind in respect of working on fundamental 'skills.' As referred to earlier in Chapters 2 and 3, a key purpose of physical literacy is to nurture a commitment to physical activity for life. Any work on fundamental 'skills' needs to keep this aspiration very much in mind. Fundamental 'skills' are only one element in developing physical literacy, and every effort needs to be made to engage participants in meaningful activity contexts. The real heart of developing physical literacy lies in experiences that have the potential to develop confidence and self-belief alongside stimulating interest and commitment. Zimmerman and Saura (2017) discuss the notion of meaningful experiences (see explanatory glossary) in an activity context. Working from an existentialist perspective, they describe the close relationship between the mover and the world as realising a 'harmony between the athlete's movements and their challenges from the particular environments' (p. 159). Furthermore, they argue that ways in which individuals respond to challenges guide them to new possibilities of being themselves and thus play a part 'in the development of human potential' (p. 162).

As has been indicated above, the development of physical competence rests on the application of movement patterns in increasingly challenging and varied contexts. It falls to the practitioner to provide these contexts, as appropriate. Dewey (1938: 45), referred to in Standal (2015), describes this well in writing that the duty of an educator is to:

> determine that environment which will interact with the existing capabilities and needs of those taught, to create a worthwhile experience. That means that it is the obligation of the teacher to construct an environment by manipulating the objective conditions so that the learner can have experiences which match his or her capacities and desires.
>
> *(p. 113)*

It is worth noting that Dewey is concerned with matching environments with individuals. This aligns with the desirability to respect each individual as unique – a view strongly held by proponents of physical literacy.

Fundamental movement skills and assessment

Another concern in relation to a fundamental movement 'skills' approach is that where replication of an ideal model is the goal, the use of norm-referenced assessment procedures may be applied. This form of assessment issues in comparison with others and a sense, for some participants, of not matching up to expected standards. In addition, comparison with others is often used as stimulus to work to be the 'best'. However, as the majority of participants will never be the highest achievers, the perception of many learners leaving a session of this nature is likely to be that they have not succeeded, and that physical activity is not for them. This threatens confidence and the development of self-belief. It is proposed that normative assessment, inevitably involving comparison with others, is less appropriate than charting an individual's personal physical literacy journey (see Chapters 6 and 17). This can be seen as a fairer way of judging an individual's progress, as each participant will be at a different place in his or her journey. Ipsative assessment, being a method that records achievement from the standpoint of personal progress, can legitimately celebrate success for all and can have a positive effect on motivation.

There are also contextual concerns about assessment in respect of a focus on fundamental movement 'skills'. Pot et al. (2018) question the value of assessment of isolated 'skills' out of context, in that of themselves they have no meaning. Where progress is made in respect of isolated 'skills', this has no necessary connection to, or bearing on, effective participation in an activity. Robinson et al. (2015) carried out research in this area and concluded that there is little conclusive evidence of a relationship between early 'skill' development and long-term participation. Barnett et al. (2016), however, suggest one possible relationship between isolated 'skills' and their context, in writing that 'The psychological effects of perceiving oneself as competent … may have a tangible impact on an individual's desire to engage in other physical activities' beyond the fundamental 'skill' practised (p. 221). This positive relationship will, however, only accrue where individuals feel they have been successful.

Physical competence in context

Notwithstanding the above concerns, there is absolutely no doubt that movement patterns play a key part in developing physical literacy. However, the critical aspiration of physical competence within physical literacy is effective interaction with the world, and this needs to be kept in mind at all times.

Acquiring physical competence may start with emulating an 'ideal' model of a 'skill', but the longer this somewhat mechanical repetition continues, the less relevant the 'skill' becomes in participation in physical activity. The development of movement patterns is only the very first step to effective and meaningful interaction with the world. Pot et al. (2018) concur with this in expressing the view that some form of fundamental movement 'skill' experience can be a valuable short-term focus in the early stages, but this is far from an end in itself, both in respect of physical competence and, following from this, physical literacy.

As argued above, fundamental movement 'skills' do not represent the totality of physical competency, nor, in their current form, do they include the numerous movement patterns that underpin a wide range of physical activities. It is highly debatable if there is one ideal method of performing a 'skill'; indeed, use of a 'skill' will always be subject to the endowment of the individual, the purpose of the activity, the activity setting and the parent culture. The notion of developing movement patterns aligns more closely to physical literacy than fundamental movement 'skills'. A seminal aspect of physical literacy is effective interaction within a range of activity settings. This calls for practitioners to provide progressively challenging contexts and for participants to explore, apply and adapt movement patterns to effect meaningful and satisfying experiences.

Clarification of aspects of physical literacy

There have been a number of other misunderstandings in relation to physical literacy. Space does not permit detailed consideration of all of these. However, some key questions will be discussed briefly in the final part of this chapter. These refer the nature of physical literacy as a process or a goal, the relevance of physical literacy across the lifespan, and the relationship of the concept to some current practice.

Is physical literacy a goal or a process?

Physical literacy is neither a process nor a goal. Physical literacy per se is not a goal, as this implies that it is a clearly identified objective that, once attained, is sustained thereafter; rather, it is a disposition or attitude. Physical literacy as a disposition cannot be established 'once and for all', but needs to be nurtured, as appropriate, through all phases of life. The aspiration of practitioners is to establish a secure and robust disposition in all participants with whom they work. An individual's ongoing commitment or otherwise to participation in physical activity is often referred to as a physical literacy journey. The concept of a journey describes the interface between attitudes, abilities, opportunities and circumstances that together affect a person's way of life. The journey is not another description of physical literacy; rather, it is a narrative of a life pattern (see Chapter 17).

Physical literacy in itself is not a process. As originally conceived, physical literacy is described as a desirable personal disposition – a commitment to physical activity for life. Fostering this disposition will, of course, generate recommended practices that practitioners might undertake. These in themselves might be interpreted as being a process. However, this is a facilitative process that has the potential to support individuals on their physical literacy journey. This process is best designed to foster the development of a well-established disposition in respect of lifelong participation. These processes will provide a series of experiences that will have an impact on the physical literacy journey; they will shape the journey, but they are not in themselves the journey. This facilitative process should take into account both the nature of the disposition, being a commitment to physical activity for life and the means by which it is suggested it can be fostered, as well as showing respect for the underlying philosophy. This will be taken up in Chapter 5, which addresses the implications of working to establish a secure and robust disposition in respect of participation in physical activity for life. In brief, this process will comprise a logically planned series of opportunities, all experienced in a supportive environment that will foster the development of a commitment to an active lifestyle. This should not be understood as 'teaching' physical literacy; rather, the process should provide meaningful experiences (see explanatory glossary) through which participants will grow in respect of the motivation, confidence, physical competence, knowledge and understanding to value and take responsibility for engaging in physical activities for life. Jurbala (2015) proposes an insightful 'journey type process' representing the development of physical literacy (p. 378).

Is physical literacy relevant throughout life?

Physical literacy is relevant to all, whatever age and endowment. Some early work in physical literacy in countries such as Canada and Wales was focused on young people of school age, and in addition particular attention in Canada was given to long-term athletic development of these young people. While it is correct to suggest that fostering physical literacy at this age is very important and may have a strong influence on participation in later years, it is a misunderstanding to associate physical literacy particularly with these young people.

Set out in Table 3.1 is a brief description of characteristics of a positive disposition to physical activity through different periods of life. A fuller chart can be found on the IPLA website (see IPLA, 2019).

TABLE 3.1 Physical literacy for life

Physical literacy for life
This table identifies the broad general framework of a physical literacy journey to demonstrate how physical literacy develops through the different phases of life.
Preschool 0 to 3–5 years. These young children begin their physical literacy journey as they grow and develop while exploring the world. Inquisitiveness, exploration and imagination are evident. They exhibit a natural tendency to observe and copy others and take great pleasure in their new-found abilities.
Early years and primary school 3–5 to 9–11 years. In this phase, children's physical development continues alongside growth in confidence in respect of physical competency. Knowledge and understanding about the nature of movement and physical activities grow, as does appreciation of the health benefits of physical activity.
Secondary school 9–11 to 16–19 years. Here, challenges of physical development in adolescence are worked through as confidence is developed in respect of physical competence. Participants begin to take more responsibility for setting goals and choosing activities. Knowledge and understanding of holistic health benefits of physical activity are evident, and participants are motivated take the initiative to be involved in physical activity beyond the school.
Young adulthood 16–19 to 30–35 years. Participants now take full responsibility for engagement in physical activity. They are enthusiastic about physical activity and may wish to specialise in one area of activity or take part in a range of settings, novel or familiar. Appreciation of the value of physical activity is acknowledged and decisions to take part are rationally determined.
Older adulthood 30–35 to 70–80 years. Physical activity is established as a part of lifestyle. Participants are proactive in taking part in physical activities. Appreciation of the value of physical activity is acknowledged. Commitment to physical activity and its holistic benefits is shared with others.
Older age 70–80 to 100–110 years. Physical activity is sustained as a regular aspect of life. New activities are taken up as appropriate. These individuals appreciate the importance and value of keeping active.
Note: There is no intention in this table to suggest norms in respect of progress or expectation, as individuals will each be on their unique physical literacy journey. In general, an individual's development will demonstrate progressively more secure and reliable behaviours that match the attributes. The characteristics presented in this table do not address all attributes, but are those features that are specific to a phase. The notion of unique journeys, together with examples and causes of particular journeys, is addressed in Chapter 17.

Fostering physical literacy has the potential to enrich all lives. Commitment to physical activity is relevant and valuable across all ages and whatever endowment people display. This issue will be developed further in Chapter 4. The corollary of this is that the responsibility of fostering physical literacy does not rest solely on teachers of physical education in school. All practitioners working in the area of physical activity, as well as significant others such as peers, parents and colleagues, can have an impact on fostering physical literacy.

What is the relationship between physical education and physical literacy?

Physical literacy and physical education are discrete concepts. There is no competition between them. Physical education is the name of an area of the school curriculum. It labels a school-specific event. Physical literacy identifies a value and purpose of this aspect of schooling, being the fostering of a positive attitude to participation in physical activity throughout life. The role of teachers of physical education is to nurture individuals' progress on their unique physical literacy journeys. It should be noted that nurturing physical literacy is not only relevant in schooling, but is of value throughout life.

Is physical literacy a pedagogical model?

Physical literacy is not a pedagogical model. The philosophical roots of the development of physical literacy and the aspiration inherent in the concept differ from the rationale behind pedagogical models. One of the intentions of the creation of pedagogical models is to develop well-founded models of teaching related to specific goals (e.g. sport education, health-based physical education, games for understanding, cooperative learning). This enables clarity of purpose in planning and enacting teaching. These models provide a pool of approaches that can be clearly identified and delivered. When a teacher or practitioner selects a particular goal, the pedagogical model can be referred to and operationalised. Significant in these recommendations are ways in which teaching or instruction are best conducted. Pedagogical models are a valuable addition to rational practice; however, they are options that practitioners can select as appropriate. However, it could be true to suggest that it was not intended that a particular model should be the single focus of a whole series of units of work or of an entire physical education curriculum. In contrast, it is proposed that promoting physical literacy should underpin all work in the field of physical activity. Physical literacy has the potential of encouraging all participants to be active for life. The concept is based on monism, existentialism and phenomenology, and adopts a particular view of the human being. It is fundamentally a participant-centred, inclusive concept that, it is advocated, should influence all aspects of 'managed' physical activity. These include the ambience of sessions, interpersonal interactions, task-setting and modes of feedback. All recommendations to foster physical literacy can be realised in working to any pedagogical model. There is no doubt that pedagogical models have the potential to make a valuable contribution to fostering commitment to lifelong participation. However, they are options. Physical literacy, it is argued, is not an option where long-term participation is an objective. It is suggested that each individual's physical literacy journey is most effective when appropriate practices permeate all physical activity experiences and settings.

Is being physically educated the same as developing physical literacy?

The answer to this question depends on what the physical education profession understands as being 'physically educated'. If the description of being 'physically educated' is that individuals, on completing schooling, have made progress on their unique physical literacy journey, so that participation throughout life seems a strong possibility, then there would be a close relationship between the two notions. However, if being physically educated has strong connotations with achieving a certain level of 'attainment' or a desirable end state, there is a clear difference between being physically educated and having a robust disposition to activity. Physical literacy is not judged against levels/performance norms. It is a disposition, not a battery of movement techniques/skills that need to be performed accurately.

How does physical literacy relate to high-quality physical education?

There has often been an observation or criticism that promoting physical literacy is the same as effecting high-quality physical education, and therefore physical literacy brings nothing new to the field of physical education. This has been a concern in the UK and the United States. In principle, for an activity to be labelled 'high quality', it would seem that there needs to be: first, a specified intention or goal for the activity; and, second, criteria generated by that goal against which to judge the quality/effectiveness of any manifestation or example of the activity. In respect of physical literacy, the intention is the development of lifelong commitment to participation in physical activity. The criteria against which a session would be judged as high quality, in this case, would include how far the incidence demonstrates the fostering of motivation, confidence, physical competence, and knowledge and understanding to enable all individuals to value and take responsibility to engage in physical activities for life.

Where teachers of physical education have an intention different to that described above, their interpretation of high quality would align with this aspiration. For example, if the goal was to foster talent, the criteria for high-quality physical education could well be the development of successful school teams and individuals who are working at a high level in situations beyond school.

Where teachers of physical education share the same long-term aspiration as advocates of physical literacy, high-quality physical education will be the same as providing experiences that foster physical literacy. It is certainly acknowledged that many teachers, as well as other practitioners in the field of physical activity, have long adopted high-quality teaching of this nature. It is hoped that considered reflection on the purpose of work in this area can generate agreement that long-term participation is a priority aspiration, and practice can be adapted accordingly. In this scenario, high-quality physical education would be that which generates lifelong commitment. There is no such thing as 'high quality' per se. This accolade depends on a clearly stated intention. An answer to the question 'Is high-quality physical education the same as physical literacy?' cannot be given without identifying the underlying purpose of the activity.

Conclusion

It was felt important to give space to some of the misunderstandings surrounding physical literacy.

The reflections herein have one overriding goal, this being to encourage all practitioners to engage participants in experiences that are designed to foster motivation, confidence, and knowledge and understanding, as well as physical competence. In some cases, established practices are well intentioned but carry potential disadvantages. Where practitioners align themselves with promoting physical literacy, it is valuable for them to reflect on their practices to ensure the outcomes match those to which they aspire.

References

Barnett, L., Stodden, D., Cohen, K.E. Smith, J.J., Lubans D.R., Lander, N.J., Brown, H., Dudley, D., Lenoir, M., Morgan P.J., Laukkanen, A., Miller, A.D. and Iivonan, S. (2016) Fundamental movement skills: an important focus. *Journal of Teaching Physical Education*, 35(3): 219–225.

Dewey, J. (1938) *Experience and Education*. New York: Macmillan.

Durden-Myers, E.J., Whitehead, M.E. and Green, N.R. (2018) Implications for promoting physical literacy. *Journal of Teaching in Physical Education*, 37: 262–271.

International Physical Literacy Association (IPLA) (2019) *Physical Literacy across the World: Resources and References*. Available at: www.physical-literacy.org.uk/plaw-resources-and-references/ (accessed 14 March 2019).

Jurbala, P. (2015) What is physical literacy, really? *Quest*, 67: 367–383.

Kirk, D. (2010) *Physical Education Futures*. London: Routledge.

Mauss, M. (1934) Les techniques du corps. *Journal de psychologie normal et pathologique*, 32(3–4): 5–10.

Murdoch, E. and Whitehead, M.E. (2010) Physical literacy, fostering the attributes and curriculum planning. In M.E. Whitehead (ed.), *Physical Literacy throughout the Lifecourse*. London: Routledge, pp. 175–196.

Pot, N., van Hilvoorde, I., Afonso, J., Koekoek, J. and Almond, L. (2018) Meaningful movement behavior involves more than the learning of fundamental movement skills. *International Sports Studies: Journal of the International Society for Comparative Physical Education and Sport*, 39(2): 5–20.

Robinson, L.E., Stodden, D.F., Barnett, L.M., Lopes, V.P., Rodrigues, L.P. and D'Hondt, E. (2015) Motor competence and its effect on positive developmental trajectories of health. *Sports Medicine (Auckland NZ)*, 45(9): 1275–1284.

Standal, O.F. (2015) *Phenomenology and Pedagogy in Physical Education*. London: Routledge.

Standal, O.F. and Aggerholm, K. (2016) Habits, skills and embodied experiences: a contribution to philosophy of physical education. *Sport, Ethics and Philosophy*, 10(3): 269–282.

Standal, O.F. and Moe, V.F. (2011) Merleau-Ponty meets Kretchmar: sweet tensions of embodied learning. *Sport Ethics and Philosophy*, 5(3): 256–270.

Sellinger, E.M. and Crease, R.P. (2002) Dryfus on expertise: the limits of phenomenological analysis. *Continental Philosophy Review*, 35(3): 245–279.

Whitehead, M.E. (ed.) (2010) *Physical Literacy throughout the Lifecourse*. London: Routledge.

Whitehead, M.E. (2016–2018) *Physical Literacy: Philosophical Roots, Definition, Value and Implications*. Available at: www.physical-literacy.org.uk/resources/library/download-info/physical-literacy-philosophical-roots-definition-value-and-implications/ (accessed 6 December 2018).

Zimmermann, A. and Saura, S. (2017) Body, environment and adventure: experience and spatiality. *Sport, Ethics and Philosophy*, 11(2): 155–168.

4

IN SUPPORT OF PHYSICAL LITERACY THROUGHOUT LIFE

Margaret Whitehead

Introduction

This chapter will consider the value of physical literacy, and will cover reference to the philosophical underpinning of the concept and the justification for attention to be paid to the concept arising from the perspective of social justice. The issue of physical literacy being an end in itself, rather than a means to other ends, will be addressed, and this will be followed by a brief reference to the specific value of physical literacy at different broad 'phases' in life.

Philosophy

Considerable space was devoted to philosophy in Whitehead (2010). This served as an explanation of the background to the development of the concept. Another presentation of the philosophy can be found in Whitehead (2016–2018). In this chapter, philosophy will be referred to briefly, specifically in relation to reinforcing the value of physical literacy. This will remind readers of the grounding of physical literacy in monism, existentialism and aspects of phenomenology.

With reference to monism, it was suggested by Whitehead (2010) that the low esteem in which physical activity is generally held is the result of deeply entrenched beliefs in dualism. On this view of the bipartite nature of human being, the body was always cast as inferior to the mind. While many still accept dualism without question, the academic study of the human condition has moved beyond this debate, with much work now being concerned with the way that monism operates. It seems generally agreed that there is no schism in respect of the human condition, and debate now includes a consideration of the role of human embodiment in life (see explanatory glossary). The notion of monism is, however, complicated by the fact that human embodiment has two forms of presentation, one being the body as an object or instrument, sometimes known as the living body, and the other being the embodiment as lived at a preconceptual level, referred to as the lived body. Monism accepts these two forms of presentation but is principally concerned with the lived body (see explanatory glossary). With reference to the lived body as a significant feature of human nature, new concepts are being developed such as embodied cognition and enactivism. Embodied cognition refers to the essential role that embodiment plays in shaping the mind (Claxton et al., 2010), while Valera et al. (1993) explain that the use of the term enactivism emphasises:

> the growing conviction that cognition is not the representation of a pre-given world by a pre-given mind but is rather the enactment of a world and a mind on the basis of a history of the variety of actions that a being in the world performs.
>
> *(p. 9)*

Clark (2001) entitled his book *Supersizing the Mind*, and argues that cognition should be considered as permeating the human organism as a whole. In support of these views, Maiese (2016) refers to the 'essentially embodied self' and Archer (2000) asserts that being human is characterised by the primacy of practice over consciousness and thought. The work of these scholars, and others, makes fascinating reading. Overall, the perspective they take is that human embodiment is far from a trivial detail of human existence, but rather is the ground of being human. These developments would seem to endorse the importance of human embodiment and vindicate the belief in the value of physical activity, and thus physical literacy. This issue is also referred to in Chapter 19. It would be valuable for proponents of physical literacy to keep abreast of these potentially significant developments.

A second arm of a philosophically based justification for physical activity, and by implication physical literacy, concerns a particular perspective on human life that is identified by some existentialists and phenomenologists. Philosophers from these schools of thought not only broadly support monism as related to the individual person; they also argue against perceptions of dualism that see the individual and the world as separate free-standing features. Existentialists in particular reject this outlook as a second dualistic fallacy, and strongly support the notion that humans are essentially beings in the world and rely on interaction with the world to realise their potential. They champion the view that existence precedes essence. As humans interact with the world, they are stimulated to respond, and in so doing they gradually develop a myriad of abilities. This urge to realise potential is driven by a seemingly innate need to interact with the world through a human characteristic known as intentionality. Broadly speaking, this refers to a restless directedness towards the world, a hunger to explore. As a result of this interaction, individuals not only come to know themselves, but also come to know the world. It is explained that without the world of animate and inanimate features, there would be no human life as we know it, and without human life there would be no world. Johnson (1987) writes:

> It is a mistake … to think of an organism and its environment as two entirely
> independent and unrelated entities: the organism does not exist as an organ-
> ism apart from its environment … the environment and the organism
> codetermine each other …
>
> (p. 207)

It follows from this that all aspects of human nature that afford contact with the
world are highly significant in human development. Our embodied dimension
alongside other senses creates a key avenue of contact with the world, and therefore plays an important role in developing our personhood. In this respect, human
embodiment is an indispensable feature of human life, and fostering physical literacy is worthy of serious consideration.

Phenomenologists build from this view of the fundamental significance of our
interaction with the world, and assert that what we perceive is not an objective
truth, but reflects an individual's understanding of that which is perceived, as a
result of previous experience. In this sense, the objects of perception are phenomena. On account of our embodied presence in the world, a majority of all
phenomena include properties accrued from our proprioceptive feedback from
previous interaction. In fact, all perception is imbued with our embodied nature,
and again, as such, this affirms the contribution that human embodied nature makes
to life as we know it. The writings of Polanyi (1966; see also Gill, 2000) set out the
notion of tacit knowledge or embodied wisdom, and are valuable references here.
The notion of knowing ourselves and knowing the world is closely associated with
what are known as affordances (see explanatory glossary).

Set out above briefly are pointers to the way philosophy legitimates attention
to the human embodied dimension, and thus physical literacy. Legitimacy rests to
a considerable extent on the rejection of dualism. This is supported by Claxton
(1997), who dismisses mind–body dualism as 'philosophically bankrupt and scien-
tifically discredited' (p. 223).

Physical literacy as a human capability

The notion of capabilities was referred to briefly in Whitehead (2010). Further
consideration has been given to this concept, and it is now suggested that there are
grounds for physical literacy to be a capability in its own right. Justification here
is considered not from a philosophical stance, but in the context of social justice.
Capability theory proposes that humans have the right to capitalise on all aspects
of human potential. There are a range of texts that consider capabilities, such as
Sen (1992, 1994), Robeyns (2003), Bloodworth et al. (2012) and Standal (2015).
All these texts are valuable and relevant to read; however, this short section of the
chapter will build from Whitehead (2010) and focus on the work of Nussbaum
(2000, 2011). In relation to capabilities, Nussbaum (2011) indicates that the key
question is 'What is each person able to do and to be?' (p. 18). In this context,
she argues that capabilities represent freedoms that all humans should have the

opportunity to exercise. Nussbaum identifies 10 central capabilities: life, bodily health, bodily integrity, sense/imagination, emotions, practical reason, affiliation, other species and the natural world, play, and control over one's environment (see Table 4.1). Each of these capabilities exhibits common features as well as having their own distinctive characteristics. The common features are threefold. First, they rely on innate abilities, such as talking, seeing and walking. Second, they can be interpreted as internal abilities. These are described as ways of doing and being that humans acquire as they interact with the world, such as appreciating poetry, engaging in debate, and rock climbing. Third, for humans to realise a particular capability, appropriate opportunities must be provided and be accessible. These should facilitate the development of the innate and internal capabilities that, when developed, issue in central capabilities. For example, opportunities could be in the form of appropriate schooling, and facilities such as libraries, art galleries and climbing walls. Other opportunities might be the provision of debating societies, openings to apply for a variety of jobs, and freedom to capitalise on preferred capabilities. Without the opportunity to build on innate and internal abilities, central capabilities will not develop into significant ways of doing and being. It is also important that individuals are free to choose which capabilities to develop and have confidence to select and activate their choices.

In setting out her list of capabilities, Nussbaum (2000, 2011) would seem to acknowledge the holistic nature of the human condition. Thus, involvement of embodied potential is presumed in most capabilities. This is particularly evident in the capabilities of bodily health and bodily integrity, although these would seem to focus on the living body (see explanatory glossary). Involvement of the lived body would seem to be assumed in the capabilities concerned with senses and imagination and play. While the presumption of involvement of embodied acuity is evident in respect of most of the other capabilities, thus implying a commitment to monism, it can also be read as assigning human embodiment to a secondary facilitative role.

Moving on from the observation of presumed involvement, the role of embodied acuity can be highlighted as making a valuable contribution to other capabilities in respect of enriching particular human potential and experience. This proposal is set out in Table 4.1. The right-hand column identifies suggestions of the way that embodied potential can be seen to add breadth and richness to the realisation of most capabilities.

For example, in respect of senses and imagination, experiences of physical activity in the form of some dance genres will broaden the development of sensitivity and creativity. In respect of affiliation, social interaction can be enhanced in participation in group physical activities. Regarding other species and the natural world, development of a concern for nature can be broadened in physical activities that involve exploration and challenge in the outdoors.

While there is some evidence that human embodiment is respected by Nussbaum in her work on capabilities, the lack of a specific capability that highlights this human dimension would seem to disregard the importance of this feature of human nature. Given that interaction with the world, from an existentialist perspective, is the

TABLE 4.1 Capabilities and physical literacy

Central capability	Rights from Nussbaum (2000, 2011)	Suggested contribution of embodied acuity
Life	Right to life of a normal length	Right to be involved in physical activity to prolong life
Bodily health	Right to adequate food and shelter	Right to be involved in physical activity to maintain health
Bodily integrity	Right to freedom of movement and having body boundaries treated as sovereign	Right to freedom to move from place to place Right to ownership of own living body/body as lived Right to have embodiment respected
Senses, imagination	Right to use senses to imagine, think and reason Right to freedom of expression	Right to be involved in physical activity to use embodied dimension to develop creativity, imagination and rationality
Emotions	Right to have attachments to things and people Right to love, grieve, and show gratitude and anger Right not to have emotional development blighted by abuse or neglect	Right to show expression of emotion through all aspects of non-verbal communication Right to have freedom for emotional development in participating in physical activity
Practical reason	Right to decide oneself on what is good and to engage in critical reflection regarding planning one's own life	Right to be involved in physical activity as an option for lifestyle planning
Affiliation	Right to engage in various forms of social interaction Right to develop self-respect as of equal worth as others	Right to engage with others in physical activity contexts and to be respected for this involvement Right to engage in culturally valued physical activities
Other species and the natural world	Right to demonstrate concern for nature	Right to be involved in physical activity to experience interaction with the world of nature
Play	Right to laugh, play and enjoy recreational activities	Right to be involved in physical activity as a rewarding, self-affirming experience and as a recreational activity
Control over one's environment	Right to participate in political choices, including free speech Right to own property Right to seek employment	Right to have a say in decisions about provision of facilities and practitioner support in relation to physical activity
Physical literacy	Right to develop embodied acuity, embracing embodied potential as of value in its own right, affording the interaction with the world that is unique to this human domain	

foundation of the realisation of human nature, it follows, as indicated above, that all those potentials that play a key role in interaction should be nurtured and celebrated. The human embodied dimension is one such avenue, and warrants serious consideration. The interaction this dimension affords is unique to human experience. To omit this aspect of potential would seem to negate the possibility of realising the full richness of human nature. In support of this observation, it is of note that physical potential could be seen to align with named capabilities in that it shares the features listed above. These describe capabilities as being grounded in innate abilities and internal abilities. There is no doubt that as humans, we both come into this world with a range of innate physical abilities and that these abilities are developed in interaction with the environment. In addition, the blossoming of a capability springing from embodied potential will depend on the provision of accessible and affordable facilities and opportunities. This too is apposite to physical literacy.

It might be argued that physical potential is adequately accommodated in the way that involvement of this human potential is assumed in most other capabilities. It could also be argued that physical potential is addressed in relation to the capability of play. The first justification for omitting physical potential deprives the individual of recognition of a distinctive area of experience, while the second justification casts involvement in the physical aspects of being human as principally a diversionary leisure pursuit. This last designation of physical activity is, at the very least, disappointing, as it fails to embrace the fundamental importance of human embodied nature and the rich benefits of fostering this human asset.

The case has been outlined above for physical literacy, as the expression of a significant human potential, to be accepted as of value in itself and to be a recognised capability in its own right (see Table 4.1). It is argued that each individual should be supported in the fostering of this area of potential. As has been indicated above, this means that there is an onus on those in authority, such as those in government, to give serious consideration to providing adequate opportunities for fostering physical literacy. This issues in wide-ranging responsibilities, including facility and practitioner provision to accommodate the needs and interests of individuals of all ages. These recommendations are set out in Whitehead (2010: Chapter 16).

Value of physical literacy as an end in itself

The foregoing sections have made a case for physical literacy as of value in its own right, both when addressed from a philosophical perspective and from the background of social justice. This justification for respect being shown to the human embodied dimension underwrites the aspiration of the IPLA to promote physical activity for life, for all, whatever age, endowment or country in which they live. This having been acknowledged, it cannot be denied that, on account of the holistic nature of the individual, working to this aspiration will have an impact on very many other facets of human potential. For example, in fostering confidence in a physical activity context, the individual may demonstrate a growth of self-respect in other areas of life. This is indicated in the section above, where the contribution of physical literacy to other capabilities was outlined. However, these contributions were not seen as the primary rationale for involvement in physical activity; rather, they were the outcome of the significance in human embodied capabilities in respect of very many aspects of a holistic human life.

It is unfortunate, however, that these assets, extrinsic to the core involvement in physical activity, have all too often been championed as being where its principal value lies. Much has been written about physical activity delivering on ends extrinsic to its core purpose (i.e. being seen as a means to other ends rather than being of value in itself). However, the IPLA is very clear in asserting that the fundamental purpose of engagement in physical activity is to foster physical literacy, and that extrinsic values will only be realised in situations where this capability is respected as significant and is authentically fostered and celebrated. Where physical literacy is championed principally as a means to other ends, less attention may be given to developing this distinct capability, with more focus being on human potentialities outside the principal remit of physical activity. This is likely to affect aspects of planning, promoting learning and evaluating outcomes. Attention may well be taken away from the prime concern of work in this area. In addition to this concern, there are two further problems of focusing on legitimising physical activity as principally of value to meet extrinsic ends. The first relates to the all but impossible task of attributing, with any certainty, participation in physical activity to the realisation of extrinsic ends. In many cases, there are numerous situations that can affect broader goals. For example, in relation to creativity, a wide range of experiences can help to foster this ability, and it would be highly dubious to attribute growth in this area specifically to involvement in physical activity. The second problem is that many other areas of activity will contribute to wider goals, such as communication skills and interpersonal skills. In this case, participation in physical activity would not seem to embrace a particular and significantly unique asset. Extrinsic goals in physical literacy can be easily covered elsewhere. On these grounds, this area of activity may be seen as less important, if not dispensable. In summary, the dangers of reliance on extrinsic aspirations are that they can have a detrimental effect on fostering physical literacy, cannot with any confidence be attributed to physical activity per se, and could make this area of experience redundant.

It is accepted that there is a very fine line between physical literacy per se offering rich opportunities for holistic development and using physical activity as a means to promote a range of non-physical human assets. In their work with participants, advocates of physical literacy should aim to hold fast to their principal focus of promoting lifelong physical activity. However, on account of the holistic nature of the human condition and the breadth and potential of their field, practitioners may at the same time make a significant impact on all-round human development. Arnold (1979), writing from an educational perspective, devotes a good deal of attention to the value of physical activity in the context of schooling. In his work, he attempts to embrace three areas of benefit for physical activity. He labels these as 'education about movement', 'education through movement' and 'education in movement'. A chapter devoted to Arnold's proposal can be found in Whitehead (2013). Here, it is suggested that 'education about movement', which is principally concerned with scientific knowledge, while being an aspect of experience in physical activity, is only a very small constituent of the work and probably does not deserve recognition as a key goal. With reference to 'education through movement', which champions physical activity as a means to wider ends, Whitehead raises questions concerning the devaluation of the physical in deference to broader goals and the potential risks set out above. The third value, 'education in movement', is seen as identifying the core purpose of physical education/physical activity. This area of Arnold's (1979) work builds from substantial and valuable debate concerning human nature and meaningful movement. However, this section needs to be read as embracing all participants rather than focusing on the peak experiences of the talented athlete, as set out by Arnold. The work of Arnold has recently attracted renewed attention, and is being used, in most instances, to support physical education in the school curriculum. Proponents of physical literacy are concerned that this triad of values takes attention off the richness and breadth of the potential of physical activity as of value in itself.

Physical activity as offering unique and widespread value to life

As suggested above, where experiences in physical activity are appropriately presented and enacted, there is the potential to make a contribution to wider goals. However, these wider goals can only be realised on account of the particular nature of the activity and the holistic nature of the participant. To demonstrate this point, the notion of life skills will be presented, alongside the way that physical activity, by its very nature, if engaged in authentically and if providing meaningful experiences, can contribute to the development of these 'extrinsic' competencies.

There is no definitive list of life skills worldwide. For the purposes of this short section, life skills have been clustered into groups under the following headings: personal skills, organisational and management skills, interpersonal skills, cognitive skills, creative, imaginative and aesthetic appreciation skills, and skills as an agent. It will be suggested that in the context of holistic human being, such is the nature of physical literacy that in fostering this area of human potential, the individual will encounter challenges and experiences that, in and of themselves, can contribute to the development of a range of life skills. This is a very significant point that warrants repetition. Participation in physical activity is not engaged in, first and foremost, to develop broad life skills; rather, in developing physical literacy, participants can confront, work on and master a wide range of life skills. Each group of life skills will now be considered in the context of fostering physical literacy.

Personal skills

Seminal to fostering physical literacy is development of personal skills such as commitment, confidence, determination, self-awareness and self-evaluation. Significant elements of practitioner guidance include encouragement, recognition of progress, and appreciative, constructive feedback alongside the setting of achievable but challenging tasks. Participants are guided to reflect on their own performance and set their own goals. In addition, practitioners will applaud application and determination. The outcome of these procedures and expectations can result in the development of self-respect and self-confidence. This foundation of positive and rewarding experiences lays the ground for future interest and participation, as expressed by the IPLA – choosing physical activity for life. There is no doubt that fostering of physical literacy depends on the development of personal skills, and these personal assets can permeate other areas of life.

Organisational and management skills

On account of the practical nature of physical literacy, participants will be challenged to develop effective organisation and management in a number of areas. For example, any participation will require particular clothing and equipment. In addition, time and transport issues will need to be addressed, as well as other relevant information. Within any activity session, organisation of space, time and equipment will feature. Surrounding the actual participation in most activities will be the demands to plan, practise, execute and evaluate performance. This may be concerned with, for example, set moves in a game, map-reading in orienteering, weather conditions in sailing, and choreographic issues in dance. There is no doubt that in the fostering of physical literacy, there are inherent needs and ample opportunities in which organisational and management skills are called on and developed, and these personal assets can permeate other areas of life.

Interpersonal skills

In many ways, working with others is integral to involvement in physical activity. This is evident in the basic requirement to share space and equipment. Working with others is a characteristic feature of much physical activity, in smaller or larger groups and in both cooperative and competitive situations. This group work will often rest on the use of communications skills such as listening, negotiating, leading and following. Group skills are challenged further if tasks involve problem-solving or creative solutions. There is no doubt that interpersonal skills lie at the heart of much physical activity and are essential for realising rewarding and meaningful experiences that will be an incentive to future participation. In other words, these skills are an integral aspect of physical literacy and are personal assets that can permeate other areas of life.

Cognitive skills

Those being guided to develop physical literacy will be involved in a range of tasks in which they will need to consider, deliberate and reflect. Significant here is the expectation that participants will develop a knowledge of the nature of movement and movement patterns, and will be able to use this knowledge to self-assess progress and plan future goals. In addition, participants will be expected, on occasion, to gather data, draw on existing material, and demonstrate understanding about issues concerned with health and well-being. There is no doubt that developing cognitive skills is a facet of fostering physical literacy. Not least, intelligent and thoughtful application is called for to appreciate the value of physical activity. These personal assets accrued regarding cognitive skills can permeate other areas of life.

Imaginative, creative and aesthetic appreciation skills

Problem-solving, discovery learning and creativity lie at the heart of much physical activity. This is most obvious in choreographic tasks, but also pertains to responding to novel challenges in rock-climbing, to adjusting to unfamiliar environments, and to outwitting opponents in competitive situations. Where creativity is called for, participants are very often asked to reflect on their own and others' presentations, thus beginning to exercise aesthetic judgements. In addition to these skills being an inherent part of much movement, such is the importance in fostering physical literacy of devolving responsibility to participants that it is highly recommended that this open-ended approach features in as much task-setting as possible. The differentiation that this offers is very valuable as it recognises each participant as a unique individual. There is no doubt that imaginative, creative and aesthetic appreciation skills are called on in the fostering of physical literacy, and these personal assets can permeate other areas of life.

Skills as an agent

A key aspect of physical literacy is the individual's ability to make independent decisions both about establishing a commitment to physical activity and about the type of activity in which they wish to take part. To support this area, in all instances of managed physical activity, responsibility is best devolved as far as possible to the participants. Open debate about the value of, and opportunities afforded by, physical activity are welcomed. The confidence developed within the aforementioned skills outlined above should issue in this assured attitude to options, benefits and personal planning. There is no doubt that developing skills as an agent is critical in the nurturing of physical literacy. The self-sufficiency, independence and resilience that are part of physical literacy are valuable assets and can permeate other areas of life.

As can be seen above, where participants are involved in meaningful experiences (see explanatory glossary) that foster physical literacy, the very nature of these activities can enrich life as a whole. If practitioners are true to the founding philosophy underpinning physical literacy and hold to the mission of the IPLA to promote physical activity for life, significant benefits can accrue. These benefits are not pre-planned extrinsic goals, but corollaries of the holistic nature of humans.

Value of physical literacy across the age ranges

While all the values that have been considered in this chapter are pertinent across the lifespan, it is useful to reflect, briefly, on some specific values that relate to particular groups of participants. These are sketched out below.

Children in the preschool/early years will benefit from a regime that embraces physical literacy on account of the focus on active play. Physical activity at this age both reflects physical development as well as stimulating this development. The focus on exploration and experiment as children become familiar with the world is essential for helping them to come to know themselves and understand their surroundings. Experiences in different settings and with different resources are very desirable for early movement competence. Many believe that all development springs from embodied interaction with the world. Thus, this is a key period in which to ensure that these children have the best possible start.

Pupils in primary school years will benefit from a regime that embraces physical literacy on account of the respect shown for each participant as a unique, holistic individual with particular potential and interests. Self-esteem will be sensitively nurtured. Natural curiosity and exuberance will be built on as these young people continue to explore a wide variety of movement contexts and build a bank of movement patterns. In addition, new experiences will be introduced that challenge the young person to work with others in a variety of ways and begin to take some responsibility for planning and evaluating their own goals. Important understanding will be fostered with respect to the value of physical activity in maintaining holistic health and well-being.

Learners in the secondary school years will benefit from a regime that embraces physical literacy on account of the respect shown for each participant as a unique, holistic individual with particular potential and interests. The focus on fostering motivation and confidence, as well as physical competence, can counteract fear of embarrassment and failure, and pave the way to lifelong commitment. The coverage of a range of activities can be an asset to informing participants of the very wide variety of physical activities in which they can participate. The opportunity to take some responsibility of aspects of the work is valuable both to enhance self-esteem and to empower them to make their own decisions. The consideration of the value of physical activity to holistic health will also be an asset.

Talented athletes will benefit from a regime that embraces physical literacy on account of its holistic, empathetic and personalised approach, with a focus on motivation and ipsative judgements on progress. Also of value will be the commitment to share decision-making with practitioners regarding, for example, training and goals, and the consideration of long-term participation. In a physical literacy context, the positive relationship between the practitioner and the participant is paramount. This is critical in respect of the athlete/coach relationship.

Those with particular needs will benefit from a regime that embraces physical literacy on account of the respect shown for the holistic individual and the caring, inclusive approach. The welcome and empathy shown to all should open the door to exploring new physical experiences and challenges. The focus on carefully managed progressive mastery will enhance the development of self-esteem and the strengthening of self-worth. Focus on ability rather than disability can empower these individuals to adopt a positive, confident attitude to life. Planning, creating and competing with others in a physical activity context can also add to the development of self-respect.

Adults will benefit from a regime that embraces physical literacy on account of the respect shown for each participant as a unique, holistic individual with particular potential and interests. The non-judgemental, inclusive atmosphere should foster motivation and confidence to explore new activities. These new experiences can open up avenues of activity that can be invigorating and rewarding, and strengthen self-awareness and self-confidence. Regular involvement in physical activity can be a significant asset in creating a balanced life pattern that mitigates against stress. Reflecting on and evaluating the effect of active participation on holistic health can help to maintain physical activity as an established feature of their lifestyle.

The older adult population will benefit from a regime that embraces physical literacy on account of the respect shown for the holistic individual and the caring, inclusive approach that is created. Motivation to continue to be active is a significant asset that can help to protect older people from falls, can contribute to sustaining independence, and can make a positive contribution to general health and well-being.

Conclusion

The value of physical literacy has been presented from both a philosophical stance and from a social justice perspective (see also Whitehead et al., 2018). In relation to the former, a range of newer thinking was shared. In respect of the latter, a case was made for physical literacy to be a distinct capability in its own right. In addition, the notion of fostering physical literacy as of value in itself or as a means to wider goals was discussed. Here, potential dangers of claiming wide-ranging benefits were outlined, and a case made that authentically planned and practised experiences with a clear physical literacy focus have the potential in and of themselves to enrich life as a whole. Finally, some key values in respect to different groups of people were outlined.

It is of note that there appears to be a growing consensus of opinion across the world that supports the value of lifelong participation in physical activity. This increase of awareness provides a valuable context for the development of the concept of physical literacy. The chapters written by colleagues from eight different countries in Part II demonstrate this promising development as they recount the way their countries have adopted the concept.

References

Archer, M.S. (2000) *Being Human: The Problem of Agency*. Cambridge: Cambridge University Press.

Arnold, P.J. (1979) *Meaning in Movement, Sport and Physical Education*. London: Heinmann.

Bloodworth, A., McNamee, M. and Bailey, R. (2012) Sport, physical activity and well-being: an objectivist account. *Sport, Education and Society*, 17(4): 497–514.

Clark, A. (2001) *Supersizing the Mind*. Oxford: Oxford University Press.

Claxton, G (1997) *Hair Brain Tortoise Mind*. New York: Ecco Press.

Claxton, G., Lucas, B. and Webster, R. (2010) *Bodies of Knowledge*. London: Edge Foundation.

Gill, G.H. (2000) *The Tacit Mode: Michael Polanyi's Postmodern Philosophy*. Albany, NY: State University of New York Press.

Johnson, M. (1987) *The Body and the Mind*. Chicago, IL: University of Chicago Press.

Maiese, M. (2016) *Embodied Selves and Divided Minds*. Oxford: Oxford University Press.

Nussbaum, M.C. (2000) *Women and Human Development: The Capabilities Approach*. Cambridge: Cambridge University Press.

Nussbaum, M.C. (2011) *Creating Capabilities: The Human Development Approach*. London: Belknap Press.

Polanyi, M. (1966) *The Tacit Dimension*. Garden City, NY: Doubleday.

Robeyns, I. (2003) *The Capability Approach: An Interdisciplinary Introduction*. Available at: http://citeseerx.ist.psu.edu/viewdoc/download?doi=10.1.1.196.14798&rep=rep1&type=pdf (accessed 14 March 2019).

Sen, A. (1992) *Inequality Re-Examined*. New York: Oxford University Press.

Sen, A. (1994) Capability and well being. In M. Nusbaum and A. Sen (eds), *The Quality of Life*. New York: Clarendon Press, pp. 30–53.

Standal, O.F. (2015) *Phenomenology and Pedagogy in Physical Education*. London: Routledge.

Valera, F.J., Thompson, E. and Rosch, E. (1993) *The Embodied Mind*. Cambridge, MA: MIT Press.

Whitehead, M.E. (ed.) (2010) *Physical Literacy across the Lifecourse*. London: Routledge.

Whitehead, M.E. (2013) What is the education in physical education? In S. Capel and M.E. Whitehead (eds), *Debates in Physical Education*. London: Routledge, pp. 22–36.

Whitehead, M.E. (2016–2018) *Physical Literacy: Philosophical Roots, Definition, Value and Implications*. Available at: www.physical-literacy.org.uk/resources/library/download-info/physical-literacy-philosophical-roots-definition-value-and-implications/ (accessed 6 December 2018).

Whitehead, M.E., Durden-Myers, E.J. and Pot, N. (2018) The value of physical literacy. *Journal of Teaching in Physical Education*, 37: 257–261.

5

WHAT DOES PHYSICAL LITERACY LOOK LIKE?

Overarching principles and specific descriptions

Margaret Whitehead

Introduction

'What does physical literacy look like?' is a question that is often asked alongside enquiries about how to operationalise physical literacy. The underlying concern is 'What are the implications for practitioners if the promotion of physical literacy becomes the rationale behind working with individuals and groups in respect of physical activity?' These questions have in fact been answered in a number of publications (Whitehead and Almond, 2013; Durden-Myers et al., 2018; Pot et al., 2018). However, these explanations have not always been seen as helpful. The reason for this could be that what seems to be wanted are model activities, sessions and programmes. This expectation poses significant problems, as in promoting physical literacy, the key determinant in planning is the participants. Much of the work of practitioners needs to be guided by the specific needs of the participants, rather than following a predetermined detailed plan. In other words, the practitioner 'teaches the participants, not a planned session'. This means that no one model example of a session or programme will accommodate all situations. However, there are clear guidelines that can be adopted to promote physical literacy, which can be drawn on to provide a structure for work appropriate to individuals in, for example, younger, older, very able or disabled groups. It is the role of the practitioner to use the recommendations in the guidelines to devise learning experiences for sessions with a particular group.

This chapter will set out these guidelines and exemplify broadly how these can be used in practice. The guidelines are grounded in the foundation philosophical principles underpinning the concept of physical literacy. They also relate to the definition and the attributes of physical literacy that are generated by the philosophy. The chapter continues with a consideration of planning issues in the context of physical literacy. After the conclusion and the references, there is an annex to the chapter comprised of guidance pertinent to practitioners working in different contexts. These refer to: parents and carers of preschool children; teachers and parents of primary school children aged 5 to 10–11 years; teachers of physical education at secondary level with learners aged 11 to 16–18 years; practitioners involved in coaching; practitioners working with participants with particular needs; personnel in the leisure industry; and practitioners working with the older adult population. While these recommendations are more practically based, they are developments of the principles laid out in the body of the chapter. Many of these include suggestions from practitioners who are working with the participants under discussion.

Answers to the question 'What does physical literacy look like?'

'What does physical literacy look like?' This is a frequently asked question. However, before giving an answer, further clarification about the nature of the question is needed, as it could refer to the participant, the nature of a physical activity session/programme, or to the broader context of a county, state or country. The question could therefore be asking, 'What does an individual who is making progress on a physical literacy journey look like?', 'What does a session or programme with the goal of promoting physical literacy look like?', or, 'What does a country, state or region that has adopted a policy of promoting physical literacy look like?'

The answer to the first question, 'What does an individual who is making progress on a physical literacy journey look like?', can be given with reference to the attributes set out in Chapter 2. The attributes were described as behaviours symptomatic of an individual who is making progress on a physical literacy journey. In short, a description based on the attributes might read:

> The individual takes part enthusiastically in physical activity, secure in the knowledge that the experience will be rewarding. The individual will have accrued a sound bank of movement patterns that can be drawn on in interaction with a range of physical activities. The individual can deploy imagination in solving problems in interaction with different physical environments, and can participate alone and alongside others. The individual understands the nature of movement and the value of participation in physical activity for well-being, and takes the initiative to be regularly involved in one or more activities.

This statement should be understood as an overarching description, which will need modification in relation to particular groups, such as those in the early years.

The answer to the second question, 'What does a session or programme with the goal of promoting physical literacy look like?', is best given with reference to alignment of practice to the philosophical principles underpinning the concept, the definition and the attributes of physical literacy. The definition has been described as setting out both the aspiration of physical literacy, being participation

TABLE 5.1 Relationship between the philosophical foundations, the definition and the attributes of physical literacy and physical literacy in practice

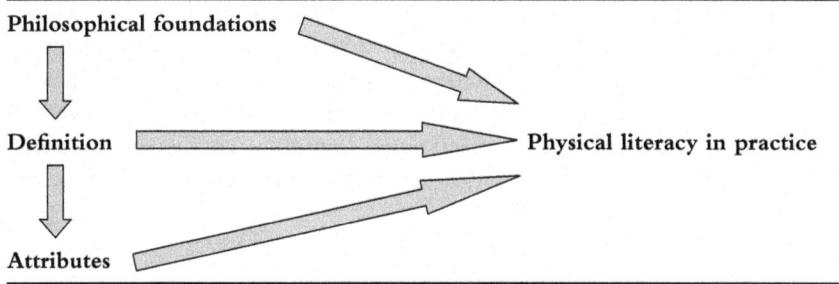

in physical activity for life, and the proposed means whereby progress can be made. These means are motivation, confidence, physical competence, and knowledge and understanding. The definition is further clarified in the attributes of physical literacy. To be true to the concept of physical literacy, the nature of sessions and the programme opportunities to promote physical literacy are best based on the relevant philosophy, the definition and the attributes. This is indicated in Table 5.1, and will be the main focus of this chapter.

The answer to the third question, 'What does a country, state or region that has adopted a policy of promoting physical literacy look like?', is that quality opportunities for physical activity for all sections of the population are evident. Policies from national and local government would be in place that articulate the value of physical activity, and this will have been followed up by strategies ensuring there are sufficient trained practitioners, adequate well-managed facilities for a wide range of physical activities, and provision of transport so that all have access to these facilities. In addition, the production of publicity material will be in evidence, as well as evaluation to ascertain that the desired outcomes of these various strategies are being achieved. This goal will be supported not only by those in the physical activity professions, but also by those working in other relevant fields (e.g. medicine and social care). All sections of the population would be catered for, inter alia, parents and carers of young children, teachers, coaches, instructors, those working with individuals with disabilities, and those working with the older adult population.

Key recommendations for working with participants

Before going into detail in respect of addressing the second question in greater depth, two points need to be stressed.

First, physical literacy is not taught. Physical literacy is fostered via participants accumulating meaningful, positive experiences, experiences that are likely to issue in lifelong participation (see explanatory glossary).

Second, the philosophical basis of physical literacy, far from being an impenetrable aspect of the concept, actually serves to clarify the nature of the work.

There is nothing mystical about the philosophy; rather, it provides clear guiding principles. Simply put, these principles are the need to treat each participant as a whole (springing from monism), the need to engage participants in a variety of activities (arising from existentialism), and the need to respect each participant as unique (a corollary of phenomenology). Where the practitioner works to these principles, they are likely to foster physical literacy. The fact that these are based on monism, existentialism and phenomenology should not confuse practitioners. The discussion in the next section of the chapter considers recommendations underpinned by these principles.

Unpacking the key recommendations for practice

With regard to practice, there are three aspects that need to be considered:

- the nature of the activity (i.e. the material or content);
- the type of learning/teaching approaches used, such as providing opportunities for participants to experiment or asking participants to replicate a given model; and
- the characteristics of the relationship between the participant and the practitioner, sometimes referred to as the overall ambience or atmosphere of the session.

Table 5.2 adds these three aspects to Table 5.1, indicating their relationship to the philosophy, definition and attributes of physical literacy.

An overarching checklist of key recommendations is presented below, and this is followed by three tables (Tables 5.3, 5.4 and 5.5), each of which sets out a more detailed consideration of each recommendation.

These identify the relationship of the proposals to the underpinning rationale from philosophy, the definition and the attributes. Some references are cited after the tables, most of which provide some background and detail of the nature of the recommendations given.

TABLE 5.2 Relationship between the philosophical foundations, the definition and the attributes of physical literacy and the key aspects of physical literacy in practice

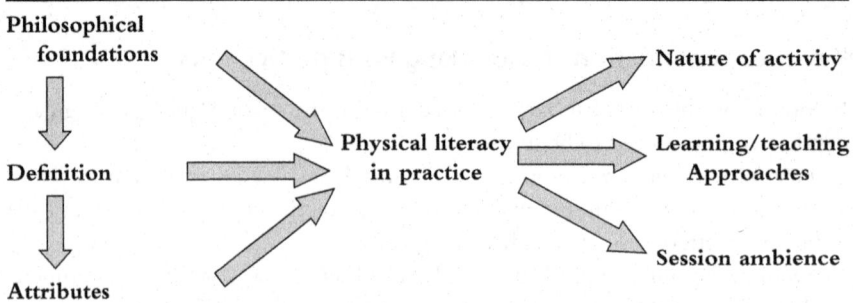

Checklist of key recommendations

Key recommendations for session content/activity/material

✓ Breadth of content covered
✓ Sufficient time given to develop competence
✓ Tasks/situations designed to match potential
✓ Explanation of the structure, protocols and value of material/activities given

Key recommendations for learning/teaching approaches

✓ Materials/tasks differentiated
✓ Individual formative feedback given
✓ Opportunities for problem-solving and creativity provided
✓ Expectation of personal goal-setting addressed

Key recommendations for session ambience or participant/practitioner interaction

✓ Knowledge of participants as individuals
✓ Each individual appreciated as a holistic feeling, moving and thinking person
✓ Work carried out in partnership/consultation with participants
✓ Overall atmosphere welcoming and experiences rewarding

Recommended texts related to Tables 5.3, 5.4 and 5.5

Session content/activity/material (Table 5.3)

Potentially valuable references include: Whitehead (2010) and Whitehead and Murdoch (2013) on breadth of coverage; Bressan and Weiss (1983) on developing competence; and Cale and Harris (2018) on promoting knowledge and understanding.

Learning/teaching approaches (Table 5.4)

Potentially valuable references include: Mosston and Ashworth (2002) on different teaching approaches and devolving responsibility to participants; Whitehead (2015) on pupil-centred teaching; Durden-Myers et al. (2018) on the range of teaching approaches; Kirk and MacPhail (2002) on situated learning; Capel et al. (2013) and Petty (2014) on differentiation; Deci and Ryan (1985), Standage et al. (2003) and Chen and Wang (2017) on self-determination theory and achievement goal theory; Holt et al. (2002), Forrest et al. (2006) and Rovegno

TABLE 5.3 Guidance on session content/activity/material covered

Session content/activity/material

Key recommendations	Underpinning rationale from philosophy, definition and attributes
Provide breadth of experience across all movement forms.	*Existentialist theory*: Individuals create themselves in interaction with the world. The richer the range of environments experienced, the greater the contribution to personal development. Breadth of experience caters for the potential/interest of all participants. *Physical competence* enhanced by breadth of experience. This relates to *attributes* C, D and E (see Chapter 2).
Give enough time to work on a particular activity to ensure well-founded growth in competence.	*Phenomenological theory*: Meaningful experiences will significantly influence future perception of similar situations (see explanatory glossary). *Physical competence* fostered where sufficient time is given for establishing movement patterns. This relates to *attributes* C, D and E.
Select tasks of an appropriate level of challenge to cater for all participants. Provide different tasks as needed.	*Phenomenological theory*: Every participant is different, and this needs to be borne in mind in challenges set. All should experience progress. *Physical competence* enhanced where tasks match participant potential. This relates to *attributes* C, D and E.
Set out and discuss the structure, protocols and value of activities.	*Monist theory*: All domains/faculties should be considered, including the cognitive. *Knowledge and understanding* fostered. Meaningful and effective engagement, and subsequent valuing, depends on understanding the nature of activities and relevant movement patterns. This relates to *attributes* F and G.

TABLE 5.4 Guidance on learning/teaching approaches

Learning/teaching approaches

Key recommendations	*Underpinning rationale from philosophy, definition and attributes*
Deploy differentiated approaches as appropriate to cater for each individual.	*Phenomenological theory:* Every participant is different, and each will make most progress if demands match potential. *Physical competence* will be enhanced. This relates to *attributes* C, D and E.
Employ informative individual feedback and assessment for learning to aid understanding.	*Phenomenological theory:* Every participant is different, and each will benefit from guidance that relates to individual need. *Physical competence* will be enhanced by individual feedback. This feeds into *attributes* C, D and E. *Knowledge and understanding* will be enhanced by informed observation and discussion. This relates to *attributes* F and G.
Involve participants in their own learning, solving problems and creating solutions, particularly in novel environments – this ensures that they take ownership of their own learning.	*Existentialist theory:* Experiences are richer where individuals have engaged in the practicalities of working in different environments. *Physical competence* will be enhanced with a heightened awareness of the different challenges set through working in a variety of environments. This relates to *attribute* D. *Valuing and taking responsibility.* Beginning to devolve responsibility to participants lays the ground for independent decision-making in the future. This relates to *attributes* F, G and H.
Involve participants in setting own goals and evaluating outcomes – this ensures that they develop a realistic appreciation of their personal potential.	*Monist theory:* Involvement of all domains/faculties should be addressed. *Physical competence* will be enhanced by individual's involvement in planning. This feeds into *attributes* C, D and E. *Knowledge and understanding* will be enhanced by informed observation reflection and discussion. This relates to *attributes* F and G.

TABLE 5.5 Guidance on session ambience or practitioner/participant interaction

Session ambience or participant/practitioner interaction

Key recommendations	Underpinning rationale from philosophy, definition and attributes
Know participants as individuals. Use participants' names and be aware of their interests and potential. Use ipsative judgement on progress	*Phenomenological theory:* Every individual is unique. *Monist theory:* Development of relationships with others is an aspect of the affective domain. *Motivation.* Participants will thrive in situations in which they feel known and valued. *Motivation* enhanced by positive non-judgemental guidance. This relates to *attributes* A and H.
Appreciate each participant as a holistic feeling, moving and thinking person. Create a 'can-do' climate and celebrate effort, progress and achievement. Set tasks that are challenging but realistic.	*Monist theory:* Refutes dualism and highlights the need to treat each person as a whole, rather than comprised of separate aspects. *Confidence.* Practitioners' confidence in participants fosters their self-confidence. This is backed up by appropriate use of praise. Practitioners' appreciation of effort is reassuring. The atmosphere is encouraging, and experiences are anticipated as being self-affirming and building self-confidence. This relates to *attributes* B and H.
Create a way of working in which the views of each individual are welcomed. The views of participants are valued, discussed and, where possible, acted upon.	*Phenomenological theory:* Every individual is valued as unique. *Confidence.* Practitioner respect for the value of contributions from the participant is empowering and encourages self-esteem and self-worth. *Knowledge and understanding* will be enhanced via involvement of reflective and reasoned discussion. This relates to *attributes* B and H.
Create an ambience in which participation is rewarding and invigorating. Participants feel cared for and welcome. Participants helped to look ahead in making physical activity a chosen aspect of life.	*Monist theory:* Supports consideration of the affective, physical and cognitive domains, and the need to respect each person as a whole. *Motivation.* Participants feel secure with no danger of embarrassment. *Knowledge and understanding* will be enhanced via involvement of reflective and reasoned discussion. This relates to *attributes* A and H.

and Dolly (2006) on participant involvement in learning; Vealey (1986) on mastery learning; and Newton and Bowler (2015) and Zwozdiak-Myers (2015) on feedback and assessment for learning.

Session ambience or participant/practitioner interaction (Table 5.5)

Potentially valuable references include: Whitehead (2015) on learner-centred teaching; Morgan and Carpenter (2002) and Appleton and Duda (2018) on motivational climate; Oliver (2009), Oliver and Hamzeh (2010) and Hellison (2011) on participant involvement in planning sessions; Bandura (1977) and Feltz and Chase (1998) on self-efficacy; and Magyar and Feltz (2003) and *Physical Education Matters* (2018) on motivating girls.

Reflection on Tables 5.3, 5.4 and 5.5

In many cases, the above descriptions may be in line with the nature of current sessions, and practitioners may feel that they are already exemplifying these recommendations. However, in some cases, alignment with the characteristics outlined could involve some modifications to practice. These modifications may be very small; however, subtle as they might be, they are critical in developing a positive attitude to participation. For physical literacy to be developed, the experience of participants is best aligned with the suggestions above. Each and every participant needs to leave a session having made some progress, feeling valued, and with enhanced self-belief and self-esteem. Positive experiences of this nature can lay the foundation to lifelong participation.

The role of planning and reflection in working to promote physical literacy

In indicating earlier that practitioners should perhaps 'teach participants, not sessions', this is not to infer that planning is no longer needed. Planning is crucial to achieve the goal of fostering physical literacy. However, this planning may need to exemplify a slightly different approach, not least as participant responses cannot always be predicted with accuracy.

Guidelines for planning

- *Introductory and plenary/concluding elements* of the session are likely to retain their standard characteristics, being a preparation for the session and a résumé/ discussion of the experiences of the session. Concluding episodes can be very valuable in the context of physical literacy as participant perceptions can be gathered and considered in respect of future planning.

- *An intended outcome of the session* is, of course, necessary, and will have been identified on consideration of the needs of the group. However, this should be seen as provisional, and may need to be modified in the light of participant response. During the course of the session, the intended outcome may need to be modified – to be less or more challenging, or to be diversified to accommodate the variety of participant responses. This may mean an adjustment in the success criteria for the session.
- *A series of tasks, exploratory movement situations* and smaller and larger group challenges designed to facilitate progress towards realising the intended outcome will need to be identified. However, it is advisable to have considered additional alternative activities should they be needed, either to simplify or to increase the challenge of the work. This aspect of sessions is essential given that each participant is unique and differentiation of activities is likely to be needed. A range of equipment needed should be earmarked and prepared, keeping in mind the potential need for modifying some of the activities.

Practitioner reflection

As indicated above, the actual course taken in a session is dependent on the responses of the participants. Any plan will provide a broad outline of the session, but its actual nature will depend on the participants. It is seen as important, therefore, that throughout the session, the practitioner is monitoring participant behaviour, reflecting on what is observed and making modifications to match needs. In an educational context, this is referred to as 'reflection in action'; that is, reflection during the session (Zwozdiak-Myers, 2012, 2015). These texts also consider the role of 'reflection on action', being reflection after the completion of the session. In the context of physical literacy, this second mode of reflective practice is critical as it focuses in on the participants, and addresses whether the learning outcomes have been achieved in a session and what aspects of the guidance given were particularly effective. Alongside the session-specific reflection on action, it is valuable for the practitioner to consider how far the work has addressed the philosophical principles and has fostered the elements of physical literacy, viz. motivation, confidence, physical competence, and knowledge and understanding. In a physical literacy context, where the interests of the participants are paramount, these two types of reflection are essential. While the references to reflection come from an educational setting, they are pertinent to all practitioners. Participants are the focus of work to foster physical literacy, and wherever possible their needs should be addressed.

Implications for programme structure

Designing programme structure is relevant to all practitioners, and importantly needs to consider depth and breadth. In respect of planning in an educational context, curricular constraints have to be considered. This is not an easy task. The dilemmas and possibilities of this planning have been debated by Whitehead and Murdoch (2010, 2013). These texts should be referred to for more detail, but in essence the recommendation is to provide experience across all movement forms in curriculum time. As advised above, experience in a particular activity is best given over a number of weeks, thus giving time for participants to become familiar with an activity and develop movement patterns that facilitate effective participation. With an overall structure of this nature, participants will only be able to experience a few examples from each movement form. To provide a breadth and depth of experience, it is recommended that all participants are encouraged to take part in further activities in extracurricular time. Extracurricular work is best designed for all, rather than being solely an opportunity for the most able to further develop their potential.

Conclusion

The chapter was concerned to address the question of what physical literacy looks like. Having considered the nature of the question posed, attention focused on what physical literacy looks like in situations where participants are working with practitioners.

The fundamental answer that provided the scaffold for this discussion was that participants are best considered as holistic individuals who will benefit from a rich variety of experiences and who are respected for their uniqueness. These are the characteristics that are essential to fostering physical literacy, and they arise from the philosophy that underpins the concept. It was stressed that the philosophy underpinning the concept, far from complicating the situation, actually provides the rationale for practice.

It was suggested that work with participants had three aspects, being the material covered, the nature of the methods used to promote progress, and the ambience of the session. Each of these aspects generated four key recommendations. These recommendations were listed and then presented in tabular form to show how each was related to the philosophy, the definition and the attributes of physical literacy. The chapter concluded with some thoughts on how working to an aspiration of developing physical literacy has implications for the nature of planning sessions, for practitioner reflection on the effect of their work with participants, and for the design of programmes or opportunities for activity.

Set out after the References is an Annex to Chapter 5 that looks at the implications of working to promote physical literacy in a range of settings. These build from the material in the body of the Chapter but comprise more practical ideas relevant to different groups of participants.

References

Appleton, P. and Duda, J. (2018) Empowering motivational climates in physical education and school sport. *Physical Education Matters*, 13(3): 46–47.

Bandura, A. (1977) Self-efficacy: toward a unifying theory of behavioral change. *Psychological Review*, 84: 191–215.

Bressan, E.S. and Weiss, M.R. (1983) A theory of instruction for developing competence, self-confidence and persistence in physical education. *Journal of Teaching in Physical Education*, 2: 38–47.

Cale, L. and Harris, J. (2018) The role of knowledge and understanding in fosterng physical literacy. *Journal of Teaching in Physical Education*, 37: 280–287.

Capel, S., Leask, M. and Turner, T. (2013) *Learning to Teach in the Secondary School*. London: Routledge.

Chen, A. and Wang, Y. (2017) The role of interest in physical education: a review of research evidence. *Journal of Teaching in Physical Education*, 36: 313–322.

Deci, E.L. and Ryan, R.M. (1985) *Intrinsic Motivation and Self Determination in Human Behavior*. New York: Plenum.

Durden-Myers, E.J., Green, N.R. and Whitehead, M.E. (2018) Implications for promoting physical literacy. *Journal of Teaching in Physical Education*, 37: 262–271.

Feltz, D.L. and Chase, M.A. (1998) The measurement of self-efficacy and confidence in sport. In J.L. Duda (ed.), *Advances in Sport and Exercise Psychology Measurement*. Morgantown, WV: FIT Press, pp. 65–80.

Forrest, G.J, Webb, P.I. and Pearson, P.J. (2006) *Teaching Games for Understanding: A Model for Pre-Service Teachers*. Available at: http://ro.uow.edu.au/cgi/viewcontent.cgi?article=1075&context=edupapers (accessed 14 March 2019).

Hellison, D.R. (2011) *Teaching Personal and Social Responsibility through Physical Activity*, 3rd edn. Champaign, IL: Human Kinetics.

Holt, N.L., Stream, W.B. and Bengoechea, E.G. (2002) Expanding the teaching games for understanding model: new avenues for future research and practice. *Journal of Teaching in Physical Education*, 21: 167–176.

Kirk, D. and MacPhail, A. (2002) Teaching games for understanding and situated learning: rethinking the Bunker and Thorpe model. *Journal of Teaching in Physical Edicatiion*, 21: 177–192.

Magyar, T.M. and Feltz, D.L. (2003) The influence of dispositional and situational tendencies on adolescent girls' sport confidence sources. *Psychology of Sport and Exercise*, 4: 175–190.

Morgan, K. and Carpenter, P. (2002) Effects of manipulating the motivational climate in physical education lessons. *European Physical Education Review*, 8(3): 209–232.

Mosston, M. and Ashworth, S. (2002) *Teaching Physical Education*, 5th edn. San Francisco, CA: Benjamin Cummings.

Newton, A. and Bowler, M. (2015) Assessment for and of learning in PE. In S. Capel and M.E. Whitehead (eds), *Learning to Teach Physical Education in the Secondary School*, 4th edn. London: Routledge, pp. 140–155.

Oliver, K.L. (2009) Girly girls can play games. *Journal of Teaching in Physical Education*, 28(1): 90–110.

Oliver, K.L. and Hamzeh, M. (2010) 'The boys won't let us play': fifth grade mestizas challenge physical activity discourse at school. *Research Quarterly for Exercise and Sport*, 81(1): 38–51.

Petty, G. (2014) *Teaching Today: A Practical Guide*, 5th edn. Oxford: Oxford University Press.

Physical Education Matters (2018) 13(1) (whole section on articles consdering empowering girls).

Pot, N., Whitehead, M.E. and Durden-Myers, E.J. (2018) Physical literacy from philosophy to practice. *Journal of Teaching in Physical Education*, 37: 246–251.

Rovegno, I. and Dolly, J.P. (2006) Constructivist perspectives on learning. In D. Kirk, D. Macdonald and M. O'Sullivan (eds), *The Handbook of Physical Education*. London: Sage, pp. 242–261.

Standage, M., Duda, J.L. and Ntoumanis, N. (2003) A model of contextual motivation in physical education: using constructs from self-determination and achievement goal theories to predict physical activity intentions. *Journal of Educational Psychology*, 95: 97–110.

Vealey, R.S. (1986) Conceptualization of sport-confidence and competitive orientation: preliminary investigation and instrument development. *Journal of Sport Psychology*, 8: 221–246.

Whitehead, M.E. (ed.) (2010) *Physical Literacy throughout the Lifecourse*. London: Routledge.

Whitehead, M.E. (2015) Learner centred teaching: a physical literacy approach. In S. Capel and M.E. Whitehead (eds), *Learning to Teach Physical Education in the Secondary School*, 4th edn. London: Routledge, pp. 171–183.

Whitehead, M.E. and Almond, L. (2013) Creating learning experiences to foster physical literacy. *Physical Education Matters*, 8(1): 24–27.

Whitehead, M.E. and Murdoch, E. (2010) Physical literacy, fostering the attributes and curriculum planning. In M.E. Whitehead (ed.), *Physical Literacy throughout the Lifecourse*. London: Routledge, pp. 175–188.

Whitehead, M.E. and Murdoch E. (2013) What should pupils learn in physical education? In M.E. Whitehead (ed.), *Debates in Physical Education*. London: Routledge, pp. 55–73.

Zwozdiak-Myers, P. (2012) *The Teacher's Reflective Practice Handbook*. London: Routledge.

Zwozdiak-Myers, P. (2015) Teacher as a researcher/reflective practitioner. In S. Capel and M.E. Whitehead (eds), *Learning to Teach Physical Education in the Secondary School*, 4th edn. London: Routledge, pp. 233–255.

ANNEX TO CHAPTER 5

Recommendations for practitioners working in different contexts

Work to promote physical literacy is presented in respect of the following practitioners:

1. Parents and carers of preschool children
2. Teachers and parents of primary school children aged 5 to 10–11 years
3. Teachers of physical education at secondary level with learners aged 11 to 16–18 years
4. Practitioners involved in coaching
5. Practitioners working with participants with particular needs
6. Personnel in the leisure industry
7. Practitioners working with the older adult population

While these recommendations are more practically based, they are developments of the principles laid out in the body of the chapter. Most of these short pieces of guidance include suggestions from practitioners working in the field under discussion. It would be valuable in the future to gather models of best practice in respect of working with each of the following groups of participants. Recommended texts are included with each section.

1. Parents and carers of preschool children

What are the implications for parents and carers of preschool children in relation to fostering the foundation of physical literacy? While the general principles outlined in the first half of the chapter are significant and relevant, young children of this age have very particular characteristics and needs. These young people are developing very rapidly, and their characteristics will change from month to month. However, throughout these early years, they are 'movement-hungry', and it is principally through movement that they make contact with the world and come to realise their physical capabilities. These children are readily fascinated by the effect they can make on the environment and will happily spend many hours exploring. This exploration is not inconsequential play, but the essential trigger to holistic development. It is important that as they use movement to find out about the world, this is a rewarding pleasurable experience. In this learning to interact with their surroundings, children begin to build up a bank of movement memories. In addition, young children are astute observers and learn a great deal from copying the movement of other children and adults.

In the light of these characteristics, the recommendations to parents and carers are grouped under the headings of: maximise movement opportunities; provide opportunities to interact with a range of settings; encourage exploration; and be active with the young child.

Maximise movement opportunities

✓ *Enable* babies to move freely and to maximise physical activity during every waking hour (e.g. leg-kicking, arm-waving and grasping when back-lying, pushing up to raise the head and chest in tummy time, reaching and rolling over).

✓ *Encourage* progression to pushing up to hands and knees, crawling, sitting, standing, walking, toddling, balancing and climbing.

✓ *Promote* movement development by encouraging free play, movement exploration and discovery. Limit use of restraints and keep sedentary time to a minimum.

✓ *Promote* physical development with young children through their use of large muscles needed for locomotion, core and upper body strength, and smaller/finer muscles needed for manipulation.

Provide opportunities to interact with a range of settings

✓ *Introduce* babies and young children to all available environments, indoors, outdoors and in water, and encourage active play.

✓ *Provide* a wide variety of toys and other resources (including in the natural environment) of varying texture, shape, size and colour to encourage and stimulate physical activity and development of physical competence.

✓ *Include* moving with music to extend movement experiences. Encourage activities such as clapping, swaying and waving, and movements such as bending, stretching, wobbling, shaking, twisting and turning. Encourage rhythmical movement and travelling such as stepping, jumping and bouncing.

Encourage exploration

✓ *Encourage* inquisitiveness, trial and error, and safe experimentation in movement to help to embed movement vocabulary and movement memory, and to aid the development of movement confidence.

✓ *Express* enthusiasm for inventiveness and initiative.

✓ *Facilitate* repetition and celebrate growing balance, control and coordination.

✓ *Share* in the excitement of discovering the world around.

✓ *Describe* in language what the child is doing.

Be active with the young child

✓ *Engage* in frequent contact play with babies, on the floor, in arms, in water and outdoors.

✓ *Encourage* other children and carers to play with babies and young children, and together explore movements, environments, a range of toys and other stimuli.

✓ *Promote* physical development with young children through participating with them in activities that develop both the large muscles, needed for locomotion, core and upper body strength, and the fine muscles, needed for manipulation.

✓ *Provide* models of simple movements as you play with the child.

✓ *Describe* in language what you are doing and applaud the child emulating the adult.

The support and encouragement described above have the potential to lay the foundations for the motivation, confidence, physical competence, and knowledge and understanding that will facilitate the development of rewarding participation in physical activity. It cannot be stressed too strongly that these early experiences are absolutely crucial to physical literacy and to holistic future development.

Recommended reading

Brodie, K. (2018) *The Holistic Care and Development of Children from Birth to Three*. London: Routledge.

Conkbayir, M. (2017) *Early Childhood and Neuroscience: Theory, Research and Implications for Practice*. London: Bloomsbury Academic.

Goddard-Blythe, S. (2005) *The Well Balanced Child*. Stroud: Hawthorn Press.

With thanks to Patricia Maude.

2. Teachers and parents of primary school children aged 5 to 10–11 years

What are the implications for teachers and parents of children aged 5 to 10–11 years in relation to fostering physical literacy? This is an important period in the individual's physical literacy development, linking the preschool years to the adolescent years. This period is sometimes seen as pivotal to the development of physical literacy, as these children are naturally inquisitive, active and keen to be involved in a wide variety of experiences. Steady physical growth continues to underpin physical competence while affective and cognitive development is marked, making these children impressionable, enquiring and reflective. As a result, it is imperative that attention is paid to all aspects of physical literacy. However, as these children grow towards adulthood, they become ever-more unique, and it is important that this is taken into account in promoting physical literacy. In line with these characteristics and needs, the implications are set out under the following headings: facilitate development of physical competence; provide a wide range of environments; enable all participants to develop motivation and confidence; promote effective interaction with other learners; and foster perceptive learners.

Facilitate development of physical competence

✓ *Provide*, for the younger child, frequent active movement/play throughout each day while keeping sedentary time to a minimum.
✓ *Encourage* the younger child to explore a wide range of activities, such as running, jumping, leaping, skipping, climbing and swinging.
✓ *Capitalise* on opportunities for each child to develop physically in strength, dexterity and endurance.
✓ *Guide* children in increasing their movement vocabulary, extending their movement memory, and enhancing their movement quality.
✓ *Establish* a range of movement capacities and movement patterns.
✓ *Set* tasks that challenge each child within their own potential and help them to make progress.

Provide a wide range of environments

✓ *Provide* a wide range of safe indoor, outdoor and water-based environments.
✓ *Engage* younger children in play in these environments.
✓ *Introduce* the older learner to a range of movement forms.
✓ *Discuss* and explore physical activity demands in each of these different environments.
✓ *Set* challenges to work in and explore a range of environments – familiar and novel.
✓ *Set* challenges across all areas of activity that progress from individual practice to small group situations, through to larger group planning, choreography and game play.
✓ *Encourage* children to learn by experience in interacting with different environments.

Enable all participants to develop motivation and confidence

✓ *Use* encouragement and praise to build motivation and confidence.
✓ *Get to know* each child and be able to respond to individual progress.

✓ *Develop* self-esteem by showing care and respect for each child.
✓ *Celebrate* application, progress and achievement.
✓ *Provide* optimistic feedback and use assessment for learning.
✓ *Adopt* a positive 'can-do' approach.
✓ *Help* children to be realistic in relation to their potential.
✓ *Encourage* learners to set appropriate goals and learn from their mistakes.
✓ *Help* children to manage ways of learning through winning and losing.

Promote effective interaction with other learners

✓ *Develop* cooperation, competitiveness and respect for others.
✓ *Set* an example in respecting all learners, appreciating their different interests and potential.
✓ *Encourage* mutual respect among learners.
✓ *Provide* opportunities for learners to work together to support learning, solve problems and debate outcomes.
✓ *Encourage* working together, listening to each other and sharing ideas.
✓ *Facilitate* sharing views of favourite activities, particular challenges and personal goals.

Foster perceptive learners

✓ *Encourage* children to become independent learners who question, think, rethink, reflect, problem-solve and evaluate their progress in all domains of physical literacy.
✓ *Involve* children in observing movement and articulating strengths and areas for development.
✓ *Discuss* types of physical activity and resultant challenges and expectations.
✓ *Debate* and reinforce the value and importance of frequent activity for physical development and lifelong health.
✓ *Consider* issues relating to choosing physical activity for life.

The support and encouragement described above have the potential to build from the foundation laid in the preschool years to create a springboard for developing an ever-more secure and robust attitude to physical activity. This will facilitate further development of physical literacy in the later years of schooling. As indicated above, it is important that throughout this stage of life, every young person experiences growth in the motivation, confidence, physical competence, and knowledge and understanding in relation to physical literacy. Valuing and taking responsibility for participation in physical activity should be well on the way to being established at this stage, and thus commitment to lifelong participation should be a real possibility.

Recommended reading

Maude, P. (2001) *Physical Children, Active Teaching*. Buckingham: Open University Press.
Pickard, A. and Maude, P. (2014) *Teaching Physical Education Creatively*. London: Routledge.
Whitebread, D. and Coltman, P. (2015) *Teaching and Learning in the Early Years*, 4th edn. London: Routledge

With thanks for contributions from Patricia Maude.

3. Teachers of physical education at secondary level with learners aged 11 to 16–18 years

What are the implications for teachers of learners in the secondary age range (11 to 16–18 years of age) in relation to fostering physical literacy? The general principles outlined in the main body of the chapter are all relevant to learners of this age. Ideally, these teachers will be building on from the learners' previous experiences and will be concerned to help these young people make further progress in respect of all domains – affective, physical and cognitive. This time in schooling is particularly significant as it will be the last time that every young person will take part in physical education lessons taught by qualified specialist teachers. On leaving school, there is no guarantee that these young adults will be involved in physical activity. It is therefore critical that these teachers address all areas of physical literacy and reach every young person, enhancing their motivation, confidence, physical competence, knowledge and understanding, and commitment to choose physical activity for life. Considering these needs, recommendations for these teachers are grouped under the following headings: ensure that motivation and confidence are enhanced; provide opportunities for the development of physical competence; extend knowledge and understanding of movement and physical activities; enhance appreciation of the value of physical activity; and develop a commitment to participation in physical activity and the ability to take responsibility for holding to this intention.

Ensure that motivation and confidence are enhanced

- ✓ *Maintain* an enthusiastic and encouraging approach.
- ✓ *Create* a 'can-do' ambience in which learners experience success, satisfaction and enjoyment.
- ✓ *Use* praise as appropriate with all learners.
- ✓ *Recognise* application, effort, progress and achievement.
- ✓ *Plan* to ensure all can succeed by recognising personal strengths and needs.
- ✓ *Build* self-confidence and self-respect by showing empathetic concern for each learner as an individual.
- ✓ *Ensure* all learners feel valued and avoid their experiencing any embarrassment.

Provide opportunities for the development of physical competence

✓ *Plan* differentiated tasks that cater for all abilities.
✓ *Plan* a series of progressive tasks to engage and challenge learners in line with their potential.
✓ *Use* mastery learning as appropriate.
✓ *Balance* establishing routines with keeping sessions lively and varied.
✓ *Provide* sufficient time for practice.
✓ *Provide* for appropriate feedback in the form of 'assessment for learning'.
✓ *Apply* movement techniques to competitive and cooperative group situations, and to solo activity sequences and challenges.
✓ *Ensure* that learners have opportunities to experience examples of all movement forms for a length of time sufficient to experience meaningful engagements.

Extend knowledge and understanding of movement and physical activities

✓ *Use* a rich and wide vocabulary of human movement descriptors.
✓ *Describe* clearly the nature of the movement being worked on and encourage learners to use this language.
✓ *Clarify* key observation points and steps to make progress.
✓ *Create* posters and work cards to set out aspects of movement.
✓ *Underpin* the involvement in forms of activity with clear rubrics, rules and procedures.
✓ *Welcome* questions and dialogue about all aspects of human movement.

Enhance appreciation of the value of physical activity

✓ *Work* to involve learners in movement and physical activity experiences that are meaningful, rewarding and self-affirming (see explanatory glossary).
✓ *Make links* with areas of holistic health as appropriate in the course of the sessions.
✓ *Welcome* discussion about the benefits of physical activity.
✓ *Encourage* reflection on the nature of their own experiences, preferences and goals.

Develop a commitment to participation in physical activity and the ability to take responsibility for holding to this intention

✓ *Build* learner involvement into each part of the session as appropriate.
✓ *Set* tasks involving discovery and problem-solving.
✓ *Allow* learners to set their own goals and evaluate their own progress.
✓ *Encourage* group discussion regarding planning and evaluation.

✓ *Devolve* responsibility as appropriate for session and unit planning.
✓ *Share* and debate the wide range of opportunities for participation beyond school.
✓ *Help* learners to look ahead in respect of making physical activity integral to their life.
✓ *Debate* the problems they might meet in holding to their intentions.

As set out above, it is very important that all areas of physical literacy are covered and established in this final period of schooling. The overall aspiration with these young people would be to establish a robust and secure disposition in respect of choosing physical literacy for life. It would seem to be essential that those practitioners working in this stage engage with each learner as a unique individual. It is suggested that practitioners need to demonstrate their respect for all individuals – and acknowledge that they may have particular potentials, personal interests and/or individual needs. Experiences in physical activity will be more likely to issue in lifelong commitment: first, where individuals develop their self-respect and self-confidence as a result of participation; and second, where there is a clear understanding that they are on their own physical literacy journey that will be particular to them and will not be 'matched' against that of others.

Recommended reading

Almond, L. and Whitehead, M.E. (2012) Translating physical literacy into practice for all teachers. *Physical Education Matters*, 7(3): 67–70.
Ames, C. (1992) Achievement goals, motivational climate and motivational processes. In G.C. Roberts (ed.), *Motivation in Sport and Exercise*. Champaign, IL: Human Kinetics, pp. 161–176.
Petty, G. (2014) *Teaching Today: A Practical Guide*, 5th edn. Oxford: Oxford University Press.
Whitehead, M.E. (ed.) (2010) *Physical Literacy throughout the Lifecourse*. London: Routledge.
Whitehead, M.E. (2015) Learner centred teaching: a physical literacy approach. In S. Capel and M.E. Whitehead (eds), *Learning to Teach Physical Education in the Secondary School*, 4th edn. London: Routledge, pp. 171–183.
Whitehead, M.E. and Almond, L. (2013) Creating learning experiences to foster physical literacy. *Physical Education Matters*, 8(1): 24–47.

4. Practitioners involved in coaching

What are the implications for those working in the field of coaching with respect to fostering physical literacy? It is suggested that consideration of the underpinning philosophy of physical literacy, as well as the definition and its constituents, could be of benefit to the coaching profession in at least two ways. Coaches would wish to promote a commitment on the part of the participant to a particular physical activity and the processes that help the athlete to make progress in this activity. In addition, coaches would hope that once elite participation comes to an end, participants would continue with involvement in some form or forms of physical activity.

Coaching creates a unique scenario for involvement in physical activity, and any recommendations for practice need to be set in this context. Where valuing commitment to physical activity is concerned, the broad principles set out in the main body of the chapter provide a sound framework to practice.

However, the coaching scenario presents a range of particular challenges that can mitigate against some aspects of the framework. This is a significant area of study that cannot be addressed in full here. However, five key concerns will be identified and some recommendations will be listed. These areas relate first to avoiding a dualist attitude in which attention to the physical domain can preclude sensitivity to the affective aspect of being human. Second, there is danger of somewhat rigid models of practice being employed and a disregard of the unique nature of each participant. Third, there can sometimes be a tendency for coaches to be overcritical of performance and progress, with less recognition of improvement. Fourth, a coach may take responsibility for all planning and goal-setting without discussion with the athlete. Finally, closely related to the fourth issue may be a coach's adoption of a style of self-presentation that presumes total authority. In the light of these issues, recommendations are grouped under the following headings: appreciation of the holistic nature of each participant; recognition that each participant is on their unique physical literacy journey; promotion of motivation by creating an optimistic and positive environment; work in partnership with participants; and establish an appropriate learning/coaching context.

Appreciation of the holistic nature of each participant

✓ *Show* a genuine interest in each participant in respect of all aspects of their nature – physical, affective and cognitive – in and beyond their sport(s).
✓ *Take time* to understand participants' previous experiences.
✓ *Understand* the wider context(s) around your participants (e.g. school sport pressures, work environments, NGB talent/performance contexts to avoid burnout and dropout).
✓ *Take time* to get to know their aspirations, hopes and fears.
✓ *Understand* how maturation cycles affect performance both positively and negatively, and therefore realise that performance measurement is not always an accurate articulation of effort.
✓ *Appreciate* the importance of significant others (parents, siblings, etc.) and engage with those within participants' support network(s).

Recognition that each participant is on their unique physical literacy journey

✓ *Value* every individual by showing belief in and respect for them.
✓ *Guide* participants, interacting with sensitivity with each individual.
✓ *Be flexible* to adapt session(s) intensity, content and context relative to changing personal circumstances (e.g. school exams, performances, work pressures).

✓ *Set* tasks that are challenging but realistic, allowing participants to negotiate aspects of task development in line with personal and collaborative objectives.

✓ *Develop* participant self-belief and self-esteem via showing acceptance of their particular characteristics/unique nature.

Promotion of motivation by creating an optimistic and positive environment

✓ *Create* a supportive 'can-do' atmosphere to promote confidence.

✓ *Use* appropriate feedback to reward effort, progress and achievement.

✓ *Foster* motivation via ipsative assessment – judgements being made against previous performance.

✓ *Avoid* comparison with other participants.

✓ *Recognise* individual and collaborative successes (even within losing scenarios) – what did you/we do well/learn? Do this both personally and corporately.

Work in partnership with participants

✓ *Develop* mutual respect.

✓ *Adopt* the role of facilitator.

✓ *Collaborate* to agree long-term and short-term goals.

✓ *Encourage* participants to contribute to discussions about planning individualised programmes.

✓ *Promote* participant understanding of the nature of challenges and empower them to share responsibility for planning tasks.

✓ *Ensure* they are clear about the nature of the whole programme journey, outlining expectations and what sessions may involve, emphasising a culture of mutual support.

✓ *Communicate* regularly and clearly with each individual about their developmental journey.

Establish an appropriate learning/coaching context

✓ *Adopt* pedagogical approaches that empower participants.

✓ *Use* leadership styles that allow your participants to grow into leaders.

✓ *Model* prosocial behaviours to establish a supportive culture.

✓ *Explain and articulate* your philosophy and coaching approaches to ensure participants understand the principles underpinning your work.

✓ *Establish/negotiate* a vision and values that all your participants buy into.

Recommended reading

Cassidy, T., Jones, R. and Potrac, P. (2008) *Understanding Sports Coaching*. London: Routledge.
Jones, R. (ed.) (2006) *The Sports Coach as Educator*. London: Routledge.
Martens, R. (2012) *Successful Coaching*. Champaign, IL: Human Kinetics.

With thanks to Simon Padley.

5. Practitioners working with participants with particular needs

What are the implications for those working with participants with particular needs in relation to fostering physical literacy? The general principles outlined in the main body of the chapter are all relevant to these participants across the age range. At root, physical literacy is an inclusive concept. All individuals can make progress on their physical literacy journey. While every participant is unique, it is suggested that those with special needs may also share some common characteristics. It can be the case that these individuals lack self-confidence and self-belief. They can be resigned to their situation and seldom consider new avenues or goals. It might be the case that involvement in physical activity has never been considered an option in respect of their participation. In addition, these individuals may have very many of the decisions about their activities and lifestyle made by others. Clearly, others have their best interests at heart, but lack of autonomy can be depressing and debilitating. In addition, there are often a series of challenges to meet when new projects are considered. Sometimes these barriers can mitigate against participation.

Taking into account the particular characteristics and needs of these participants, the recommendations are set out under the following headings: work to enhance self-belief, motivation and confidence; respect participants as individuals; ensure that each session is rewarding, with progress being made; offer a wide range of activities to cater for all; provide opportunities to give participants autonomy; and be alert to barriers to participation.

Work to enhance self-belief, motivation and confidence

✓ *Create* a positive supportive ambience/culture.
✓ *Ensure* participants are valued and feel that they belong.
✓ *Be aware* of potential low self-esteem and fear of bullying.
✓ *Develop* a 'can-do' ambience and reward effort as well as progress.
✓ *Handle* failure with empathy.
✓ *Use humour* as appropriate and with sensitivity.

Respect participants as individuals

✓ *Take* steps to welcome each participant.
✓ *Know* participants as individuals, using their names and showing interest in their particular aspirations.
✓ *Maintain* consistent practitioner/participant relationships.

Ensure that each session is rewarding, with progress being made

✓ *Ensure* activities are purposeful and meaningful.
✓ *Create* situations in which participants succeed and are proud of their progress.

✓ *Employ* differentiated approaches to cater for all and create an inclusive climate.
✓ *Provide* individualised feedback.
✓ *Display patience* as participants explore involvement.
✓ *Show genuine delight* when there is evidence of growing competence.

Offer a wide range of activities to cater for all

✓ *Include* group, individual, competitive and cooperative activities.
✓ *As appropriate,* have activities on or in water and outdoors.
✓ *Use modified* activity forms as well as activities designed for those with a disability.
✓ *Include aesthetic* activities as an option.

Provide opportunities to give participants autonomy

✓ *Take time* to discuss opportunities and possibilities with participants.
✓ *Involve* participants in all decisions concerning choice of activities.
✓ *Work* with participants to set individual schedules and goals.
✓ *Plan* for the long term with the participants.
✓ *Always be open* to listen to participants' views and ideas.

Be alert to barriers to participation

✓ *Take steps* to make the physical environment welcoming.
✓ *Be proactive* to accommodate practical issues such as travel arrangements and provision of assistance.
✓ *Address individual barriers,* such as previous unsatisfactory experiences or bullying, with sensitivity.
✓ *Ensure consistency* in the pattern of sessions for autistic participants.
✓ *Counteract apprehensions* of parents by reassuring them regarding safety and underlining the value of participation.
✓ *Involve parents* in encouraging participants to attend regularly.

There is no doubt that people of all ages with particular needs can benefit greatly from participation in physical activity. All can build on their abilities to make progress on their physical literacy journey. Their individual development, and the recognition this brings, can have a significant influence on their quality of life and provide additional purpose, pleasure and meaning. If the recommendations set out above are carefully considered and appropriately applied, it can often be the case that these participants can find physical activity engaging and rewarding, and grow in self-esteem and self-respect. In addition, this involvement can enhance understanding of movement and of the value of physical activity for holistic health.

Recommended reading

Arbour-Nicitopoulos, K.P., Boross-Harmer, A., Leo, J., Allison, A., Bremner, R., Taverna, F., Sora, D. and Wright, V.F. (2018) Igniting fitness possibilities: a case study of an inclusive community-based physical literacy program for children and youth. *Leisure/Loisir*, 42: 69–92.

Coates, J. (2011) Physically fit or physically literate? How children with special educational needs understand physical education. *European Physical Education Review*, 17: 167–181.

Muir, A. (2013) Developing physical literacy in children and youth with a disability. *Physical & Health Education Journal*, 78(4): 44.

Rimmer, J.H., Padalabalanarayanan, S. and Malone, L. (2017) Fitness facilities still lack accessibility for people with disabilities. *Disability and Health Journal*, 10: 214–221.

Withers, A.J. (2012) *Disability Politics & Theory*. Nova Scotia: Fernwood.

World Health Organization (WHO) (2011) *World Report on Disability*. Geneva: WHO.

With thanks to Stuart MacReynolds and colleagues in the Abilities Centre in Ottawa, Canada.

6. Personnel in the leisure industry

What are the implications for personnel in the leisure industry in relation to promoting physical literacy? How can they make a positive impact on promoting life-long participation? All the general principles outlined in the main body of the chapter will be pertinent; however, the implications for those in the leisure industry will need to take account of their particular customers/participants. These people come voluntarily and pay for involvement in physical activities. In a sense, practitioners in the leisure industry are involved in marketing. Those people with a sound commitment to physical activity are likely to use leisure facilities readily and regularly; however, there will be many who will need to be coaxed, encouraged and even persuaded to take part. Some of these in the latter group may not have had altogether positive experiences in respect of physical activity in the past, and could be labelled 'hard to reach'. There may be some potential for the leisure service to collaborate with the medical services in the locality.

What can personnel in the leisure field do to attract more people to take part? There are perhaps five areas to consider. These are: be alert to potential barriers to participation; provide a welcoming ambience; cater for a wide range of interests; provide positive rewarding experiences; and ensure that participants feel valued and respected. Each leisure provider across the world will have particular roles and opportunities, and the suggestions set out below represent just some of the constituents of these five areas that might be apposite. Recommendations to consider in practice will be clustered under the areas identified above.

Be alert to potential barriers to participation

This could include consideration of ease of travel to the centre, cost of participation, availability and clarity of publicity material, provision of childcare facilities, and family-friendly schedules.

Provide a welcoming ambience

This could include ensuring there is a warm and caring contact with all staff. It is the case that some people come to an activity centre as much for the social contact as the activity, and their interaction with others can make a significant impact on their returning. The centre itself should have a welcoming ambience with, for example, good lighting and signage.

Cater for a wide range of interests

This could include opportunities for participation in a wide range of activities (e.g. competitive, cooperative, in groups, as an individual). Provision of classes at different levels of challenge and links with other activity providers can be assets. The message that physical activity is for all, and not just the highly skilled, can be reassuring for many participants

Provide positive rewarding experiences

There could well be two types of participant: those who come for the positive experience of being active with others, and those that attend with a goal of enhancement of physical competence. The first group will benefit from encouragement, support and maybe a variety of programmes on offer. The second group may welcome a more 'hands-on' relationship with practitioners, involving specific praise, advice and individual feedback. In classes such as these, consistent staffing is valuable to ensure participants are known and can be guided to make appropriate progress. All progress in respect of both groups can be celebrated, however small.

Ensure that participants feel valued and respected

This could include participants being known by name and being respected as having very different needs, interests and aspirations. Individuals with particular needs should be welcomed with appropriate programmes offered wherever possible. Sincere concern for problems raised by participants and a willingness to work with them to find solutions demonstrates that client views are valued. Again, a willingness to listen to clients' suggestions for developments can create a partnership that might help to retain participation.

Through addressing a range of the above suggestions, there is significant potential to promote motivation, confidence, physical competence, and knowledge and understanding to an extent that participants become committed to physical activity for life.

Recommended reading

VTCT World Class Qualifications (n.d.) *Customer Services in the Sport and Active Leisure Industry. Level 4 course, UV 30577 H/6901/7676.* Available at: http:// qualifications.vtct.org.uk/finder/unitpdf/UV30577.pdf (accessed 19 March 2019).

7. Practitioners working with the older adult population

What are the implications for those working with the older adult population in relation to promoting physical activity, and thus fostering physical literacy?

All the general principles outlined in the body of the chapter will be pertinent; however, the implications for practitioners working with the older adult are likely to have to address needs particular to those in this age range. These needs are well documented in, for example, UK Active (2017). This document identifies barriers that include 'lack of motivation or perceived ability, lack of opportunities or a lack of confidence regarding what activity is appropriate and the positive impact it can have on health' (p. 8). Identified here are the key elements of physical literacy being motivation, confidence, physical competence, and knowledge and understanding. Recommendations to consider in practice will be clustered under the above four areas.

Promote motivation

✓ *Show* pleasure in seeing participants at the session.
✓ *Get to know* your participants and use their names.
✓ *Take time* to understand participants as unique individuals.
✓ *Use* encouragement and praise, both of which are powerful motivators.
✓ *Create* a relaxed atmosphere and an ambience of enjoyment.
✓ *Use* music as appropriate, for stimulation, relaxation and scaffolding movement tasks.

Foster confidence

✓ *Give* individualised feedback to recognise effort, progress and achievement.
✓ *Use* language that is readily understood, repeating guidance as needed.
✓ *Repeat* activities frequently to develop confidence.
✓ *Recognise* and respond appropriately to the different potentials and restrictions displayed by the class.
✓ *Celebrate* participation, progress and success – however small.
✓ *Reassure* participants, wherever possible, on the good quality of their movement participation.
✓ *Respect* each participant as a valuable member of the group.

Maintain physical competence

✓ *Include* activities that enhance strength and flexibility in different joints and muscles.
✓ *Include* activities that are designed to prevent falls.
✓ *Repeat* activities frequently to promote progress.
✓ *Increase* challenge as appropriate, for the whole class or for individuals.
✓ *Devise* sessions that include a variety of activities.
✓ *Use* a range of equipment, such as balls, scarves and small dumb-bells.

Encourage knowledge and understanding

✓ *Share* with participants the value of the session, and how the exercises will help them carry out everyday tasks and sustain their independence.

✓ *Explain* the nature of the focus of the session.

✓ *Use* simple, clear instructions explaining the purpose of each activity.

✓ *Recap* what you have done and why at the end of the session.

✓ *Provide* opportunities for participants to reflect on and discuss the impact and value of the sessions.

✓ *Invite* participants to suggest other activities.

As appropriate, participants should be encouraged to repeat some of the movement challenges between sessions. Where possible, it can be useful to enable participants to be in contact with the practitioner between sessions. Some participants may be happy to keep a diary of their activities. It can be helpful to encourage participants to share their experiences with their doctor and others in the medical professions.

Through addressing a range of the above suggestions, there is significant potential to promote motivation, confidence, physical competence, and knowledge and understanding to an extent that participants value physical activity and maintain participation.

Recommended reading

ACC (2003) *Otago Exercise Programme to Prevent Falls.* Available at: www.acc.co.nz/assets/injury-prevention/acc1162-otago-exercise-manual.pdf (accessed 14 August 2018).

Extend (n.d.) *Movement to Music for the Over Sixties and Less Able People.* Available at: www.extend.org.uk (accessed 14 March 2019).

Jones, G.R., Stathokostas, L., Young, B.W., Wister, A.V., Chau, S., Clark, P. Duggan, M., Mitchell, D. and Norland, P. (2018) A physical literacy model for older adults: a consensus process by the collaborative working group on physical literacy for older Canadians. *BMC Geriatrics* 18(3), doi: 10.1186/s12877-017-0687-x.

UK Active (2017) *Moving More, Ageing Well.* Available at: https://110percent.co.uk/wp-content/uploads/2017/12/UK-Active-Life-Fitness-Active-Ageing-Report.pdf?x12015 (accessed 14 August 2018).

With thanks to Steve Clark, Kenny Butler and Tracy Levy.

6

CHARTING THE PHYSICAL LITERACY JOURNEY

Margaret Whitehead

Physical literacy as a journey

As has been stressed in this text, physical literacy is not a state that is attained and then maintained thereafter. Therefore, the question, 'Are you physically literate?' is not appropriate. Physical literacy is a disposition or attitude, and can be understood as a personal perspective on an aspect of life. This perspective develops as the individual accrues experiences in interacting with the world and thus is a perspective that can change throughout the course of life.

Notwithstanding the somewhat ephemeral nature of physical literacy as a disposition, it is a feature of life and can be reflected on and described. Any description of this disposition will represent a considered response to the question, 'What is your current perception of participating in physical activity?' As life experiences are unique to the individual and as each experience will modify perception, attitudes to participation in physical activity will take a course specific to that individual. Hence, the IPLA proposes that the notion of charting a journey rather than assessing any form of 'progress' is better aligned to the concept of physical literacy.

Charting progress in line with the philosophical principles underpinning physical literacy

As was described in preceding chapters, work to promote physical literacy should at all times relate to and build from the philosophical basis of the concept. Reference to this grounding is essential to be true to the beliefs that are fundamental to physical literacy. Clear alignment to the philosophical basis both highlights the specific nature of the concept and maintains the integrity of physical literacy. Charting an individual's journey is a very significant aspect of fostering physical literacy, and the design of any procedure needs to acknowledge and address the underlying philosophy.

Physical literacy is founded on the *monist principle* that, as humans, we are a whole, a whole comprised of a range of essentially interrelated and interdependent domains. Whatever the nature of experiences in which individuals are involved, it is the case that very many of these domains will be involved. In respect of physical literacy, the affective, physical and cognitive domains will play a part in any experience. To address this monist view, it is recommended that all three domains are taken into consideration and given equal status in the gathering of data on an individual's journey. No one domain is privileged over another. The IPLA would want to ensure that nothing stands in the way of a commitment to physical activity for life. Less than sound motivation and robust confidence within the affective domain, less than broadly based physical competence in the physical domain, or less than secure knowledge and understanding in the cognitive domain can, in their different ways, threaten future participation. It is perhaps valuable to stress that given the importance of motivation in respect of fostering physical literacy, any process used to chart a journey should be seen as an opportunity to enhance motivation. Wherever possible, these procedures should celebrate personal success.

Physical literacy is also grounded in the philosophical theories comprising *existentialism*, where richness of experience is advocated in order to provide varied and challenging environments to promote personal development. It is through working within and responding to different situations that individuals will 'craft' their uniqueness and develop their potential to thrive. It is therefore recommended that information gathered concerning a physical literacy journey should include reflections on involvement in physical activity in the widest range of situations in which it is feasible for participants to be involved. This range includes varied environments, different movement forms (Whitehead, 2010) and alternative ways of interacting with other people. The notion of 'literacy' within the concept of 'physical literacy' arises from the importance of interaction as described by existentialists. This physical interaction is, principally, that which takes place in participation in movement forms. The recording of progress concerned with interaction in movement forms should constitute a very important aspect of charting progress in respect of physical competence. It is suggested that the acquisition of techniques that lay the ground for effective interaction should only constitute a small part of any charting process.

The third philosophical pillar on which physical literacy is founded is *phenomenology*. Put simply, phenomenology celebrates the uniqueness of each individual. Each person accrues a specific set of experiences that colour perception of and response to the situations encountered. Where charting a physical literacy journey is concerned, it is felt important that all changes identified in respect of an individual should be judged against the previous behaviours of that person. Comparison with others is not relevant as each individual has specific endowments and brings a unique set of previous experiences to an activity setting. The imprint of these earlier experiences will affect how participants view and respond to the challenges set. For example, the level of motivation and confidence (affective domain) shown will be indicative of the nature of previous experiences and the physical competence (physical domain) evident will reflect both individual endowment and previous

TABLE 6.1 Relationship between philosophical principles underpinning physical literacy and instruments to chart progress on an individual's physical literacy journey

Philosophy	Implications for charting a physical literacy journey
Monism	Information captured from across all three domains, affective, physical and cognitive. All procedures designed to promote motivation.
Existentialism	Information captured in a wide variety of situations, including those involving different environments, different physical activity protocols and different relationships to others. Judgements regarding constituent aspects of participation (e.g. techniques) are a relatively small consideration.
Phenomenology	Individuals treated as unique. No comparison made with others. Judgements ipsative (i.e. set against previous personal data).

opportunities to develop movement patterns (Whitehead, 2010). Knowledge and understanding (cognitive domain) will, in the same way, reflect individual endowment and opportunities to appreciate processes and values inherent in physical activity. In the context of respecting each individual, it is recommended that any benchmarks used in charting the journey should be criterion-referenced, not norm-referenced, and, importantly, be viewed as formative rather than summative. For data collection to be true to phenomenological principles, any gathering of information should be ipsative (i.e. judged against previous information concerning the individual).

The impact of philosophy on charting a physical literacy journey is summarised in Table 6.1.

Charting progress in line with the definition of physical literacy

Keeping the principles arising from philosophy in mind, the design and use of a scheme to chart a physical literacy journey will require clarification of the nature of the information to be collected. This will characteristically be in the form of descriptors. Indeed, all the schemes that will be referred to in this chapter have created categories of descriptors against which to judge aspects of physical literacy. To retain the integrity of the concept, it would seem to follow that the descriptors created need to address all aspects of the definition of the concept.

In line with this need to accommodate the aspects referred to in the definition, the IPLA has drafted descriptors that address the elements of motivation, confidence, physical competence, and knowledge and understanding. In creating the descriptors, attention was also given to the attributes, which, as was explained in Chapter 2, are designed to give further clarification to the definition. The IPLA matrix can be seen in Table 6.2.

The horizontal rows in the matrix feature these four elements. Each of these sections is expanded into three subsections:

- Evidence of motivation identifies: (1) motivation to participate in physical activity; (2) sustained application and engagement with motivation to apply self; and (3) motivation to take steps to include physical activity in a life pattern.
- Evidence of confidence identifies: (1) confidence to engage; (2) self-perception of ability and a belief that progress can be made; and (3) confidence to interact and engage with a range of environments.
- Evidence of physical competence identifies: (1) evidence of the foundation movement patterns that constitute the basis of all movement/physical activity; (2) movement within a wide range of environments in individual and group contexts; and (3) sensitive perception of, and perceptive action in, physical activity environments.
- Evidence of knowledge and understanding identifies: (1) knowledge and understanding in respect of reflection on and improvement of performance; (2) knowledge and understanding of planning, interacting and creativity; and (3) knowledge and understanding of well-being in relation to the value of physical activity.

Further development of the IPLA matrix

Following addressing the philosophical issues and the parameters of the definition, the IPLA debated the broad principles that should be recognised in the use of the matrix. It is suggested that the following should be seriously considered.

It is recommended that the matrix should:

- make a positive contribution to fostering physical literacy;
- create a holistic 'picture' of the participant;
- provide an opportunity to celebrate progress;
- be applicable for use with participants of all ages;
- be easy to use;
- involve completion, wherever possible, by the participant;
- use best-fit self-reflective descriptors in simple language;
- enable all participants to engage in constructive self-reflection throughout life;
- accommodate realistic expectations that respect changing life patterns; and
- be in a form that could be completed online.

With these broad principles in mind, a matrix was drawn up with five columns creating an overarching structure. The columns are headed: unaware of or dismissing potential; exploring potential; developing potential; consolidating potential; and maximising potential. The matrix is designed for charting a lifelong journey, accommodating people of all ages. While the headings are not tied to a particular age group, in most cases descriptors under the headings of exploring potential and developing potential will be evident in childhood and adolescence, and descriptors under the heading of consolidating potential will generally be characteristic of adults. It would be true to say that the underlying aspiration of physical literacy is

TABLE 6.2 IPLA draft instrument to chart a physical literacy journey

Characteristics of physical literacy journeys		*Unaware of or dismissing potential*
Motivation	Motivated to participate in physical activity	I seldom want to engage in physical activity.
	Sustained application and engagement – motivated to apply oneself	I do not apply myself fully when engaged in physical activity.
	Motivated to take steps to include physical activity in my life pattern	I take steps to avoid physical activity.
Confidence	Confident to engage	I am not confident to take part in physical activity.
	Self-perception of ability and belief that progress can be made	I am not confident that I can make progress in phsyical activity.
	Confident to interact and engage with a range of environments	I am generally not at ease in physical activity environments.
Physical competence	Movement patterns that constitute the foundation of all movement/physical activity	I have limited movement vocabulary related to physical activities.
	Movement within a wide range of environments, both individually and with others	I am seldom able to move effectively in movement environments.

Exploring potential	Developing potential	Consolidating potentail	Maximising potential
I am physically active because I enjoy it.	I participate in physical activity for the joy of it and because it is important to me.	I maintain being physically active because it is part of who I am and because I value it.	I am motivated to try new activities and challenge my capabilities.
I apply myself during physical acitvity.	I do not give up easily and keep going. I am persistent and resilient.	I sustain my engagment and involvement in regular physical activity.	I am determined to challenge myself in a range of environments.
Physical activity is included in my life pattern.	Physical activity forms an increasingly regular part of my life pattern.	Physical activity is a secure part of my life pattern.	I seek new ways to include physical activity in my life pattern.
I look forward to taking part in physical activity.	I am confident that I can fulfil the tasks set and that others will support me.	I am certain that participation will be rewarding and enhance my self-confidence.	I am confident that with practice/effort, I can fulfil the challenges set by myself and others.
I am confident that I can make progress in physical activity.	I am aware that I have made progress in some activities and confident that I am capable of making further progress.	I know I can have rewarding experiences in physical activities, and this enhances my self-esteem.	I appreciate my movement abilitiy, and am confident that I can enhance my expertise and learn from future challenging experiences.
I am at ease engaging in physical activity in varied indoor and outdoor situations.	I look forward to new settings and activities with the confidence that I can engage effectively within these environments.	I am confident to explore a range of settings, more or less familiar to me, with the assurance that I can respond to the demands they make on me.	I relish new and challenging environments and set myself ambitious goals.
I am developing my movement vocabulary associated with a wide variety of physical activities.	I am developing general and refined movement patterns and linking them into sequences associated with a range of physical activities.	I continue to apply and adapt my movement patterns that form more complex sequences related to the physical activities in which I participate.	I am able to move effectively using specific movement patterns in one or more challenging physical activities.
I am starting to engage a wide variety of physical activity environments, both individually and with others.	I am succesfully engaging in physical activity in an increasing range of varied environments, both individually and with others.	I continue to engage effectively and efficiently in a variety of physical activity environments, both individually and with others.	I seek out opportunities to challenge myself in a range of physical activity environments, both invidually and with others.

(continued)

TABLE 6.2 *(continued)*

Characteristics of physical literacy journeys		Unaware of or dismissing potential
	Sensitive perception of and perceptive action in interaction with physical activity environments.	I am not aware of movement requirements related to most physical activity environments
Knowledge and understanding	Reflecting on and improving performance	I find it difficult to describe what I am doing well and where I need to improve.
	Planning, interacting and creativity	I find it hard to work by myself or with others when I participate in physical activity.
	Well-being and valuing physical activity	I am not conviced of the importance of physical activity for my holistic health and well-being.

Exploring potential	Developing potential	Consolidating potentail	Maximising potential
I am starting to develop my awareness of the movement requirements of varied physical activity environments.	I am becoming more aware of and sensitive to the demands presented by varied physical activity environments.	I show heightened sensitivity to and awareness of my physical competence when interacting perceptively in physical activity environments.	I am perceptive in appreciating all aspects of challenging physical activity environments, anticipating movement needs or possibilities and responding appropriately to these with perception and imagination.
I can identify movements that I am working on and think about what I need to improve.	I can describe movements that I am working on, suggesting where I am being successful and targets that I could work towards.	I can evaluate movements that I am working on, identifying where I am being successful, setting realistic targets and devising ways in which I can work towards these targets.	I can analyse all aspects of movement that I am working on, describing my strengths and aspects that require improvement. I challenge myself by devising strategies through which I can reach targets.
I can work individually and with others in planning and adapting movement sequences and physical activities, contributing ideas and listening to the views of others.	I can work individually and with others, in a range of settings, creating and refining movement sequences and physical activities, contributing ideas, listening to and respecting the views of others.	I can work individually and with others in reflecting on, creating and refining movement sequences and physical activities. I contribute ideas, listening to and respecting the views of others and play my part in different roles in competing and cooperating with others.	I work individually and with others, in challenging physical activity environments, creatively planning my own and others' responsibilities in competitive and cooperative situations.
I understand that physical activity helps me to keep well so that I can enjoy life.	I understand that participating in physical activities will have a beneficial effect on my holistic health and provide opportunities for me to thrive in physical activity settings alone and/or with others in a variety of different environments.	I understand that participating in a range of physical activities will have a positive impact on my holistic health and enable me to maintain my quality of life.	I understand that participating in a range of physical activities opens up a world of opportunity for challenging myself in worthwhile experiences in a wide variety of settings that will contribute to my holistic health, as well as enhance my quality of life.

that all adults should identify themselves as aligned with descriptors in the consolidating potential column.

The IPLA has included an unaware of or dismissing potential column to accommodate those who, for a variety of reasons at any age, are not involved in physical activity. This may be caused by a lack of opportunity to become aware of embodied potential, or a rejection of involvement in physical activity as a result of negative experiences or as a consequence of unavoidable changes in a life pattern. These changes could be the result of serious illness or injury, the imperative to take on caring responsibilities, or the necessities related to employment expectations (see Whitehead, 2010: 7; regarding physical illiteracy, see also the explanatory glossary). Where unaware of or dismissing potential is recorded, the goal would be to work towards re-engagement, in which case the individual may need to address expectations in the exploring potential and developing potential columns before hopefully aligning with consolidating potential descriptors. The fifth heading of maximising potential has been included to accommodate those who set themselves the goal to reach their full potential, typically, but not exclusively, in a competitive situation. Personal goal-setting of this nature may feature at almost any age and may last a longer or shorter time. While most people maximising potential will be in the young adult age range, adults of any age could well set themselves a particularly challenging target. These individuals will position themselves in the maximising potential descriptor column. Later, they are likely to return to the consolidating potential. Given that lives are full of twists and turns, it is highly likely that in every journey, there will be movement to the right and the left of the matrix.

Detailed descriptors have been created that indicate the changes that can be made looking horizontally across the five columns, from unaware of or dismissing potential to maximising potential, in respect of each of the elements. This gives 60 descriptors. These descriptors outline characteristics that represent how individuals perceive themselves at the time of completing the matrix. The selection of descriptors made can be read to indicate where, for example, motivation or physical competence have been enhanced, and can thus provide the opportunity to celebrate progress. The descriptors can also give guidance about the nature of future goals towards realising an ever-more robust disposition to choose physical activity for life.

To signal the long-term aspiration of taking responsibility for self-evaluation and forward planning, the matrix is a self-report instrument completed by the participant. The task of the participant is to select the 12 best-fit descriptors, identifying one from each horizontal row/element subsection. The IPLA has tried to create a simply worded and easy-to-use instrument. All the descriptors/boxes selected do not necessarily need to fall under one column, such as developing potential or consolidating potential. The IPLA is considering whether to include an additional judgement once a 'descriptor/box' has been identified. This could take the form of completing a simple Likert scale or the addition of one of the following descriptors: *sometimes, often* or *frequently*. It is anticipated that an individual may identify the same 'box' over a number of charting situations, and the possibility of making this extra judgement gives individuals the opportunity to record progress within a single descriptor.

The IPLA is also currently working on ways that information from the charting matrix can be recorded, retained and displayed in a way that 'paints a picture' of the participant, and over time tells an individual story. In addition, the IPLA plans to develop software to record the outcome of individuals' matrix use online.

Issues concerning the use of the IPLA instrument

The underlying purposes of the IPLA matrix are to record and celebrate developing physical literacy at the same time as encouraging individuals to take responsibility for their own physical literacy journey. It is appreciated that in the early years, a parent or carer will be responsible for completing the matrix with increasing discussion with the young person. In the years of schooling, the teacher, coach or other practitioner may well provide support and guidance until the individual can take on full responsibility. With respect to the older adult population, another adult may need to be involved. It is indeed the case that throughout life, the involvement of another person in reflecting on the story revealed by the matrix can be very valuable on at least two counts. First, parents, teachers, coaches and carers might become aware of ways that they themselves can play a part in promoting an individual's physical literacy. Indeed, it could well challenge practitioners to consider the content and pedagogy for which they are responsible. Second, a peer, doctor, friend or family member may be able to discuss reasons for the nature of the records and consider possible ways forward. In broad terms, the IPLA matrix represents a resource to support progress or, as referred to in literature, a tool to effect 'assessment for learning' (Black and Wiliam, 2002).

The matrix has been shared widely for discussion but has yet to be trialled. It is expected that descriptors may need to be clarified and language use may need modification for different age groups. The IPLA intends to keep colleagues up to date, via the IPLA website, on developments of the matrix, and will be pleased to hear from anyone who has used aspects of the matrix. It is important to recognise that the IPLA matrix has been designed to align closely with both the underlying philosophy related to the concept and the IPLA definition. The intention was also to create a manageable resource that can be used by the participant and can play a valuable role in the development of physical literacy.

Some practical issues concerning charting a physical literacy journey

This section looks briefly at the importance of charting physical literacy journeys and some misunderstandings that have problematised charting physical literacy journeys.

Apart from a triad of instruments created in Canada and one in the United States, systems of assessment of physical literacy, which the IPLA refers to as systems to chart an individual's progress on a physical literacy journey, have been slow to develop. Reference to the definition and/or attributes is a useful starting point. The IPLA based its proposal on the elements of the definition being motivation, confidence, physical competence, and knowledge and understanding. However, attributes are also a very useful focus as they are designed to describe behaviours symptomatic of developing physical literacy. Linking charting progress with the definition and/or the attributes is valuable in that this signposts the relationship of these aspects of physical literacy with participant practice. In this way, the credibility of the concept is enhanced.

Without a tool to capture relevant information, those promoting physical activity have been unable to demonstrate progress in respect of physical literacy and unable to verify ways of modifying learning approaches and experiences to effect the desired behaviour change. This has damaged the acceptance and credibility of the concept. There are a number of issues here.

At the heart of the problem has been the monist nature of the concept set against the need to gather information concerning a variety of behaviours or symptoms. It is felt that charting progress needs to take account of the affective, physical and cognitive domains involved in physical literacy. While this gives the impression of a form of dualism and a 'segmented' individual, it is considered essential that information on each of the feeling, acting and thinking strands of the concept needs to be addressed separately. One justification of this separation may be that behaviour change related to each domain is best gathered in particular ways in line with the discipline involved. As will be seen from the schemes referred to below, data and other information are captured in a wide variety of ways. Amalgamating all this information into a coherent picture has, in some cases, been challenging. Multiple descriptors arising from different perspectives can prove unwieldy, while attributing scores that are simply added up into one total would seem to lose critical information about different domains. Where 'scores' are given, it is all too easy to make comparisons between individuals rather than to focus on differences in an individual's 'score' over time. The IPLA has tried to solve this problem in that the outcome of working from the proposed matrix is a series of descriptive personal pictures that the individual has seen and currently sees as the best fit for him or herself. Another corollary of attributing 'scores' can be the all-too-ready identification of norms that are to be expected at different ages and stages. Norm-referencing, in the context of charting a journey, is not recommended. Every individual is on a unique journey. Where pressure is put on practitioners to create norms, it is imperative that these are used sensitively, ideally in relation to personal goals. As far as possible, messages of 'not making the grade' or 'failure' should be avoided, as this can be demotivating and put future participation at risk.

Some misunderstandings concerning physical literacy and how these can affect procedures to chart a physical literacy journey

There have been a number of misunderstandings concerning physical literacy alongside some perceptions of assessment processes that have made charting progress problematic. These are set out in Table 6.3 alongside consequences with reference to charting physical literacy journeys.

TABLE 6.3 Misunderstandings and their consequences in respect of charting a physical literacy journey

Misunderstanding	Outcome in relation to charting a physical literacy journey
1. 'Literacy' understood as intellectual acuity is viewed as the key aspect of the concept	Only information concerning intellectual change is captured (cognitive domain)
2. The affective domain is viewed as of little importance	The affective domain is all but ignored
3. Information has to be quantifiable to be valid	Only readily quantifiable information is collected
4. Physical education and physical literacy are interchangeable	Systems in use to assess physical education have been maintained, presuming they are relevant to physical literacy
5. Developing foundation movement techniques (or FMS) believed to be the same as fostering physical literacy	Data on physical competence only gathered in a 'practice/drill-like' situation, and no attention given to the meaningful interaction in varied physical activity contexts to which physical literacy aspires
6. Clear evidence of changes in respect of physical literacy can be evident in a short space of time	Unrealistic expectation of significant change over a very short space of time (e.g. 5 or 10 weeks)

Misunderstandings 1–5 in are unfortunate, and each in their different way threaten the integrity of the concept of physical literacy. Misunderstanding 6 – the expectation of rapid change – fails to appreciate that modifying a disposition is a slow process. The aspiration of promoting physical literacy is a lifelong challenge and can only be fully realised in life as a whole.

Instruments across the world

To update colleagues on work being carried out across the world, this section contains a brief outline of five systems to chart/measure physical literacy – some of which have been used over a number of years and some that are still being tri-alled. There are three fully developed schemes from Canada and one in the United States. The scheme referred to in Australia is in the planning stage. All the schemes have involved a great deal of investment and work, and the IPLA is grateful for this endeavour. It needs to be understood that each scheme has been developed as apposite to a specific country and has built from a particular version of the definition of physical literacy. Most of the schemes have been designed for use in a school or coaching context. Some of the schemes have a substantial aspect referring to movement competence, and this has resulted in the development of detailed continua of descriptors setting out incremental movement mastery. Continua of descriptors are also evident in some schemes in relation to affective and cognitive domains. Some of the schemes involve the participant in the assessment, and most include advice regarding what can be worked on to build on current strengths and remedy weaknesses. Some of the schemes require qualified observers to gather the data. Most schemes involve grading and the amalgamation of these grades in different ways. Access to further detail of each scheme is signposted where possible.

Canada: Canadian Assessment of Physical Literacy (CAPL)

The definition of physical literacy used to underpin this assessment scheme is described as 'the motivation, confidence, physical competence, knowledge and understanding to value and take responsibility for engagement in physical activities for life' (Tremblay et al., 2018: 1).

Discussion in the Healthy Active Living and Obesity Group at the Children's Hospital of Eastern Ontario Research Institute in Canada concerning an assessment tool for physical literacy began in 2007 and resulted in the CAPL-1 (Longmuir et al., 2015).

The rationale for measuring physical literacy using the CAPL is to identify areas of weakness so that interventions can be targeted and ultimately be more successful at improving physical literacy over time (Longmuir, 2013).

The CAPL has been used across Canada since 2014, and has recently been subject to comprehensive testing on over 10,000 Canadian schoolchildren. This study was funded by the Royal Bank of Canada (RBC), the Public Health Agency of Canada and Mitacs, and was delivered in partnership with ParticipACTION within their Learn to Play Project, and has been recorded in 14 refereed journal articles.

As a result of this foundational research, there have been significant modifications made to the measurement protocols producing the CAPL-2 (see www.capl-ecsfp.ca). Principal among these modifications were shortening and simplifying the content, the redesign of the Motivation and Confidence domain, and the reweighting of the scoring for each domain. For example, prior to the recent modifications, Motivation and Confidence were weighted 18%. This domain is now weighted 30%.

Working from a definition of physical literacy very close to that of the IPLA, the CAPL-2 is designed to measure physical literacy levels in 8- to 12-year-olds and addresses four domains:

- *Physical Competence*, which includes measures of fitness and dynamic movement skills. These aspects of physical literacy were designed to be assessed by qualified observers.
- *Knowledge and Understanding*, which includes coverage of areas such as recommended participation in physical activity, cardiovascular fitness, muscle strength and endurance, and improvement of sport skill. This domain of the CAPL is completed by the participant and can be administered in paper form or online.
- *Motivation and Confidence*, which assesses intrinsic motivation, competence, predilection and adequacy. This is a self-report tool completed by the participant in paper form or online.

- *Daily Behaviour*, which includes an average daily step count using a pedometer and a self-report element regarding active participation in physical activity through a week.

Physical Competence, Daily Behaviour, and Motivation and Confidence each attract 30 marks, while Knowledge and Understanding is attributed 10 marks.

All data are entered into a web-based database and results are automatically totalled, culminating in a score out of 100.

The individual scores and their total can be used in a number of ways:

1. For individuals to know how they are progressing. Involvement of the participants is seen as preparation for future responsibility for their own participation.
2. For individuals and significant others to consider the nature of future challenges. This is supported in the documentation through the inclusions of suggestions of how current levels can be built on to promote progress.
3. For the practitioner to clarify if the teaching is achieving identified goals.
4. For parents and those in positions of responsibility to gauge the quality and success of programmes and interventions. Scores can be compared with the target range of marks based on normative and criterion-based evidence.

In relation to each measure, domain and total score, descriptors are provided to explain how participants are progressing. These descriptors are categorised in sequence as: Beginning, Progressing, Achieving or Excelling. These can be used to help monitor, inform and motivate personal and population physical literacy journeys.

The custodians of the CAPL are cautiously optimistic that the scheme is being effective in changing practice and encouraging participation in physical activity.

With thanks to Mark Tremblay (references can be found at the end of the chapter).

Canada: Passport for Life (PFL) – Physical and Health Education Canada

Physical and Health Education Canada (PHE Canada) developed the physical literacy educational assessment resource entitled Passport for Life (PFL) to support the awareness, assessment and advancement of physical literacy among physical education students and teachers (see http://passportforlife.ca/what-is-passport-for-life). The definition used by PHE Canada describes physical literacy as referring to an individual who is moving 'with competence and confidence in a wide variety of physical activities in multiple environments that benefit the healthy development of the whole person' (Lodewyk and Mandigo, 2017: 442).

PFL is designed to assess four components: *Movement Skills*, which addresses Locomotion, Object Control and Object Manipulation; *Fitness Skills*, which addresses Cardiovascular Endurance, Balance and Core Strength; *Living Skills*, which considers Feeling, Thinking and Interacting, and also examines living skills such as confidence, autonomy, enjoyment, problem-solving, cooperation and social skills; and *Active Participation*, which focuses on the range of physical activity experiences in which the student participates, and their motivation to take part in these activities across different environments.

PFL is an online platform where both students and teachers have personalised accounts. The Living Skills and Active Participation components are self-reported questionnaires completed online by the student. The K–3 students are assisted by the teacher in completing the self-reported assessments. Movement and Fitness Skills are assessed by the teacher, who enters the results online. Each student receives an individualised passport, which includes an overview of their assessment results for learning. Teachers also have access to a class passport to guide programme development.

The resources are unique in that there are four separate sets of assessment instruments: one each for grades K–3, 4–6, 7–9 and 10–12. All assessments include the same components, but the activities are modified to cater to the different developmental levels. PHE Canada is very clear in stating that PFL is not to be used as a report card grade, and that results should be used to support student awareness and improvement. In this way, the role of the resource is to progress the students' physical literacy journey. Included in the tool are goal-setting lessons designed to advance the physical literacy journey.

The assessment levels are set out in a progressive format as a guide of where students are expected to be at each grade level. Students' results are reported within target ranges of Emerging, Developing, Acquired or Accomplished. The curricular-based goal is to have all children attain the recommended level or higher.

The development of PFL began in 2006, and continues to include research, pilot studies, revisions and evaluations. Findings and feedback have resulted in minor changes to a range of elements, including the addition of accommodations for persons with a disability. Currently, PHE Canada has received funding from Heritage Canada to ensure PFL is inclusive of the diverse Canadian population. Recently published papers have provided evidence for the validity of the assessments relative to the aims of Passport for Life in grades 4–9.

While PFL has not been in use long enough to give evidence of individual progress, cross-sectional data indicate that there has been steady improvement. National data analysis reports are produced each year, and provide helpful insights into the active participation levels, competencies and living skills of Canadian children and youth.

With thanks to Ken Lodewyk and Tricia Zakaria (references can be found at the end of the chapter).

Canada: Physical Literacy Assessment for Youth (PLAY)

The definition used to underpin this tool reads: 'Individuals are physically literate when they have acquired the movement skills and confidence to enjoy a variety of sports and physical activities' (Kriellaars, 2013: 4).

In 2008, Canada Sport for Life adopted a suite of tools developed by Dean Kriellaars from the University of Manitoba to assess physical literacy. These are known as PLAY tools (see https://play.physicalliteracy.ca/what-play) and comprise a suite of six assessments. PLAY tools are designed to improve the Canadian population's level of physical literacy and can be used by people of all ages. The tools aim to determine the status of physical literacy development in key domains such as cognitive, psychological, behavioural and motor competence. Each booklet is designed for use by particular players in the field of physical literacy, these being the teacher, the child, the parent, and professionals from the coaching and paramedical communities. The six booklets are named *PLAYfun, PLAYbasic, PLAYparent, PLAYcoach, PLAYself* and *PLAYinventory*. Recent developments have seen the introduction of *PLAY Creativity, PLAY PE teacher* and, for special populations, *A-PLAY*.

The PLAY tools have been used with children across Canada since 2013. Since then, they have been deployed to assess over 41,000 Canadian children in relation to in-school and after-school programmes. They were not originally designed for use in school; however, teachers have found them valuable. This has been in part on the grounds that aspects of the assessment are in line with national and global outcomes in physical education and beyond.

PLAYfun is a comprehensive tool, and assesses motor competence, confidence and comprehension of 18 movement skills. There are four aspects of movement tested, being Locomotor, Transport, Upper and Lower body object control, and Balance and body control. Each is given a score using an innovative 100 mm visual analogue scale with four category sections: 1 for Developing – Initial; 2 for Developing – Emerging; 3 for Acquired – Competent; and 4 for Acquired – Proficient. *PLAYfun* comprises 18 tasks. There is also the opportunity to judge if the participant has low, medium or high confidence prior to and during execution of each task, at whatever stage they demonstrate.

PLAYbasic is a shorter version of *PLAYfun*, and addresses five tasks, one for each of the five categories of movement. Both of these tools are designed to be administered by someone with a good knowledge of movement.

PLAYparent and *PLAYcoach* are questionnaires whereby the parent or coach provides their perspective on the child's physical literacy.

PLAYparent has five areas of physical literacy to consider. These are Physical Literacy Visual Analogue Scale, Cognitive Domain, Motor Competence, Environment, and Fitness. Relevant levels and scoring are set out. *PLAYcoach* is similar to *PLAYparent*, but is more comprehensive, and is directed at coaches, physiotherapists, athletic therapists, exercise professionals and recreation professionals. Both *PLAYparent* and *PLAYcoach* address aspects of the affective, physical and cognitive domains.

PLAYself is a self-evaluation tool to be used by the child to determine their perception of their physical literacy. This has four subsections: Environment, which looks at participation in different activities; Physical Literacy Self-description, which addresses the affective, the physical and the cognitive domains in physical literacy; Ranking of literacies; and Fitness. Participants score themselves in the different areas.

PLAYinventory is a form that helps a parent or child track and record their activity participation over a period of time. Throughout many of the booklets, there are descriptions of examples of behaviours that may be expected to be evident at different ages, as well as 'Calls for Action' to consider how progress might be achieved (for further details, see https://play.physicalliteracy.ca/what-play).

Research into aspects of *PLAYfun* is reported in Cairney et al. (2018a) and Stearns et al. (2108). Research into the preschool tool is reported in Cairney (2018b).

With thanks to Dean Kriellaars (references can be found at the end of the chapter).

United States: National Standards for K–12 Physical Education and PE Metrics – Society of Healthy and Physical Educators America (SHAPE America)

The definition of physical literacy used to underpin this instrument reads that physically literate individuals 'have the knowledge, skills and confidence to enjoy a lifetime of healthful physical activity' (SHAPE America, 2014).

In 2014, a task force appointed by the Society of Health and Physical Educators (SHAPE America) revised the National Standards for Physical Education and created the Grade-Level Outcomes for K–12 Physical Education (SHAPE America, 2014). In 2018, SHAPE America used these standards as the foundation to create PE Metrics, which comprises examples for assessing student performance (SHAPE America, 2018).

The 2014 National Standards for Physical Education are described as a tool for those in the physical education profession to use in designing curricula and planning units and lessons. As referred to in the National Standards and Grade-Level Outcomes booklet, physical literacy is described as 'the ability to move with competence and confidence in a wide variety of physical activities in multiple environments that benefit the healthful development of the whole person' (Mandigo et al., 2012: 28).

The 2014 National Standards manual sets out a very comprehensive analysis of five standards in formulating Grade-Level Outcome descriptors arising from each Standard. These descriptors are presented for Elementary School (grades K–5), Middle School (grades 6–8) and High School (grades 9–12) so that students can be tracked through their years of physical education. The Standards are carefully crafted to be readily usable to assist the accuracy of assessment of student performance. The standards and the number of related Grade-Level Outcomes are listed in Table 6.4.

Grade-Level Outcomes of the Standards display a detailed analysis of progressive expectations, which are characterised as moving from Emerging to Maturing and on to Applying. The Outcomes form a logical blueprint of student progress and also provide broad expectations of student development through the Grades.

PE Metrics is a comprehensive manual of assessment tasks. The featured assessments are linked to the National Standards for Physical Education, with mastery of each Grade-Level Outcome judged as Developing, Competent or Proficient. The purpose of the assessment in using the matrix in the Standards publication is both formative and summative, focusing on student growth towards mature patterns

TABLE 6.4 US Standards and the number of outcomes for each group of grades

The five Standards aspire to foster physical literacy in which an individual:	Each grade has a series of outcomes for each Standard		
	Elementary school (grades K–5)	Middle school (grades 6–8)	High school (grades 9–12)
Demonstrates competency in a variety of motor skills and movement patterns	27	24	3
Applies knowledge of concepts, principles, strategies and tactics related to movement and performance	5	13	4
Demonstrates the knowledge and skill to achieve and maintain a health-enhancing level of physical activity and fitness	6	18	14
Exhibits responsible personal and social behaviour that respects self and others	6	7	5
Recognises the value of physical activity for health, enjoyment, challenge, self-expression and/or social interaction	4	6	4

Source: Reproduced courtesy of SHAPE America

of motor performance, and understanding in the cognitive and affective domains within physical education.

A range of different data collection methods, including the use of technology, are suggested. However, the authors stress that the assessments are samples, and teachers should use *PE Metrics* as a basis for creating their own descriptors and systems of data collection that match their students' needs. The use of the manual is currently undergoing trials.

Reflecting on assessment in general, the authors of the SHAPE America documents assert that:

> Just as the role of assessment has evolved, so have the uses of assessment. While the focus remains on measuring student learning, using assessment to provide feedback on student performance, making instruction-related decisions to inform teaching is just as important.
>
> (SHAPE America, 2018: 9)

With thanks to Michelle Carter, Chris Hersl and Shirley Hale/Holt (see references at the end of the chapter).

Australia: Australian Physical Literacy Standard and charting progress

Sport Australia (formerly the Australian Sports Commission) is currently working on a system to track participants on their physical literacy journeys. Sport Australia defines physical literacy as 'the lifelong holistic learning acquired and applied in movement and physical activity. It brings together the skills, capabilities and knowledge which we know contribute to well-rounded people who value and participate in an active life' (ASC, 2017).

Sport Australia is focused on developing a cross-sector national commitment to increasing physical literacy of all Australians, particularly young Australians, as part of a solution to the inactivity crisis. This work aligns to Australia's newly released national sports plan – Sport 2030 – that clearly articulates a goal to reduce inactivity by 15% by 2030.

As a first step to introducing and monitoring physical literacy, Sport Australia identified four domains: physical, psychological, social and cognitive. Each of these domains is analysed and presented in the form of a number of elements. For example, against psychological, the following are listed: Motivation, Self-regulation (Emotional), Self-regulation (Physical), Awareness, Confidence, and Engagement and Enjoyment.

In addition, Sport Australia 'has identified five levels of development that outline the stages a person can progress (or regress) through.' These levels are listed as Pre-Foundational, Foundation & Exploration, Acquisition & Accumulation, Consolidation & Mastery and Transfer & Empowerment. Development across levels may be independent from one element to another and from elements in other domains.

Following from this analysis, there are proposals in the form of tips for development that provide general and practical advice to support proficiency within an element.

This information was accurate at the time of writing, however developments are expected and reference can be made to the Sport Australia website for information on progress and future development of the instrument (www.sportaus. gov.au/physical_literacy).

With thanks to Pierre Comis (references can be found at the end of the chapter).

Conclusion

As can be seen from the examples above, a great deal of work has gone into the creation of the different instruments. The identification of stages of progression, apart from being an essential first step in creating an assessment instrument, is extremely valuable to demonstrate that physical activity practitioners are firmly grounded in clear expectations and goals. An offshoot of this development is the benefit accrued from having a shared language.

As has been signalled in the examples set out above and the lists in the references section at the end of this chapter, a range of papers have been written on charting physical literacy journeys. Most of these consider one instrument; however, papers by Giblin et al. (2014) and Robinson and Randall (2017) look across schemes and reflect on the challenges of assessing physical literacy.

Giblin et al. (2014) conducted a critique of the different ways that are used to assess the physical domain, and caution against a tendency to consider domains in isolation, seeing them as interdependent. Robinson and Randall (2017) conduct an analysis of the three Canadian schemes, and as a conclusion reflect on the nature of physical literacy as a human disposition and wonder if it can be assessed. They write, 'Perhaps in the very act of measuring physical literacy, something is lost'. They then ask, 'For what gain? Consider this; other noble life course pursuits (e.g. beauty, truth or joy) do not require measurement. Perhaps physical literacy is the same' (p. 53).

Notwithstanding Robinson and Randall's thought-provoking challenge, there are reasons to continue work in this area. Charting progress would seem to be an essential and integral aspect of effecting physical literacy. It is proposed that it is of value for:

- participants to recognise and celebrate development and identify new challenges;
- practitioners concerned to promote physical literacy, to provide evidence of the effectiveness of their work with participants; and
- advocates of physical literacy to convey information to those in government and other senior positions, which demonstrates clarity of thought, evidence-based practice and a clear sense of direction.

For proponents of physical literacy, charting journeys is currently a priority focus. The IPLA believes that developments in this area can make a significant contribution, both to fostering physical literacy for all and to having the evidence to recommend, with confidence, the ways in which this can be achieved. The establishment of an international working party to look in detail at methods of charting progress could be a valuable initiative. The fundamental question to ask would seem to be, 'Are processes concerned with charting or assessment of physical literacy enhancing motivation to participate?' In other words, 'How far is a particular assessment instrument making a positive impact on achieving the aspiration of more individuals choosing physical activity for life?'

References for the body of the chapter

Black, P. and Wiliam, D. (2002) *Working inside the Black Box: Assessment for Learning in the Classroom*. London: King's College.

Giblin, S., Collins, D. and Butler, C. (2014) Physical literacy: importance, assessment and future directions. *Sports Medicine September*, 44(9): 1177–1184.

IPLA (2019) *Physical Literacy across the World: Resources and References*. Available at: www.physical-literacy.org.uk/plaw-resources-and-references/ (accessed 14 March 2019).

Robinson, D.B. and Randall, L. (2017) Marking physical literacy or missing the mark on physical literacy? A conceptual critique of Canada's physical literacy assessment instruments. *Measurement in Physical Education and Exercise Science*, 21(1): 40–55.

Whitehead, M.E. (ed.) (2010) *Physical Literacy throughout the Lifecourse*. London: Routledge.

References/reading for Canada: CAPL

Longmuir, P.E. (2013) Understanding the physical literacy journey of children: the Canadian Assessment of Physical Literacy. *ICSSPE Bulletin: Journal of Sport Science and Physical Education*, 65 (October): 276–282.

Longmuir, P.E., Boyer, C., Lloyd, M., Yang, Y., Boiarskaia, E. and Tremblay, M.S. (2015) The Canadian Assessment of Physical Literacy: methods for children in grades 4 to 6 (8 to 12 years). *BMC Public Health*, 15(767): 1–11.

Recently, 14 papers have been written analysing aspects of the CAPL. Three examples are given below. The other papers can be accessed via the IPLA website (see IPLA, 2019).

Gunnell, K.E., Longmuir, P.E., Barnes, J.D., Belanger, K. and Tremblay, M.S. (2018) Refining the Canadian Assessment of Physical Literacy based on theory and factor analyses. *BMC Public Health*, 18(2): 1044. Available at: https://bmcpublichealth.biomedcentral.com/track/pdf/10.1186/s12889-018-5899-2 (accessed 14 March 2019).

Longmuir, P.E., Gunnell, K.E., Barnes, J.D., Belanger, K., Leduc, G., Woodruff, S.J. and Tremblay, M.S. (2018) Canadian Assessment of Physical Literacy Second Edition: a streamlined assessment of the capacity for physical activity among children 8 to 12 years of age. *BMC Public Health*, 18(2): 1047. Available at: https://bmcpublichealth.biomedcentral.com/track/pdf/10.1186/s12889-018-5902-y (accessed 14 March 2019).

Tremblay, M.S., Longmuir, P.E. , Barnes, J.D., Belanger, K., Anderson, K.D., Bruner, B., Copeland, J.L., Nyström, C.D., Gregg, M.J., Hall, N., Kolen, A.M., Lane, K.N., Law, B., MacDonald, D.J., Martin, L.J., Saunders, T.J., Sheehan, D., Stone, M.R. and Woodruff, S.J. (2018) Physical literacy levels of Canadian children aged 8–12 years: descriptive and normative results from the RBC Learn to Play–CAPL project. *BMC Public Health*, 18(2): 1036. Available at: https://bmcpublichealth.biomedcentral.com/track/pdf/10.1186/s12889-018-5891-x (accessed 14 March 2019).

References/reading for Canada: Passport for Life

Lodewyk, K.R. and Mandigo, J. (2017) Early validation evidence of a Canadian practitioner-based assessment of physical literacy in physical education: Passport for Life. *The Physical Educator*, 74(3): 1–15.

Lodewyk, K.R. (2019) Early validation evidence of the Canadian practitioner-based assessment of physical literacy in secondary physical education. *The Physical Educator*, 76: 634–660.

References/reading for Canada: PLAY/CS4L

Cairney, J., Clark, H.J., James, M.E., Mitchell, D., Dudley, D. and Kriellaars, D. (2018a) The preschool physical literacy tool: testing a new physical literacy tool for the early years. *Frontiers in Pediatrics: Children and Health*, June 2018, https//doi.org/10.3389/fprd.2018.00138.

Cairney, J., Veldhuizen, S., Graham, J.D., Rodriguez, C., Bedard, C., Bremer, E. and Kriellaars, D. (2018b) A construct validation of PLAYfun. *Medicine and Science in Sports and Exercise*, 50(4): 855–862.

Kriellaars, D. (2013) PLAYfun. In *Physical Literacy Assessment for Youth*. Canadian Sport for Life, Canadian Sport Institutes, pp. 1–38. Available at: https://play.physicalliteracy.ca/what-play (accessed 25 March 2019).

Stearns, J.A., Wohlers, B., McHugh, T.F., Kuzik, N. and Spence, J. (2018) *Reliability and Validity of the PLAYfun Tool with Children and Youth in Northern Canada.* Available at: www.tandfonline.com/doi/full/10.1080/1091367X.2018.1500368 (accessed 25 March 2019).

References/reading for United States: SHAPE

Mandigo, J., Francis, N., Lodewyk, K. and Lopez, R. (2012) Physical literacy for educators. *Physical Education and Health Journal*, 75(3): 27–30.
Society of Health and Physical Educators (SHAPE America) (2014) *National Standards and Grade-Level Outcomes for K–12 Physical Education.* Champaign, IL: Human Kinetics.
Society of Health and Physical Educators (SHAPE America) (2018) *PE Metrics.* Champaign, IL: Human Kinetics.

References/reading for Australia

Australian Sports Commission (ASC) (2017) *Draft Australian Physical Literacy Standard Development: Milestones for Lifelong Participation.* Canberra: Australian Sports Commission.
O'Halloran, P., Randle, E., Nicholson, M., Stukes, A. and Seal, E. (2018) Using the draft Australian Sports Commission Physical Literacy Standards as a design tool. *Journal of Science and Medicine in Sport*, 21(Supplement 1 Paper 3): 556–557.
Randle, E., Nicholson, M., O'Halloran, P., Seal, E. and Kingsley, M. (2018) Initial perceptions of the draft Australian Sports Commission Physical Literacy Standards from the Sport, Health and Education sectors. *Journal of Science and Medicine in Sport*, 21(Supplement 1 Paper 2): 556.

PART II

International perspectives on physical literacy

7

INTRODUCTION TO INTERNATIONAL PERSPECTIVES ON PHYSICAL LITERACY

Margaret Whitehead

Introduction

Part II comprises chapters written by colleagues in eight countries across the world. These colleagues, in their different ways, have played a leading role in the development of physical literacy in their country. The chapters are presented in alphabetical order of the countries: Australia, Canada, continental Europe, India, New Zealand, Scotland, Wales and the United States. As will be seen, these individuals come from a range of backgrounds and contexts. The authors from Australia, Canada and continental Europe work in the university sector, while the colleagues from New Zealand and Wales work in the sports sector. The colleague from the United States has a background in a professional association for teachers of physical education. The founding interest for work in India came from a national sports star, and the chapter is written by a colleague in a sports foundation. The authors from Scotland represent a partnership between public health and a university.

Careful reading and analysis of these chapters generates a series of topics, many of which were referred to by a number of authors. This introduction to these chapters will address how the concept of physical literacy came to the attention of colleagues and circumstances that facilitated interest and discussion. Also covered will be debates about the understanding, or otherwise, of the definition of physical literacy, and how the concept was initially disseminated. As a further reflection on these chapters, other common ground will be discussed in Chapter 16. This will refer to how physical literacy has been embedded in work in the different countries, the challenges encountered, and aspirations for the future.

Awareness of the concept

Awareness of the concept of physical literacy has arisen via the work of a variety of organisations and institutions. Physical literacy came to attention in both New

Zealand and Wales through work being carried out in the field of physical activity and sport, via Sport New Zealand and Sport Wales, respectively. In Australia and Holland, colleagues in the university system identified the concept as worthy of consideration. In Scotland, local government personnel recognised that physical literacy had the potential to help them meet some of their priorities, while in the United States the concept was highlighted as a valuable innovation by SHAPE, the teachers' association for Sport, Health and Physical Education. In Canada, it was a government-supported enterprise, Canada Sport 4 All (CS4L), that first promoted physical literacy, although universities in Canada were quick to pick up on the potential of the concept. India was unique in that it was a national sporting hero, Shri Pullela Gopichand, who first championed physical literacy, and who then worked with associates from sports management in Andhra Pradesh. The groups, associations and individuals identified above have been, and remain, the key drivers of the concept in their respective countries.

The particular context to the adoption of the concept

While the narratives presented necessarily reflect different cultural contexts, all share one area of concern, this being the growth of sedentary behaviours. In each case, interest in physical literacy arose against a background of worrying developments regarding the health and well-being of a significant percentage of the population. All writers refer to serious concerns about obesity, mental health problems, and ever-decreasing numbers of people engaging in active lifestyles. Countries such as Australia and New Zealand perceived worrying signs of a move away from the 'active nation' characteristic they held so dear. Colleagues in the Czech Republic voiced concerns about dropout from physical education, while those in the United States were worried that the time for physical education in schools was falling. Canadian practitioners describe the disturbing lessening of opportunities for younger children to be involved in free play, and Indian advocates report that there was little if any physical education in state schools, and only 1% of the population were involved in regular physical activity.

In addition to the differing professional backgrounds of the writers, the stories they recount necessarily reflect some of the traditions, philosophies and political priorities of their country. For example, colleagues in India and New Zealand identified closely with the holistic nature of the concept, this being very much in line with their attitudes to the nature of being. Academics in continental Europe embraced the concept as being very much in tune with their existing philosophy and welcomed the academic rigour this brought to the study of physical activity. With particular reference to trends in education, colleagues in some countries reacted positively to the concept as providing the emergence of a refreshingly new way to conceive of physical activity. Others observed that physical literacy was in tune with current trends in physical activity pedagogy. Examples given here were the incorporation of student voice and the development of reflective self-perception in encouraging participant responsibility. In some countries, physical literacy was seen as centrally relevant to preadolescent young people, and in a few instances there was an underlying interest in using physical literacy to identify and nurture talent. There was also the opposite perception, being that working within the intentions of physical literacy would counteract the prioritisation of the elite participant in physical education.

Specific opportunities for the development of physical literacy

Alongside the disturbing scenarios identified above, there were circumstances in many of the countries that provided opportunities for reflection, for effecting change, for drawing up new policies, and for the creation of innovative pro-grammes. Those in Dumfries and Galloway, Scotland, were challenged to create new strategies to promote healthy living in respect of diet and exercise, and found the concept of physical literacy valuable in this context. Colleagues in Wales, working from a government brief of *The Well-Being of Future Generations*, real-ised the potential of physical literacy as they began to map out new approaches and programmes. A colleague in Australia charged with creating a plan to 'Get Australia Moving' used physical literacy as a focus in this publication. Those in Sport New Zealand were working on a new community sports strategy when they were introduced to the concept, and Shri Gopichand in India found the concept while despairing over the almost total lack of physical competence in many young people in his country. CS4L were looking to create planned sup-port for children up to 12 years, and were also keen to map out developments for long-term athlete development. Physical literacy held promise to support this work. University colleagues in Europe and Canada, most of whom were working in physical education teacher education (PETE), and who were reviewing and updating courses, introduced physical literacy in their work with students. In a similar way, SHAPE in the United States learnt about physical literacy in drawing up policies to present to national and state legislature to make physical education more relevant to current circumstances.

The definition of physical literacy

Each chapter discusses the way that the concept of physical literacy was viewed. Debates about the nature and implications of the definition were conducted in each country. As described in Part I, while a variety of definitions have been formulated, it would seem to be true to judge that all countries interpret the concept as relevant throughout the lifecourse, and all acknowledge that in promoting progress in respect of physical literacy, attention needs to go beyond the physical, respecting the individual as a whole. Finally, most coun-tries acknowledge that treating each individual as unique is essential if all are to benefit from progress towards the aspiration of 'choosing physical activity for life' (IPLA, 2019).

At the time of writing, Wales, the Netherlands, Scotland and India are working to the IPLA definition (see Chapter 2), with Canada being closely aligned to this. The Aspen Institute in the United States, in collaboration with the physical education and sport professions, drew up their own definition, and likewise New Zealand and Australia have each put their own stamp on the concept. The United States preferred the notion of 'desire' to motivation, New Zealand added a spiritual dimension, and Australia a social dimension. Some non-English-speaking countries had difficulty translating 'physical literacy' into their own language. English speakers had a range of different views. Some were of the opinion that the notion was too complex, while others suggested that there was nothing new being suggested. Some were fearful that physical literacy might damage physical education, and others were concerned that it represented dualistic thinking and also introduced an additional focus for failure for participants, in respect of the notion of illiteracy (see explanatory glossary). Colleagues in a number of countries, such as Canada, India and the Netherlands, have had to work hard to explain that adopting physical literacy does not simply involve mounting programmes of fundamental movement skills.

Relationship between physical literacy and other literacies

A recurring trend that features in many chapters is the perceived relationship between physical literacy, other literacies and other areas of human concern. Dumfries and Galloway, Scotland, decided, in consultation with others in local government, that physical literacy could not be considered separately from food literacy, and so they developed a physical and food literacy policy. In a number of countries, physical literacy was viewed as integral to health, and Australia has placed physical education under the broad heading of health in their curriculum planning. Colleagues in New Zealand are looking at the relationship between physical literacy and health, not least in the context of health being a key perspective of Maori life. Somewhat similarly, Wales is now addressing physical literacy as contributing to policies focused on promoting healthy and confident young people. The United States is considering physical literacy as contributing to an area concerned with nutrition and mindfulness. These observations anticipate the general trend in most countries of developing partnerships in order to facilitate permeation of the concept of physical literacy across constituencies and age ranges.

Developing partnerships

Those working in the sport sector in Wales and in New Zealand are developing partnerships with both the health sector and the education sector. Approaches differ, as Sport Wales' remit includes high-level athletes while Sport New Zealand is principally concerned with whole population participation. Welsh colleagues have also developed links with universities, and both New Zealand and Wales are collaborating with specific groups such as those working with the ageing population and those with a disability. In addition, advocates in both countries are developing links with relevant government departments. In sharing their progress, they recognise that partnerships need to be handled carefully. New Zealand colleagues refer to the need for flexibility, while Welsh colleagues realise that in working with people in sectors other than sport, they need to avoid a dictatorial approach, create bespoke advocacy materials, and give presentations that show appreciation of and sensitivity to current practices. Those working in Scotland, who already had a broad remit including health, forged links with policymakers in education, sport and the environment. In addition, they have worked with schools, presenting and sharing views with school head teachers, school staff, parents and sport/activity coaches, and community groups. Those in the United States have not only targeted schools, but, together with the Aspen Institute, have collaborated with national governing bodies of sport as well as state and national health sectors. CS4L, in championing the concept early in the twenty-first century, recruited support from education, sport, recreation and health. Latterly, other areas are coming on stream in Canada, such as VIVO, which promotes adult participation, and the Abilities Centre, which caters for disability sport. The Canadian university sector is also a key player in advocating physical literacy, as is the Canadian Physical Education Association. In countries as large as the United States and Canada, collaboration is challenging and consensus is hard-won. This scenario is also characteristic of India. However, in all cases, there are initiatives in place to develop links between education, sport, recreation and health.

While government funding supported the university sector in Australia to make the first moves in respect of physical literacy, there were ready-made links with coaching, education and health, not least on account of work with students preparing to move into these sectors. As physical literacy has been developed, so have strong links with government departments and the physical education profession. In a similar way, some European colleagues are both fostering collaborative work with health and sport faculties in their universities and considering opportunities to liaise with relevant government departments.

These partnerships have proved to be extremely valuable to inform others of physical literacy and identify the relevance of the concept in a range of areas. In this work, it has been possible to support the particular work of other groups as well as providing opportunities for physical literacy advocacy and the sharing of knowledge. These partnerships have strengthened the hands of champions of physical literacy in respect of influencing government perspectives and policies. In some cases, funding has been secured, and in all cases partnerships have enabled further progress to take place, building on the successful endeavours of the key advocates. One very promising development has taken place in the United States, New Zealand and Wales, being the development of work with non-educational organisations for young people. In the United States, the American Council on Exercise and Boys & Girls Clubs of America are embracing physical literacy, while youth development organisations in New Zealand and Girl Guides in Wales are also promoting the concept.

The chapters that follow are placed in alphabetical order by country. Each is given the title suggested by the author(s). Throughout the chapters, policies and material that could be of value to readers are signposted. In fact, there is now a wealth of material written on the topic of physical literacy, of which only a very small sample can be mentioned in this volume.

Reference

IPLA (2019) *Physical Literacy across the World: Resources and References.* Available at: www. physical-literacy.org.uk/plaw-resources-and-references/ (accessed 14 March 2019).

8

A BRIEF HISTORY OF PHYSICAL LITERACY IN AUSTRALIA

Richard Keegan, Dean Dudley and Lisa Barnett

Reflecting on the history of physical literacy, the concept has multiple traceable roots in Australia, and more recently it has been supported by an array of initiatives in research, practice and policy settings. Reflecting this non-linear, multifaceted and simultaneous approach, the following chapter will trace several different narratives, as opposed to a single story arc. The following chapter will note some of the historical developments that frame the recent flourishing of the concept in Australia, as well as detailing current projects and initiatives. In particular, Australia has unique geographic and demographic characteristics that affect the interpretation and implementation of physical literacy in the country. Australia also has a unique and extremely important indigenous culture, which existed tens of thousands of years before European settlement, and which provides important clues about how humans can exist within and upon the Australian landscape. For example, broadly speaking, the culture of Australia's indigenous people – while there are many diverse traditions – reflects deep dependence on the land and climate, both for sustenance but also for central cultural reference points reflected in the dreaming, songlines and tjuringas. Any physical literacy strategy for Australia would benefit from being sensitive to these cultural traditions. Subsequently, European settlers have developed and codified a number of unique sports and activities, including Australian Rules football, surf lifesaving and bushwalking. These too provide important local contexts in shaping the meaning of physical literacy in Australia. Finally, this chapter will review recent developments in articulating a unique definition, standards framework and national strategy for physical literacy, before briefly considering the future directions and possibilities within this conceptual space for Australian contexts and systems.

In 2016, the Australian Sports Commission (ASC – now renamed Sport Australia) incorporated physical literacy into their organisational strategic plan by setting the objective to 'drive demand for lifelong participation in sport and physical activity by focusing on younger Australians through the Sporting Schools program and a *focus on physical literacy*' (ASC, 2017: 10, emphasis added). To a large extent, the activities undertaken by Sport Australia since this time have formed a focal emphasis for a number of initiatives, given their explicit attempt to engage with audiences spanning education, health and sport, including youth sport, recreational sport and elite sport. Nonetheless, before the emergence of Sport Australia as a key driver of the physical literacy agenda, important work was being conducted in education by the Australian Council for Health, Physical Education and Recreation (ACHPER), who have persistently and energetically advocated for the importance of high-quality physical education (PE) in schools. As well as offering in-service training and support for teachers, the advocacy of the ACHPER played a significant role in the shaping of the most recent Australian physical education curriculum (Australian Curriculum, Assessment and Reporting Authority – ACARA, 2016). Notably, the 2016 ACARA PE curriculum did not explicitly recognise the term 'physical literacy', preferring to only introduce one 'new' literacy (i.e. health literacy; cf. MacDonald and Enright, 2014). Hence, these initiatives and organisations laid important foundations for the Sport Australia work, and ensured that the release of Sport Australia physical literacy resources in 2017 was both timely and well received. Further to all of the above, there were ongoing and successful research programmes embedded in several Australian universities, including:

(a) The University of Canberra, producing several reports and initial overviews of physical literacy, and initiating a subsequent research programme, catalysed by the work of Telford's longitudinal studies 'Lifestyle of Our Kids' (LOOK) (Telford et al., 2009a, 2009b, 2013a, 2013b).

(b) Deakin University, the University of Wollongong, Sydney University and the University of Newcastle, where a sustained collaborative approach had highlighted the importance of fundamental movement skills (FMS) in children's health and fitness, and subsequent lifelong engagement in physical activity (Okely et al., 2001; Barnett et al., 2008b, 2009, 2010, 2016; Dudley et al., 2011; Hardy et al., 2013; Cohen et al., 2015; Hulteen et al., 2015, 2018).

(c) La Trobe University, with a clear emphasis on embodied cognition, which was well aligned to the concept of physical literacy (Stolz, 2014, 2015; Stolz and Thorburn, 2017). See O'Halloran et al. (2017) and Randle et al. (2018).

(d) The University of Queensland, where a highly influential team were contributing research evidence into policy frameworks and researching the effectiveness of such policy frameworks (Hickey et al., 2014; Hunter et al., 2014; Macdonald and Enright, 2014).

(e) Macquarie University, in Sydney, where education researcher Dean Dudley maintained a long and productive collaboration with colleagues in Canada (Dudley, 2015; Cairney et al., 2016; Dudley et al., 2016, 2017), as well as contributing to the UNESCO Quality Physical Education Guidelines (UNESCO, 2015) and the Kazan Action Plan (UNESCO, 2017).

The strong engagement between various government agencies, at federal and state levels, as well as not-for-profit organisations, advocacy groups and universities, represents a key strength of Australia's approach to physical literacy, rendering their policies and programmes evidence-based, and ensuring that their research is of applied relevance, understood by all key groups, and with the potential for immediate impact. The above organisations and research teams formed the 'critical mass' that, from 2013 onwards, allowed physical literacy to rapidly gain momentum at all levels: from individuals and families, to schools and state education departments, and even national governing bodies and the federal government. One such influential initiative was developed by the New South Wales Department for Education: in the early adoption of physical literacy and the development of a 'physical literacy continuum' that traced developmental trajectories that might be observed as learners progress through their physical literacy journeys (New South Wales Department for Education, 2015). Staff from the education department worked closely with the researchers listed above in developing, refining and promoting a resource that explicitly helped teachers in a manner that was aligned to Whitehead's (2010) intentions for physical literacy, while also adopting the language and curriculum structures with which teachers were already familiar. The combination of close collaboration between researchers, policymakers and practitioners, as well as the adoption of specific local language and norms, remains an excellent example of best-practice implementation with respect to physical literacy.

Why physical literacy has achieved 'traction' in Australia: perceived value

While education, and particularly primary education, was ostensibly the first place that physical literacy generated sustained interest, the concept also appealed to people in health settings, recreational and elite sport, and, of course, researchers. Hence, many of the initial discussions regarding physical literacy in Australia took place in relation to the preparation of a revised health and physical education curriculum (ACARA, 2016), where, as noted above, the decision was made to introduce the new term 'health literacy'. It was agreed in these discussions that introducing two 'new' literacy terms might be viewed as confusing (i.e. both physical and health 'literacies'). Nonetheless, there were numerous clear articulations of physical literacy, and its related thinking, in the renewed curriculum, with an emphasis on holistic learning across the areas of physical, emotional, cognitive and social development through physical education. There was strong agreement that physical education provides a wide range of important benefits to children. However, there were concerns about the apparent devaluing of physical education in Australian schools, as evidenced by reduced class time, lesson frequency and physical activity within the classes (van Beurden et al., 2003; McKenzie and Lounsbery, 2009; Frémeaux et al., 2011; Dudley et al., 2012a, 2012b; Carlson et al., 2013; Lounsbery et al., 2013). Around the same time, ongoing research demonstrating the importance of physical activity in supporting positive health outcomes (Goldberg and King, 2007; CDC,

2010; Kirk et al., 2010; Zhang and Chaaban, 2013) was identifying that the early development of motor proficiency – in the form of fundamental motor skills and/ or gross motor skills – appeared to be a key precursor to adolescent and adult physical activity (Barnett et al., 2008a, 2015; Stodden et al., 2008; Lopes et al., 2011; Cattuzzo et al., 2016). Related research also demonstrated that not only are objective observations of motor proficiency informative, but also that subjective perceptions of one's own motor and/or sport competence were also important predictors of participation in physical activity (Barnett et al., 2008a, 2011, 2013; Babic et al., 2014; Robinson et al., 2015). Furthermore, as well as the consideration of perceived motor competence (for a full recent discussion on the definition, see Estevan and Barnett, 2018), researchers were reinforcing the importance of motivation in determining participation in physical activity, and subsequent health outcomes (Yan & McCullagh, 2004; Rosenkranz et al., 2012; Lonsdale et al., 2013; Plotnikoff et al., 2013; Sterdt et al., 2013; Owen et al., 2014). That is, motor competence, subjective rating of proficiency (i.e. perceived competence) and motivation were all coming to the fore as key determinants of physical activity and health-promoting lifestyle choices. 'Arriving' into this historical context, physical literacy provided a neat bridge between those seeking to advocate physical education and those seeking to promote health through enhanced physical activity. Walking the line between these two complementary areas of interest, Telford's LOOK project was demonstrating that even one year of high-quality PE in primary school – delivered by a trained specialist, and importantly delivered in protected time windows to ensure the sessions took place – resulted in improvements in: (a) hand–eye coordination; (b) physical activity participation (using accelerometer data); (c) mental health scores; (d) academic achievement (using the national assessments conducted each year); (e) body composition (using a DEXA scanner); (f) blood lipids (i.e. cholesterol); and (g) insulin resistance, a precursor to diabetes (Telford et al., 2009a, 2012a, 2012b, 2013b, 2013c, 2013d; Daly et al., 2012; Olive et al., 2012). Hence, although Australia was a relatively late arrival to the physical literacy 'bandwagon' – with policy development and consultation specifically linked to physical literacy only really beginning in earnest from around 2013 – the proverbial ground was rich and fertile when the seeds were finally sown (see Figure 8.1).

Interest from sporting organisations

The potential relevance of physical literacy to promoting sporting participation, and potentially even supporting elite sport, was not lost on sporting organisations in Australia. In 2013, the Australian Sports Commission (ASC) began to keep a page on their website – 'Clearinghouse' – which became a repository for links to various papers, blogs and resources regarding physical literacy. Over time, the ASC's role in physical literacy evolved from merely reflecting what was already published and available, using the above site, to becoming a driving force in the conceptualisation, promotion and championing of physical literacy in Australia. Importantly, however, before engaging with physical literacy, the ASC had already

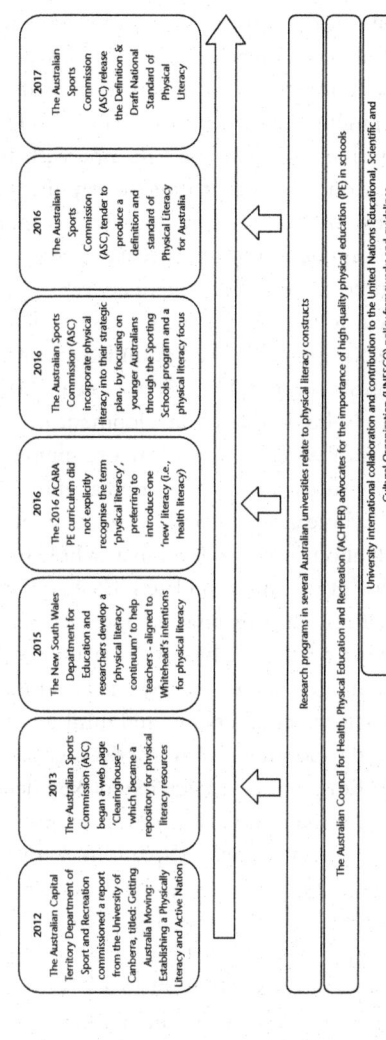

FIGURE 8.1 A timeline of key events in the development of physical literacy in Australia

devoted significant time and attention to the development of a model to inform their training pathway for elite sport: the FTEM model (Gulbin et al., 2013). The FTEM model described transitions from a *foundational* skill development phase, into a *talent* phase, when an athlete's potential and promise have been identified. Subsequently, a smaller proportion of athletes may enter onto the *elite* pathway, competing at high-level national or international events, before becoming established at this top level, and achieving *mastery*. These four phases, including a total of 10 sub-phases, appeared to describe a linear pathway from the beginning of a sporting career towards the very pinnacle where only a select few ever venture – and as such, the model was immediately criticised as: (i) being too similar to Balyi's long-term athlete development (LTAD) model (Balyi and Hamilton, 2004; Balyi et al., 2006); (ii) not catering for those who do not wish to (or are unable to) pursue top-level competition; and (iii) failing to capture the many non-linear and idiosyncratic ways that athletes reach the top level of sports (MacNamara and Collins, 2013). While the model's authors tried to clarify their position (Gulbin et al., 2014), the main source of the disagreement appears to have been the emphasis on the model's acronym implying sequential phases, when in fact much of the thinking underpinning their approach was grounded in their 'three-dimensional athlete development' framework, or 3DAD (Farrow et al., 2013). The 3DAD does indeed emphasise holistic, 'whole-athlete' development in an integrated manner, over time, within a context or system – in a manner reminiscent of physical literacy thinking. Hence, under the surface, there was good alignment between the ASC's vision of how to develop 'whole athletes', and the wider conceptualisations in education and health research about how to develop a 'whole person'. Consequently, when the Australian federal government updated the ASC's mandate to increasing participation in sport, renaming the organisation Sport Australia and bringing them under the Health Minister's portfolio, there were a number of neat alignments, both in terms of published models and resources, but also (more importantly) in the thinking of key senior managers, civil servants and ministers. Arguments regarding 'holistic' and 'integrated' development were increasingly accepted in Australian schools and many boardrooms, and to a large extent key decision-makers already understood the alignment between: (a) participation in sport and physical activity; (b) the accumulation of experiences and adaptations from this participation; (c) physical health benefits (including benefits to the economy from greater productivity); and (d) wider holistic benefits beyond physical health. Hence, when the ASC first commissioned researchers, in 2016, to develop a set of physical literacy resources for Australia, they knew exactly what to ask for.

Overall, a very important element of the progress of physical literacy in Australia has been the inclusion of, and ownership by, a wide range of stakeholders and interest groups – from the very outset, spanning education, health, sport and research. This diverse and inclusive approach mirrors the logic underpinning physical literacy itself – that development is more sustainable and meaningful when it is integrated and holistic, both for the individual but also for a whole country's physical literacy movement.

Setting the foundations: the *GAME PLAN*

In 2012, the Australian Capital Territory Department of Sport and Recreation commissioned a report from staff at the University of Canberra, looking to clarify current thinking regarding physical literacy, as well as summarising existing physical literacy programmes around the world. Published in 2013, the resulting document was titled *Getting Australia Moving: Establishing a Physically Literate and Active Nation (GAME PLAN)* (Keegan et al., 2013). With the agreement of the state government, the report was made public via the university's website, and was quickly picked up across Australia and globally. At the time, the report offered a descriptive overview of current thinking and practices, but perhaps equally as important it made the economic case for promoting physical activity and physical literacy, specifically by presenting contemporary analyses suggesting that physical inactivity poses a significant economic burden – even when separated out from obesity and smoking (e.g. Ding et al., 2016). Using Australian data, it was also clear that Australians, like their contemporaries in the United States and the UK, were living sedentary lives. At the time of writing, 54% of the Australian adult population were not getting enough physical activity to remain healthy (NPAS, 2000), and 36% of the adults sampled by the Australian Board of Statistics (ABS) in 2008 had been totally sedentary in the previous two weeks – an increase from 32% in 2001 (ABS, 2011). In the most recent statistics, less than one-third of Australian children (30%) aged 2–17 meet the physical activity guidelines, and only one in three (35%) aged 5–12 meet the sedentary screen-based behaviour guidelines (AIHW, 2018). The resulting message might be summarised as: 'Everybody else is doing it, we're being left behind, and it's costing us financially', which predictably led to a number of key stakeholders – in government and industry – taking note.

The evidence presented in the *GAME PLAN* report made it clear that physical inactivity is a significant threat to Australia – its physical and economic health – and that this threat is common across many developed nations. While many previous initiatives had appeared to focus on sport alone (often competitive sport) as a solution to the problem of inactive lifestyles, the *GAME PLAN*'s analysis of recent trends suggested that any Australian approach should recognise that not all physical activity is sporting activity. Instead, they suggested that wider, holistic physical literacy – in the form of movement proficiency, motivation to move, and appreciation of the value of moving – would be a more inclusive and holistic approach. The report argued that a physical literacy approach may reach more children, alienate and exclude fewer children, and thus ensure that more children are more active. The report also offered an analysis 'unpacking' the concept of physical literacy, which made it possible to trace potential causal chains from determinants (teachers, parents, individual attributes) through to outcomes (physical, mental and social health) in the short and long term. For example, in Figure 8.2, it was suggested that research evidence was broadly supportive of links between concepts that are close together in the figure but often lacking for 'longer' links, or the overall picture – which would, of course, require more sophisticated, longitudinal and large-scale research methodologies.

Chronological sequence →

Level of complexity →

	Determinants of physical literacy	Components of physical literacy	Short term outcomes of physical literacy	Long term outcomes of physical literacy
Socio-cultural	11) Valuing physical proficiency alongside numeracy/literacy	12) Understanding of relevance of physical activity	12) Improved understanding of relevance/importance of PA	11) Reduced health costs and economic losses
	10) Curriculum, teacher training and teaching/assessment practices	11) Emotional sensitivity and empathy	11) Better relationships and feelings of belongingness	10) Improved performance in arts and sport
	9) Cultural stereotypes around physical prowess (e.g., "dumb jocks", "all activity = sport")	10) Meta-awareness of movement capacities and physicality	10) Improved health literacy	9) More tolerant and inclusive society?
	8) Volume and quality of PE in schools	9) Elevated Physical Activity	9) Improved self-awareness and self coaching	8) Improved life-skills (communication, organisation, coping)
	7) Parental attitudes and role modelling	8) Increased motivation for physical tasks	8) Improved cognitive and academic performance	7) Healthy diet and lifestyle
	6) Early exposure and positive experiences of being active	7) Improved self-perceptions/ self esteem	7) Increased motivation towards PA (and PE)	6) Improved educational outcomes and/or career options
Psychology	5) Secure attachment	6) Higher perceived competence	6) More positive attitude towards PA/PE (willingness)	5) Improved mental health and psychological well-being
	4) Early aspects of personality – outgoing, open etc.	5) Spatial awareness and 'game reading'	5) Improved mental health and psychological well-being	4) Increased PA + energy expenditure
	3) Genetic endowment / predisposition	4) Motor competence (FMS/ GMS)	4) Increased PA participation + energy expenditure	3) Reduced sedentary behaviour
Biology and Physiology	2) Development stage	3) Motor development	3) Reduced sedentary behaviour	2) Reduced injury frequency/ severity
	1) Absence of pathology	2) Plasticity, cortical thickness, cell density	2) Reduced injury frequency/ severity	1) LT Improved individual health outcomes
		1) Physical health and immune function	1) ST Improved individual health outcomes	

FIGURE 8.2 A taxonomy detailing the proposed contributors to, and benefits associated with, physical literacy

Source: Keegan et al. (2013)

When concluding, the report sought to learn from existing programmes, developing 10 recommendations that any programme to promote physical literacy should:

1. Look beyond solely using sport as a vessel, and encourage any/all physical movement activities – including dance, creative expression and everyday travel – ensuring motivation to move and appreciation of its importance, as well as the basic ability to move.
2. Make provisions for unique aspects of Australia (e.g. explicitly considering the needs of Aborigines and Torres Straight Islanders, and city versus rural populations).
3. When focusing on primary school teachers, who are often not confident in delivering physical literacy or physical education, offer freely available, simple-to-use and well-organised resources that allow teachers to deliver fun, inspiring and effective lessons.
4. Develop the ability to monitor and assess programmes' uptake and effectiveness. The idea of a central website, such as Passport for Life (Canada), which both disseminates resources and encourages feedback and user contributions, was suggested to be promising in this respect.
5. Develop programmes that permit refinement and development (i.e. not a prescriptive 'finished product'), so that best practice can be assured in the short and long term, in response to emerging evidence.
6. Work closely with universities in order to ensure academic rigour and reliable data (i.e. evidence-based practice).
7. Recognise that the development of physical literacy, and the slow accrual of benefits from physical activity, are often long-term and untenable – despite their importance. Thus, programmes should acknowledge that slow and non-linear advancement may undermine the uptake of and adherence to physical literacy programmes by schools, teachers and children. To prevent this, it was recommended that any Australian programme should seek, wherever possible, to generate immediate and self-evident benefits to users to reinforce and encourage participation.
8. Acknowledge that the physical literacy of adults and older adults should not be overlooked, and that programmes to promote physical activity in these groups will take a very different shape, with a different message (perhaps less focused on sport and games) and different delivery mechanisms (perhaps mass media and health professionals, as school is no longer an option).
9. Seek and secure the significant funding that will likely be required to drive such programmes – for example, government investments (federal, state, or both) – as it is estimated at AU$150–200 million per annum was required to match one of the leading programmes analysed in the report. Likewise, sponsorships and partnerships with industry, not-for-profit organisations and public donations may be leveraged to form appropriate funding. It was recommended that any Australian programmes should have a clear structure for

physical literacy, and if grants are to be offered, funding should encourage adoption of this underlying model/structure, the use of the programme's resources, and (preferably) the reporting of information about uptake and effectiveness, so as to support monitoring, reporting and improvement (i.e. evidence-based practice).

10. Promote physical literacy in a positive, engaging manner, and not rely on national league tables, competitive evaluation or stringent testing regimes, which can be highly detrimental to intrinsic motivation and subsequent sustained engagement.

When reviewing recent developments in Australia (see the following section), there is evidence that the majority of these recommendations have indeed been recognised in the current physical literacy programme(s).

Australia's approach to physical literacy

In May 2016, the Australian Sports Commission recruited a team of researchers to produce, for Australia, a physical literacy definition, standards framework, assessment guidelines and implementation guidelines. Specifically, the researchers were required to develop: (1) an academically sound research base for the establishment of a physical literacy definition and standard – literature review, annotated bibliography or similar (available on request from first author); (2) develop an accepted definition of physical literacy for the Australian environment and an accompanying report outlining justification of interpretation; (3) provide a draft national physical literacy standard, which includes agreed elements, developmental advice (interventions) and advice for target audience segments (teachers, parents and community members); (4) provision of a national physical literacy standard and a visual model or framework that outlines the nature of the physical literacy standard; (5) a research report on effective measuring of physical literacy in schools, including: (a) effective measurement; (b) implementation considerations; and (c) measurement and monitoring (contained within Barnett et al., 2019); and (6) a set of guiding principles for the development of physical literacy in education settings. The resulting resources and documents were published as open-access documents on the ASC website, and can also be requested from the authors of this chapter.

The ensuing project was coordinated through the University of Canberra, which in 2015 was identified as the leading physical literacy advocacy group within Australia (Aspen Institute, 2015). The core researchers in the team (Keegan et al., 2019), conducted a wide-ranging literature review of physical literacy, followed by expert panel meetings and a Delphi consultation process involving three rounds of Delphi surveys to pursue consensus. Following this process, it was agreed that physical literacy should be theoretically separable from physical activity – a so-called 'double dissociation' wherein a person could be high or low in both, separately or together. Likewise, the group agreed that motor competency could be similarly dissociated from physical literacy, in that it may be possible for:

(i) *person A* to display highly refined motor skills without engaging in, or enjoying, frequent physical activity (e.g. after unpleasant experience of PE or youth coaching that focused too much on skill development); whereas (ii) *person B* might struggle to develop refined and sophisticated motor patterns but enjoy sampling a wide array of movement pursuits for recreational and social reasons. In terms of what is left behind or accumulated through these experiences, while both are forms of physical literacy, person B's profile might be closer to the 'spirit' of what is meant by physical literacy. After a series of workshops and Delphi rounds, the group agreed on a set of 'defining statements', making it clear that each individual has the potential to learn through participation in physical activity – and that potential can be developed to a level where it is self-perpetuating. The group agreed that it would be important to offer accessible and simple statements, and to achieve this it was agreed to separate out the core of the concept from its causes, consequences and contexts (such as health, poise, proficiency, etc.) – as very few concepts in language or science are typically defined by their associated causes and consequences. In fact, once these confounding ideas were teased out, and likewise the emphasis on what comprises physical literacy (motivation, confidence, competence and knowledge *versus* physical, affective, cognitive and social capabilities), a very simple idea was left: any learning that occurs as a result of our movement – something that any human being has, and which will take on a unique profile according to each person's experiences. Quite separately, that learning can reach a configuration wherein it becomes self-perpetuating, and the person remains highly disposed to seek out more challenging and more fulfilling movement experiences, which may include benefits for health. As a result, there were four defining statements issued by Sport Australia, with between 94 and 100% consensus recorded from an expert group of 18 leading researchers (including several international experts; see Keegan et al., 2019):

1. *Core/process*: Physical literacy is lifelong holistic learning acquired and applied in movement and physical activity contexts (94% consensus).
2. *Components/constructs*: It reflects ongoing changes integrating physical, psychological, cognitive and social capabilities (94% consensus).
3. *Importance*: It is vital in helping us lead healthy and fulfilling lives through movement and physical activity (100% consensus).
4. *Aspiration*: A physically literate person is able to draw on their integrated physical, psychological, cognitive and social capacities to support health promoting and fulfilling movement and physical activity – relative to their situation and context – throughout the lifespan (94% consensus).

Central to these defining statements was the clarification that whole-person, holistic development spans four key learning domains: the physical, psychological, cognitive and social. The physical domain includes physical competence, motor skills, health- and skill-related fitness, technique, and psychomotor skills. The psychological domain concerns itself with one's experiences of internal signals such as fatigue and exertion, as well as more emotional concepts such as motivation, confidence, self-esteem and engagement. The cognitive domain covers conscious and unconscious knowledge and understanding, including problem-solving and decision-making, awareness of rules and tactics, appreciation of healthy and active lifestyles, and processing of feedback and reflection. The social domain includes cultural sensitivity, leadership, understanding ethical principles, working with peers, coaches, teachers and more, treating others with sensitivity, and effective communication. The group heavily emphasised that development and learning must be *integrated* across all four domains, and not merely focus on the physical. The work has been well received in stakeholder focus groups and has support from the Commonwealth government, including ongoing funding of Sport Australia's work in this area across Australia, e.g. O'Halloran et al. (2018) and Randle et al. (2018).

The standards element of the work was pursued by seeking to use physical literacy as a 'lens' for understanding, and bringing meaning to, existing curricula in education and sporting body coaching guidelines. An analogy was drawn with visual illusions, such as magic eye or Gestalt switching, where a simple shift in perception allows one to see a picture in an otherwise meaningless image. The Delphi process adopted by the team was informed by an inductive content analysis of all existing curricula and standards, including those from swimming, surf lifesaving and cycling, and with important inputs from experts in indigenous games and disability and inclusion. To structure the learning progression, acknowledging that it would be important to offer non-prescriptive and non-linear developmental pathways, the Australian standard drew on Biggs' system of observed learning outcomes (SOLO) taxonomy, set out in Figure 8.3 (Biggs and Collis, 1982; Biggs and Tang, 2007). The efficacy of the SOLO taxonomy to movement-based learning had previously been reported in Australian physical literacy (Dudley, 2015) and physical education settings, and therefore made a logical starting place in this instance (Dudley and Baxter, 2009, 2013). In this approach, the unfulfilled capability to learn is represented by a dot, whereas initial accumulations of experience varying only in small degrees are represented first by a line (one area/topic/skill), and then several parallel lines (several areas/topics/skills). While those lines are, of course, linear, there are important additional aspects of learning: first, when different learnings become connected and compared/mapped, enabling the translation of ideas between them through metaphor and analogy, and ultimately a deeper understanding of the structure of a skill or task. Further, there is a level of learning where these rich and connected mental models can be abstracted and used creatively to solve new, novel and interesting problems that do not follow naturally from what was learned in the more 'linear' stage.

The learning structures and patterns outlined in the SOLO taxonomy are asserted to underlay all human learning, and it has the important implication that the highest forms of learning and skill development are not isolated, highly precise, individual skills, but rather highly integrated, richly connected and highly portable, 'abstractable' capabilities. By mapping existing curricula into the SOLO taxonomy, it became possible to offer a framework for understanding and modelling each individual's physical literacy journey. Importantly, once a person understands

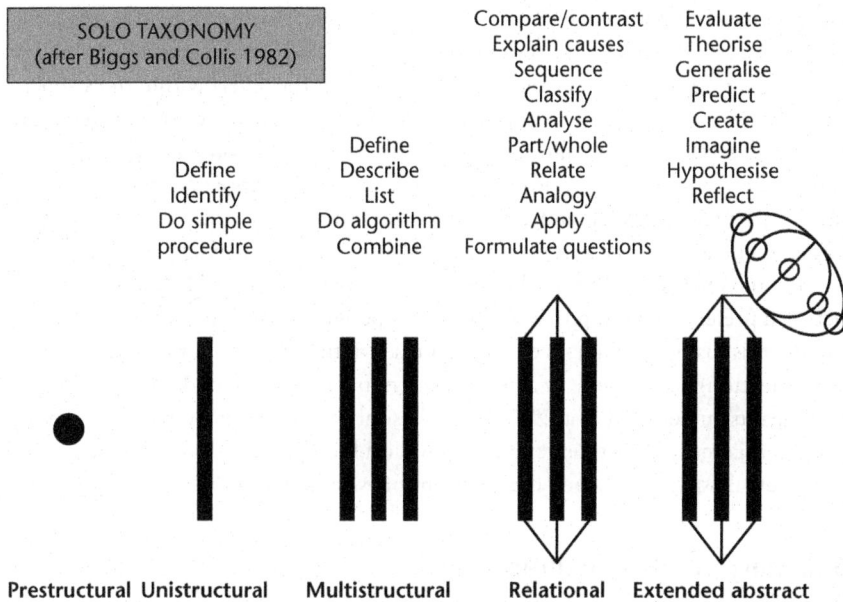

SOLO TAXONOMY
(after Biggs and Collis 1982)

Define
Identify
Do simple
procedure

Define
Describe
List
Do algorithm
Combine

Compare/contrast
Explain causes
Sequence
Classify
Analyse
Part/whole
Relate
Analogy
Apply
Formulate questions

Evaluate
Theorise
Generalise
Predict
Create
Imagine
Hypothesise
Reflect

Prestructural **Unistructural**   **Multistructural**   **Relational** **Extended abstract**

FIGURE 8.3   An overview of the proposed learning configurations in the SOLO taxonomy (1982)

Source: Reproduced courtesy of Biggs and Collis (1982)

which SOLO stage they are currently demonstrating in a particular skill or area, the next step also becomes obvious. For example, the first step of learning any skill is to accumulate experience and understand the basics (i.e. how force and speed parameters might change in a throwing or kicking movement). From there, the second stage might involve changing the context or type of skill by small degrees so that a suite of relatable skill sets is constructed (i.e. a series of parallel lines). Staying with throwing and kicking, using different sized objects, different surfaces, and instruments such as rackets and bats may be appropriate progressions. Once several 'parallel' learning structures have been accumulated, then a learner needs to be encouraged to compare, contrast, relate and transfer information between them, and this is a difficult set of skills in itself, as well as depending on the accumulation of experiences first. Finally, once a learner becomes adept at relating and catalysing learning between similar (but perhaps, over time, increasingly diverse) skills, then they should be encouraged to transfer and adapt this understanding into new, novel and challenging environments. The skill of using existing capabilities to solve new and unfamiliar challenges is important, and yet relatively rare compared to those that have preceded in the learning history. As before, over 80% consensus was reached for these key decisions, and the expert panel convened for the Sport Australia project also offered important feedback on the specific wordings of level descriptors and aspirations/aims. Specifically, 89% of the experts indicated, 'I agree with the use of the four learning domains as a way to structure the standards'; 94% indicated, 'I agree with the use of the SOLO taxonomy as a way to portray the learning of PL', and 89% indicated, 'I agree that the levels within the standards should *not* have age or grades specified'. Detailed breakdown of the standards and the visual model used to illustrate them can be accessed on the Sport Australia website (www.sportaus.gov.au). At the time of writing, Sport Australia had commissioned a team of Web and app designers to build applications that facilitate: (a) engagement with physical literacy; leading to (b) self-categorisation of capabilities and interests in life to date; leading to (c) suggested 'next steps' based on the user's personal preferences and previous learning experiences. An important aspect of this 'product' is that it encourages engagement, self-ratings (and thus self-awareness and self-reflection), and the use of a flexible and non-prescriptive coding system to help participants understand both: (a) their physical literacy journey to date; and also (b) potential next steps to extend their physical literacy development, based on the way they classify and encode their current physical literacy.

Summary and future directions

Australia is a country with many attributes that make it an ideal fit with the concept of physical literacy. It has a mostly warm and pleasant climate – in the populated areas at least – which makes outdoor activities more appealing, as well as diverse geographical features spanning bushland, beaches, lush green fields, snow-covered mountains, fresh water and the sea: it both facilitates and rewards engaging in a diverse array of movement pursuits. Furthermore, modern Australia is fiercely proud of its sporting achievements, and proactively projects this brand around the world. Historically, indigenous cultures have also placed a clear emphasis on the story and songs of the land, and humanity's intricate connection to, and reliance on, the land. This different understanding of the surroundings, and the meaning of moving through the physical world, might be viewed as complementing and extending modern Australians' understanding of physical embodiment, and potentially infuse into the Australian understanding of physical literacy. In the same way that these diverse ways of understanding the physical world enrich and strengthen life in Australia, the different approach to physical literacy that has been developed in Australia may complement, extend and ultimately strengthen the wider physical literacy movement. Indeed, recent review papers by Edwards et al. (2017) and Shearer et al. (2018) have reflected on the benefits of pluralism in approaches to physical literacy, encouraging critical comparisons, positive competition, and thus – over time – progress. The Australian Sports Commission appears to have been quite forward-thinking in this respect, proactively encouraging a new approach, and ultimately a panel of Australian experts reached consensus around a new wording and framework. This achievement suggests that there may well be 'yards left to run' in articulating and operationalising physical literacy, particularly with respect to proactively pursuing uptake, buy-in and wider understanding (explicitly emphasised in the Sport Australia work). To a large extent, the 'story' of multiple parallel narratives converging and leveraging from each other in Australia is a neat parallel for the way that physical literacy develops within each individual: rarely 'linear', often messy, interwoven and richly connected, and seemingly full of happy coincidences. Future research may seek to examine not only the nature of the concept and how best to measure or 'chart' physical literacy (cf. Green et al., 2018), but the best ways of 'marketing' and promoting understanding about physical literacy, with a view to maximising uptake and engagement. For example, the University of Western Australia has developed a unit of learning on physical literacy. Through such widening of engagement with the concept, more diverse perspectives and experiences may be engaged, leading to a richer dialogue/conversation about physical literacy, and – in the long run – a deeper understanding of how different contexts, backgrounds, dispositions and cultures influence an individual's physical literacy journey.

References

Aspen Institute (2015) *Physical Literacy: A Global Environmental Scan.* Available at: http://plreport.projectplay.us/ (accessed 12 March 2019).

Australian Bureau of Statistics (ABS) (2011) *Physical Activity in Australia: A Snapshot, 2007–08.* Available at: www.abs.gov.au/AUSSTATS/abs@.nsf/Lookup/4835.0.55.001Main+Features12007-08?OpenDocument (accessed 25 March 2019).

Australian Curriculum, Assessment and Reporting Authority (ACARA) (2016) *The Australian Curriculum Health and Physical Education.* Available at: www.australiancurriculum.edu.au/f-10-curriculum/health-and-physical-education/ (accessed 25 March 2019).

Australian Institute of Health and Welfare (AIHW) (2018) *Physical Activity across the Life Stages.* Australian Government Cat. no. PHE 225. Canberra: AIHW.

Australian Sports Commission (ASC) (2017) *Corporate Plan 2017–2021.* Available at: www.slideshare.net/PatrickRoult/asc-plan-2017-2021 (accessed 12 March 2019).

Babic, M.J., Morgan, P.J., Plotnikoff, R.C., Lonsdale, C., White, R.L. and Lubans, D.R. (2014) Physical activity and physical self-concept in youth: systematic review and meta-analysis. *Sports Medicine,* 44(11): 1589–1601.

Balyi, I. and Hamilton, A. (2004) *Long-Term Athlete Development: Trainability in Childhood and Adolescence.* Windows of Opportunity. Optimal Trainability. Victoria: National Coaching Institute British Columbia & Advanced Training and Performance.

Balyi, I., Cardinal, C., Higgs, C., Norris, S. and Way, R. (2006). *Long-Term Athlete Development.* Vancouver: Canadian Sport Centres.

Barnett, L.M., Morgan, P.J., van Beurden, E. and Beard, J.R. (2008a) Perceived sports competence mediates the relationship between childhood motor skill proficiency and adolescent physical activity and fitness: a longitudinal assessment. *International Journal of Behavioral Nutrition and Physical Activity,* 5(1), 40.

Barnett, L.M., van Beurden, E., Morgan, P.J., Brooks, L.O. and Beard, J.R. (2008b) Does childhood motor skill proficiency predict adolescent fitness? *Medicine and Science in Sports and Exercise,* 40(12): 2137–2144.

Barnett, L.M., van Beurden, E., Morgan, P.J., Brooks, L.O. and Beard, J.R. (2009) Childhood motor skill proficiency as a predictor of adolescent physical activity. *Journal of Adolescent Health,* 44(3), 252–259.

Barnett, L.M., van Beurden, E., Morgan, P.J., Brooks, L.O. and Beard, J.R. (2010) Gender differences in motor skill proficiency from childhood to adolescence: a longitudinal study. *Research Quarterly for Exercise and Sport,* 81(2): 162–170.

Barnett, L.M., Morgan, P.J., van Beurden, E., Ball, K. and Lubans, D.R. (2011) A reverse pathway? Actual and perceived skill proficiency and physical activity. *Medicine and Science in Sports and Exercise*, 43(5): 898–904.

Barnett, L., Hinkley, T., Okely, A.D. and Salmon, J. (2013) Child, family and environmental correlates of children's motor skill proficiency. *Journal of Science and Medicine in Sport*, 16(4): 332–336.

Barnett, L.M., Zask, A., Rose, L., Hughes, D. and Adams, J. (2015) Three-year follow-up of an early childhood intervention: what about physical activity and weight status? *Journal of Physical Activity and Health*, 12(3): 319–321.

Barnett, L.M., Lai, S.K., Veldman, S.L.C., Hardy, L.L., Cliff, D.P., Morgan, P.J., … Okely, A.D. (2016) Correlates of gross motor competence in children and adolescents: a systematic review and meta-analysis. *Sports Medicine*, 46(11): 1663–1688.

Barnett, L.M., Dudley, D.A., Telford, R.D., Lubans, D.R., Schranz, N.K., Bryant, A.S., Roberts, W.M., Salmon, J., Vella, S.A., Ziviani, J., Morgan, P.J., Weissensteiner, J.R., Okely, A.D., Wainwright, N., Evans, J.R. and Keegan, R.J. (2019) Physical literacy in young people: guidelines and recommendations for the selection of measures in Australian schools. *Journal of Teaching and Physical Education*, https://doi.org/10.1123/jtpe.2018-0219.

Biggs, J.B. and Collis, K.F. (1982) *Evaluating the Quality of Learning: The SOLO Taxonomy (Structure of the Observed Learning Outcome)*. New York: Academic Press.

Biggs, J. and Tang, C. (2007) Using constructive alignment in outcomes-based teaching and learning. In *Teaching for Quality Learning at University*, 3rd edn. Maidenhead, UK: Open University Press, pp. 50–63.

Cairney, J., Bedard, C. and Dudley, D. (2016) Towards a physical literacy framework to guide the design, implementation and evaluation of early childhood movement-based interventions targeting cognitive development. *Annals of Sports Medicine and Research*, 3(4): 1073–1078.

Carlson, J.A., Sallis, J.F., Chriqui, J.F., Schneider, L., McDermid, L.C. and Agron, P. (2013) State policies about physical activity minutes in physical education or during school. *The Journal of School Health*, 83(3): 150–156.

Cattuzzo, M.T., dos Santos Henrique, R., Ré, A.H.N., de Oliveira, I.S., Melo, B.M., de Sousa Moura, M., … Stodden, D. (2016) Motor competence and health related physical fitness in youth: a systematic review. *Journal of Science and Medicine in Sport*, 19(2): 123–129.

Centers for Disease Control and Prevention (CDC) (2010) *State Indicator Report on Physical Activity*. Atlanta, GA: CDC.

Cohen, K.E., Morgan, P.J., Plotnikoff, R.C., Barnett, L.M. and Lubans, D.R. (2015) Improvements in fundamental movement skill competency mediate the effect of the SCORES intervention on physical activity and cardiorespiratory fitness in children. *Journal of Sports Sciences*, 33(18): 1908–1918.

Daly, R., Ducher, G., Cunningham, R., Hill, B., Eser, P., Naughton, G., … Telford, R. (2012) Effects of a specialized school physical education program on bone structure and strength: a 4-year randomised controlled trial. *Journal of Science and Medicine in Sport*, 15: S89–S90.

Ding, D., Lawson, K.D., Kolbe-Alexander, T.L., Finkelstein, E.A., Katzmarzyk, P.T., van Mechelen, W. and Pratt, M. (2016) The economic burden of physical inactivity: a global analysis of major non-communicable diseases. *The Lancet*, 388(10051), 1311–1324.

Dudley, D. (2015) A conceptual model of observed physical literacy. *The Physical Educator*, 72: 236–260.

Dudley, D. and Baxter, D. (2009) Assessing levels of student understanding in pre-service teachers using a two-cycle SOLO model. *Asia-Pacific Journal of Teacher Education*, 37(3): 283–293.

Dudley, D. and Baxter, D. (2013) Metacognitive analysis of pre-service teacher conception
of teaching games for understanding (TGFU) using blogs. *Asia-Pacific Journal of Teacher
Education*, 41(2): 186–196.

Dudley, D., Okely, A., Pearson, P. and Cotton, W. (2011) A systematic review of the effectiveness of physical education and school sport interventions targeting physical activity,
movement skills and enjoyment of physical activity. *European Physical Education Review*,
17(3), 353–378.

Dudley, D., Okely, A.D., Cotton, W.G., Pearson, P. and Caputi, P. (2012a) Physical activity levels and movement skill instruction in secondary school physical education. *Journal
of Science and Medicine in Sport*, 15(3): 231–237.

Dudley, D., Okely, A.D., Pearson, P., Cotton, W.G. and Caputi, P. (2012b) Changes in
physical activity levels, lesson context, and teacher interaction during physical education
in culturally and linguistically diverse Australian schools. *International Journal of Behavioral
Nutrition and Physical Activity*, 9(1): 114.

Dudley, D., Kriellaars, D. and Cairney, J. (2016) Physical literacy assessment and its potential for identification and treatment of children with neuro-developmental behavioral
intellectual disorders. *Current Developmental Disorders Reports*, 3(3): 195–199.

Dudley, D., Cairney, J., Wainwright, N., Kriellaars, D. and Mitchell, D. (2017) Critical
considerations for physical literacy policy in public health, recreation, sport, and education agencies. *Quest*, 1: 1–17.

Edwards, L.C., Bryant, A.S., Keegan, R.J., Morgan, K. and Jones, A.M. (2017) Definitions, foundations and associations of physical literacy: a systematic review. *Sports Medicine*, 47: 113–126.

Estevan, I. and Barnett, L.M. (2018) Considerations related to the definition, measurement
and analysis of perceived motor competence. *Sports Medicine*, 48(12): 2685–2694.

Farrow, D., Baker, J. and MacMahon, C. (2013) *Developing Sport Expertise: Researchers and
Coaches Put Theory into Practice*. London: Routledge.

Frémeaux, E., Mallam, K.M., Metcalf, B.S., Hosking, J., Voss, L.D. and Wilkin, T.J. (2011)
The impact of school-time activity on total physical activity: the activitystat hypothesis
(EarlyBird 46). *International Journal of Obesity*, 35(10): 1277–1283.

Goldberg, J.H. and King, A.C. (2007) Physical activity and weight management across the
lifespan. *Annual Review of Public Health*, 28: 145–170.

Green, N., Sheehan, D., Roberts, R. and Keegan, R.J. (2018) Charting physical literacy journeys within physical education settings. *Journal of Teaching in Physical Education*,
37(3): 272–279.

Gulbin, J.P., Croser, M.J., Morley, E.J. and Weissensteiner, J.R. (2013) An integrated framework for the optimisation of sport and athlete development: a practitioner approach.
Journal of Sports Sciences, 31(12): 1319–1331.

Gulbin, J.P., Croser, M.J., Morley, E.J. and Weissensteiner, J.R. (2014) A closer look
at the FTEM framework. Response to 'More of the same? Comment on "An integrated framework for the optimisation of sport and athlete development: a practitioner
approach"'. *Journal of Sports Sciences*, 32(8): 796–800.

Hardy, L.L., Barnett, L.M., Espinel, P. and Okely, A.D. (2013) Thirteen-year trends in
child and adolescent fundamental movement skills: 1997–2010. *Medicine and Science in
Sports and Exercise*, 45(10): 1965–1970.

Hickey, C., Kirk, D., Macdonald, D. and Penney, D. (2014) Curriculum reform in 3D:
a panel of experts discuss the new HPE curriculum in Australia. *Asia-Pacific Journal of
Health, Sport and Physical Education*, 5(2): 181–192.

Hulteen, R.M., Lander, N.J., Morgan, P.J., Barnett, L.M., Robertson, S.J. and Lubans, D.R. (2015) Validity and reliability of field-based measures for assessing movement skill competency in lifelong physical activities: a systematic review. *Sports Medicine*, 45(10): 1443–1454.

Hulteen, R.M., Morgan, P.J., Barnett, L.M., Stodden, D.F. and Lubans, D.R. (2018) Development of foundational movement skills: a conceptual model for physical activity across the lifespan. *Sports Medicine*, 48(7): 1533–1540.

Hunter, L., Abbott, R., Macdonald, D., Ziviani, J. and Cuskelly, M. (2014) Active kids, active minds: a physical activity intervention to promote learning? *Asia-Pacific Journal of Health, Sport and Physical Education*, 5(2): 117–131.

Keegan, R.J., Keegan, S.L., Daley, S., Ordway, C. and Edwards, A. (2013) *Getting Australia Moving: Establishing a Physically Literate and Active Nation (GAME PLAN)*. Available at: www.canberra.edu.au/researchrepository/file/50f8c79c-2aca-a83f-aee8-254288c36220/1/full_text_final.pdf (accessed 12 March 2019).

Keegan, R.J., Barnett, L.M., Dudley, D.A., Telford, R.D., Lubans, D.R., Schranz, N.K., Bryant, A.S., Roberts,, W.M., Salmon, J., Vella, S.A., Ziviani, J., Morgan, P.J., Weissensteiner, J.R., Okely, A.D., Wainwright, N. and Evans, J.R. (2019) Defining and operationalizing physical literacy: a modified Delphi methodology. *Journal of Teaching and Physical Education*, https://doi.org/10.1123/jtpe.2018-0264.

Kirk, S.F.L., Penney, T.L. and McHugh, T.L.F. (2010) Characterizing the obesogenic environment: the state of the evidence with directions for future research. *Obesity Reviews*, 11(2): 109–117.

Lonsdale, C., Rosenkranz, R.R., Sanders, T., Peralta, L.R., Bennie, A., Jackson, B., … Lubans, D.R. (2013) A cluster randomized controlled trial of strategies to increase adolescents' physical activity and motivation in physical education: results of the Motivating Active Learning in Physical Education (MALP) trial. *Preventive Medicine*, 57(5): 696–702.

Lopes, V.P., Rodrigues, L.P., Maia, J.A.R. and Malina, R.M. (2011) Motor coordination as predictor of physical activity in childhood. *Scandinavian Journal of Medicine & Science in Sports*, 21(5): 663–669.

Lounsbery, M.F., McKenzie, T.L., Morrow, J.R., Monnat, S.M. and Holt, K.A. (2013) District and school physical education policies: implications for physical education and recess time. *Annals of Behavioral Medicine: A Publication of the Society of Behavioral Medicine*, 45(1): S131–S141.

Macdonald, D. and Enright, E. (2014) Physical literacy and the Australian health and physical education curriculum. *ICSSPE Bulletin*, 65: 352–361.

MacNamara, A. and Collins, D. (2013) More of the same? Comment on 'An integrated framework for the optimisation of sport and athlete development: a practitioner approach'. *Journal of Sports Sciences*, 32: 793–795.

McKenzie, T.L. and Lounsbery, M.F. (2009) School physical education: the pill not taken. *American Journal of Lifestyle Medicine*, 3(3): 219–225.

National Physical Activity Survey (NPAS) (2000) *Physical Activity Patterns of Australian Adults: Results of the 1999 National Physical Activity Survey*. Available at: www.aihw.gov.au/reports/physical-activity/physical-activity-patterns-of-australian-adults/contents/table-of-contents (accessed 12 March 2019).

New South Wales Department for Education (2015) *The NSW Physical Literacy Continuum K–10*. Available at: https://education.nsw.gov.au/teaching-and-learning/curriculum/key-learning-areas/pdhpe/physical-literacy/professional-learning#Improving3 (accessed 12 March 2019).

Okely, A.D., Booth, M.L. and Patterson, J.W. (2001) Relationship of physical activity to fundamental movement skills among adolescents. *Medicine and Science in Sports Exercise*, 33(11): 1899–1904.

Olive, L.S., Byrne, D.G., Cunningham, R.B. and Telford, R.D. (2012) Effects of physical activity, fitness and fatness on children's body image: the Australian LOOK longitudinal study. *Mental Health and Physical Activity*, 5(2): 116–124.

Owen, K.B., Smith, J., Lubans, D.R., Ng, J.Y.Y. and Lonsdale, C. (2014) Self-determined motivation and physical activity in children and adolescents: a systematic review and meta-analysis. *Preventive Medicine*, 67: 270–279.

Plotnikoff, R.C., Costigan, S.A., Karunamuni, N. and Lubans, D.R. (2013) Social cognitive theories used to explain physical activity behavior in adolescents: a systematic review and meta-analysis. *Preventive Medicine*, 56(5): 245–253.

Robinson, L.E., Stodden, D.F., Barnett, L.M., Lopes, V.P., Logan, S.W., Rodrigues, L.P. and D'Hondt, E. (2015) Motor competence and its effect on positive developmental trajectories of health. *Sports Medicine*, 45(9): 1273–1284.

Rosenkranz, R.R., Lubans, D.R., Peralta, L.R., Bennie, A., Sanders, T. and Lonsdale, C. (2012) A cluster-randomized controlled trial of strategies to increase adolescents' physical activity and motivation during physical education lessons: the Motivating Active Learning in Physical Education (MALP) trial. *Public Health*, 12(1): 696–702.

Shearer, C., Goss, H.R., Edwards, L.C., Keegan, R.J., Knowles, Z.R., Boddy, L.M., Durden-Myers, E.J. and Foweather, L. (2018) How is physical literacy defined? A contemporary update. *Journal of Teaching in Physical Education*, special issue, Operationalising Physical Literacy, 37(3): 237–245.

Sterdt, E., Liersch, S. and Walter, U. (2013) Correlates of physical activity of children and adolescents: a systematic review of reviews. *Health Education Journal*, 73(1): 1–18.

Stodden, D.F., Goodway, J.D., Langendorfer, S.J., Roberton, M.A., Rudisill, M.E., Garcia, C. and Garcia, L.E. (2008) A developmental perspective on the role of motor skill competence in physical activity: an emergent relationship. *Quest*, 60(2): 290–306.

Stolz, S. (2014) *The Philosophy of Physical Education: A New Perspective*. London: Routledge.

Stolz, S. (2015) Embodied learning. *Educational Philosophy and Theory*, 47(5): 474–487.

Stolz, S. and Thorburn, M. (2017) Aims and values in physical education: can rival traditions of physical education ever be resolved? In M. Thorburn (ed.), *Transformative Learning and Teaching in Physical Education*. London: Routledge, pp. 26–41.

Telford, R.D., Cunningham, R.B. and Telford, R.M. (2009a) Day-dependent step-count patterns and their persistence over 3 years in 8–10-year-old children: the LOOK project. *Annals of Human Biology*, 36(6): 669–679.

Telford, R.D., Bass, S.L., Budge, M.M., Byrne, D.G., Carlson, J.S., Coles, D., … Waring, P. (2009b) The lifestyle of our kids (LOOK) project: Outline of methods. *Journal of Science and Medicine in Sport*, 12(1), 156–163.

Telford, R.D., Cunningham, R.B., Fitzgerald, R., Olive, L.S., Prosser, L., Jiang, X. and Telford, R.M. (2012a) Physical education, obesity, and academic achievement: a 2-year longitudinal investigation of Australian elementary school children. *American Journal of Public Health*, 102(2): 368–374.

Telford, R.D., Cunningham, R.B., Telford, R.M., Abhayaratna, W.P. and Abharatna, W.P. (2012b) Schools with fitter children achieve better literacy and numeracy results: evidence of a school cultural effect. *Pediatric Exercise Science*, 24(1): 45–57.

Telford, R.D., Cunningham, R.B., Telford, R.M., Olive, L.S., Byrne D.G. and Abhayaratna, W.P. (2013a) Benefits of early development of eye–hand coordination:

evidence from the LOOK longitudinal study. *Scandinavian Journal of Medicine and Science in Sports*, 23(5): e263-9. doi: 10.1111/sms.12073.

Telford, R.M., Telford, R.D., Cunningham, R.B., Cochrane, T., Davey, R. and Waddington, G. (2013b) Longitudinal patterns of physical activity in children aged 8 to 12 years: the LOOK study. *International Journal of Behavioral Nutrition and Physical Activity*, 10(1): 1–12.

Telford, R.D., Cunningham, R.B., Waring, P., Telford, R.M., Olive, L.S. and Abhayaratna, W.P. (2013c) Physical education and blood lipid concentrations in children: the LOOK randomized cluster trial. *PLoS ONE*, 8(10): e76124.

Telford, R.D., Cunningham, R.B., Telford, R.M., Daly, R.M., Olive, L.S. and Abhayaratna, W.P. (2013d) Physical education can improve insulin resistance: the LOOK randomized cluster trial. *Medicine and Science in Sports and Exercise*, 45(10): 1956–1964.

UNESCO (2015) *Quality Physical Education: Guidelines for Policymakers*. Available at: http://unesdoc.unesco.org/images/0023/002311/231101E.pdf (accessed 12 March 2019).

UNESCO (2017) *The Kazan Action Plan*. Available at: http://unesdoc.unesco.org/images/0025/002527/252725e.pdf (accessed 12 March 2019).

van Beurden, E., Barnett, L.M., Zask, A., Dietrich, U.C., Brooks, L.O. and Beard, J. (2003) Can we skill and activate children through primary school physical education lessons? 'Move it groove it': a collaborative health promotion intervention. *Preventive Medicine*, 36(4): 493–501.

Whitehead, M. (2010) *Physical literacy throughout the Lifecourse*. London: Routledge.

Yan, J.H. and McCullagh, P. (2004) Cultural influence on youth's motivation of participation in physical activity. *Journal of Sport Behavior*, 27(4): 378–390.

Zhang, J. and Chaaban, J. (2013) The economic cost of physical inactivity in China. *Preventive Medicine*, 56(1): 75–78.

9

PHYSICAL LITERACY IN CANADA

Dwayne Sheehan, Daniel Robinson and Lynn Randall

As an early adopter of the physical literacy concept, Canada has enjoyed many years of discussion and action across multiple sectors, including sport, recreation and education. Moreover, Canada boasts a large body of scholarship related to physical literacy, as well as strong policy to support both regional and national physical literacy initiatives. The conditions that have set the stage for Canada to become a leader in the physical literacy movement are outlined herein. More specifically, relevant information and discussion is organised by the main sectors impacting and enacting physical literacy-related practices (i.e. sport, recreation and education). Further discussion is provided on how these sectors collaborate to enhance the lives of Canadians. A section is dedicated to measurement and assessment of physical literacy, as several notable tools have been developed by Canadian scholars. Additionally, a brief overview of Canadian scholarship is offered, as is an account of how physical literacy is viewed for and from minority/minoritised populations' perspectives. Finally, considering all this, a brief account of physical literacy's potential and future(s) is offered.

Defining physical literacy: a Canadian consensus journey

One of the earliest Canadian definitions of physical literacy came from the Canadian Sport Centre and Canada Sport for Life (CS4L), now known as Sport for Life (S4L) in *Developing Physical Literacy: A Guide for Parents of Children Ages 0 to 12* (Higgs et al., 2008). The message was that parents/guardians can help children gain 'the tools they need to take part in physical activity and sport, both for healthy life-long enjoyment and sporting success' (p. 5). Rooted in the sport domain and the long-term athlete development (LTAD) model (Balyi, 2001) – where the ultimate goal is to develop athletic success and the desire to be active for life – Higgs et al. (2008) proposed that children need to develop the fundamental movement skills and fundamental sport skills that 'permit a child to move confidently and with control, in a wide range of physical activity, rhythmic (dance) and sport situations' (p. 5). In an effort to simplify the concept and make it easily accessible and understandable for the general public, in many of their publications and promotional material, S4L has equated the development and acquisition of fundamental movement skills with physical literacy. S4L has been a huge advocate for physical literacy across the country. With support from Sport Canada, they have been able to reach and influence large sections of the population. To this end, many Canadians equate physical literacy as the acquisition of fundamental movement skills.

Sport Canada's approval of the LTAD framework as national policy has meant that every Canadian, regardless of age, ability or desired sporting outcome (i.e. recreational or competitive), who has participated in organised sport in Canada has been exposed to the above definition of physical literacy. That is, every national sport organisation (NSO) in Canada adopted the LTAD model and created their own sport-specific framework for athletic development, sport programming and strategic planning. These LTAD applications are skill-focused and are committed to providing the skills, attitudes and knowledge for healthy and lifelong engagement in physical activity, and, for those who have the talent, drive and commitment, the opportunity to achieve excellence (Higgs, 2010). While the intent is to create athletes for a specific sport, many LTAD applications suggest that a multitude of skills are needed from a variety of sports for a person to be physically literate.

The LTAD model suggests physical literacy is developed during the first three stages of athletic development: Active Start (for girls and boys ages 0–6), FUNdamentals (for girls ages 6–8 years and boys ages 6–9), and Learn to Train (for girls ages 8–11 and boys ages 9–12). These development stages take place in homes, schools, sports clubs and community recreation spaces. Those responsible for helping children develop their physical literacy at these stages include parents/guardians, coaches, teachers, sport and recreation leaders, and youth leaders (Higgs et al., 2008).

The year after the CS4L physical literacy guide for parents/guardians was published, Physical and Health Education (PHE) Canada (a national professional organisation for physical and health educators) published its own, arguably more holistic, definition of physical literacy. The rationale for having a definition apart from the one employed in the sporting realm was that educators serve different people with a different purpose (Mandigo et al., 2009). This PHE Canada definition of physical literacy was as follows:

> Individuals who are physically literate move with competence in a wide variety of physical activities that benefit the development of the whole person. Physically literate individuals consistently develop the motivation and ability to understand, communicate, apply and analyse different forms of movement. They are able to demonstrate a variety of movements confidently, competently, creatively and strategically across a wide range of health-related physical activities. These skills enable individuals to make healthy, active

choices throughout their life span that are both beneficial to and respectful of themselves, others and their environment.

(Mandigo et al., 2009: 6–7)

Soon after, PHE Canada released an updated definition that suggested 'individuals who are physically literate move with competence and confidence in a wide variety of physical activities in multiple environments that benefit the healthy development of the whole person' (PHE Canada, n.d.: para. 3). This updated definition addressed the observation that focusing solely upon fundamental skill development at the exclusion of the *process* of development diminished the pedagogical and educational components required of the teaching community (Mandigo et al., 2009). That is, school-based education includes 'the application of foundational knowledge and understanding in ethical and productive ways across a wide range of environments, tasks and situations' (Mandigo et al., 2009: 5). Moreover, PHE Canada was especially clear in stating that competency is not based on population norms, but rather is relative to each individual. Finally, PHE Canada's iteration also referred to the whole person and all developmental domains (i.e. physical, cognitive, affective and social).

While seemingly at odds with one another, the sport (and recreation), research and education sectors actually work in tandem to create opportunities for everyone to become physically literate (Mandigo et al., 2013). To provide clarity for the development of policy, practice and research, in 2015 sector leaders and stakeholders came together to create a physical literacy consensus statement (ParticipACTION et al., 2015). This consensus statement aimed to end the misuse of the terms 'physical activity', 'physical education', 'fundamental movement skills' and/or 'motor skill development' as synonyms for physical literacy. This consensus definition is as follows: 'Physical literacy is the motivation, confidence, physical competence, knowledge and understanding to value and take responsibility for engagement in physical activities for life' (ParticipACTION et al., 2015: para. 3). This definition includes four elements: affective (motivation and confidence), physical (physical competence), cognitive (knowledge and understanding) and behavioural (engagement in physical activities for life). The core principles that underlie this definition are that physical literacy is inclusive and accessible to all: it represents an individual journey, it can be experienced in multiple contexts and environments, it needs to be cultivated throughout life, and it contributes to the overall development of the whole person (ParticipACTION et al., 2015). This is also the definition that is currently used by the International Physical Literacy Association (IPLA).

Physical literacy in the Canadian sport sector

In 2002, Sport Canada created the Canadian Sport Policy 2002–2012 (CSP 2002) to make the sport system more effective and inclusive (Canadian Heritage, 2002a). The CSP 2002 recognised that sport is not only fun, but it also: builds strong individuals and strong communities through individual physical, social and character development; develops leadership skills; can lead to better health and quality of life; improves behaviour; offers economic development and prosperity; and is entertaining (Canadian Heritage, 2002a). Four broad goals were set for the CSP 2002 related to enhancing participation, excellence, capacity and interaction (Canadian Heritage, 2002a: 4). To achieve these goals, the federal and provincial/territorial (F-P/T) governments developed a four-year action plan (Canadian Heritage, 2002b). As part of this plan, the CSP 2002 adopted CS4L's LTAD model (Canadian Heritage, 2007). Each NSO and P/T sport organisation (P/TSO) was responsible for developing a unique LTAD plan based on the generic template (Canadian Heritage, 2007) as a condition of receiving funding (Dowling and Washington, 2017). A large-scale evaluation of the CSP 2002 took place in 2009, three years prior to the completion of stated priorities, in order to give F-P/T governments time to review the findings and create a new plan going forward (Canadian Heritage, 2010). At the time of evaluation, progress on physical literacy was still in the preliminary phases.

The CSP 2012 was developed based on such feedback, as well as feedback from governments, non-governmental organisations (NGOs) and communities. Designed to be carried out between 2012 and 2022, it provides guidance for F-P/T governments as well as other stakeholders who are 'committed to realizing the positive impacts of sport on individuals, communities and society' (Canadian Heritage, 2012: 2). This second-generation policy involves a more comprehensive network of groups involved in sport beyond just government, including agencies working in organised and unorganised sport, schools, colleges, universities, parks, and public and private sports centres. A 2016 review of the CSP 2012 concluded that for greater collaboration between sectors (sport, education, health and municipal recreation), a clear goal and common vision were necessary to achieve the CSP objective of enhancing physical literacy in children (Canadian Heritage, 2016).

Physical literacy in the Canadian recreation sector

Municipalities are a significant provider of recreational physical activity resources and opportunities. Nearly half of Canadian municipalities cite physical literacy as a reason for physical activity and sport programme development (Canadian Fitness and Lifestyle Research Institute, 2016a). Municipalities are highly involved in the recreation sector through a number of initiatives and programmes, including the following: infrastructure funding and maintenance (e.g. sports fields, arenas, pools); early skill development and exposure programmes (e.g. learn to swim); ongoing sport play (e.g. after-school drop-in programmes); coordination and communication for scheduling purposes; enhanced coaching capacity; allocation policies and subsidies; joint-use agreements with school districts; and sport hosting/sport tourism (Canadian Parks and Recreation Association and Canadian Sport for Life, 2013). Education is also undertaken by Canadian municipalities, which provide physical literacy information via websites, brochures, posters and resource centres

(Canadian Fitness and Lifestyle Research Institute, 2016b), although differences in resources do exist between provinces/territories and size of community.

A notable connection to physical literacy from the recreation sector in Canada is Vivo. Vivo for Healthier Generations is a Calgary charity that is using physical literacy as a pillar in its development of a new model for public health in Canada. Their journey started with a question about how they could contribute to healthier generations within the communities they serve. Physical literacy became their theory of change for a solution to pioneer a new standard for recreation in Canada. Three things they have learnt include:

- by changing the methods they used in their programming, they could shift activity levels, confidence and competence;
- by giving people personalised measurement tools, they could sustain healthy behaviours for life; and
- by co-creating and collaborating with others, they could drive larger social impact and system change.

Vivo is currently working at three levels (individual, community and systems) to bring about a movement called Generation Healthy (Gen H). Their aim is to support individuals and families to make healthier choices and physical activity connections an integral part of their day, to co-create, test and measure new types of play solutions with the community and partners across home, school, work and neighbourhood environments, and to reimagine the design and care of whole communities with citizens, diverse sectors and local government.

Community-based research has identified an imbalance between structured and unstructured play (Canadian Heritage, 2016). It has been reported that physical literacy is impacted by parents/guardians who are overly concerned about safety (e.g. while playing road hockey), which limits spontaneous play in children (Canadian Heritage, 2016). Even though children reported a preference for unorganised physical activity (21% organised, 27% unorganised, 49% both; Canadian Fitness and Lifestyle Research Institute, 2013a), most children participated in structured (79%) versus unstructured (4%) sporting activities (Canadian Fitness and Lifestyle Research Institute, 2013b). The opportunity to develop as a physically literate child should not be dependent on either structured or unstructured experiences solely. The Canadian Parks and Recreation Association recommends that elements of active play are integrated into preschool and day care programmes, and that physical literacy be a focused component of any recreation programme (Canadian Parks and Recreation Association and Canadian Sport for Life, 2013).

Physical literacy in the Canadian (physical) education sector

The CSP 2002 set the priority to increase sport and physical activity in school. This aligns with the expectations of Canadians that governments carry the bulk of the responsibility for ensuring daily physical education in schools (Canadian

Fitness and Lifestyle Research Institute, 2009a, 2013c). Action to make this happen is taken on a jurisdiction-by-jurisdiction basis in Canada (Canadian Heritage, 2007). Physical education specialist positions, however, continue to be removed from schools, which may be limiting the ability to implement physical literacy concepts into the physical education curriculum (Canadian Heritage, 2016). Only 62% of schools in Canada had a policy regarding hiring trained physical education specialists, and only 42% of these schools had implemented this policy (Canadian Fitness and Lifestyle Research Institute, 2016c). In some provinces, (elementary) physical education is one of the few disciplines in which no subject-specific teacher training is necessary. Classroom generalists have repeatedly stated that they do not feel comfortable teaching physical education, and further that they have limited knowledge of physical literacy (Decorby et al., 2005). In a recent study of physical education teachers, (some current, some now classroom teachers), 60% reported that physical literacy meant physical competence, while a further 8% showed no understanding of the concept at all, yet only 10% stated that the concept of physical literacy was unclear (Stoddart and Humbert, 2017). Teachers were missing critical pieces to the concept, despite not knowing this. This study was completed before the consensus statement on physical literacy was adopted. Perhaps now teachers will be less confused about the definition of physical literacy and be better equipped to incorporate it into their curricula.

While it may be perceived as a failure within the system that classroom generalists teach elementary school physical education, it presents an opportunity to incorporate the cognitive, affective and psychomotor components of physical literacy during classes outside of physical education with little additional training (Stanec and Murray-Orr, 2011; Lu and De Lisio, 2017). Elementary generalists spend the majority of the day with one group of children, rather than a physical education specialist who would only see the children for one class (hopefully) daily. This not only provides more opportunities for integration, but it also allows the generalist teacher an understanding of how children react and learn in different situations. Having a greater understanding of where and how children learn best provides more options for tailoring class plans. Schools with a well-defined and well-implemented school health policy are better suited to enable generalist elementary teachers to incorporate physical literacy concepts into other curricular subjects (Stanec and Murray-Orr, 2011). Indeed, the priority of the education system is placed on language, arts and mathematics. Parents do not demand physical literacy as part of the curriculum (only 10% of teachers reported parental inquiry into the topic; Stoddart and Humbert, 2017), generalist teachers are uncomfortable teaching physical education, and some do not view it as part of their mandate (Canadian Heritage, 2016). School administrators most often cited an emphasis on other subjects as a barrier to physical education, followed by competing demands for facilities (Canadian Fitness and Lifestyle Research Institute, 2017).

Despite these obstacles, educators in schools that have implemented physical literacy polices have noticed improvements in grades, attendance, engagement, the number trying out for after-school sport teams and better use of physical education time (Canadian Heritage, 2016). Positive attitudes from teachers, students and parents/guardians, as well as using physical activity as a reward and including it into other coursework were cited by school administrators as indicating supports for physical activity and physical education (Canadian Fitness and Lifestyle Research Institute, 2017). A shift in thinking from 'learning to move' to 'learning through movement' is necessary to demonstrate further positive outcomes (Kentel and Dobson, 2007).

Multi-sector collaborations

It is recognised that each sector requires policies and procedures to further its own mandate and realise the goals of that sector. However, specialisation at the exclusion of collaboration is not beneficial for the individuals that the sectors serve. To this end, collaboration between sport, recreation and education is necessary to empower Canadians to embark upon and benefit from their physical literacy journey. S4L is a national non-profit organisation made up of leaders from the business and the above-mentioned sectors that aims to specifically facilitate collaboration for improved physical literacy in all Canadians. Three pillars define S4L: improving the opportunity for more and enhanced physical literacy programming; preparing more Canadians to pursue excellence in sport; and increasing the likelihood of Canadians staying active for life. This is accomplished by supporting all sectors involved while aligning with community, provincial and national sport policy, and physical activity programming. S4L is highly involved in knowledge transmission across sectors for agencies within Canada and from around the world. The annual Canadian summit brings together delegates from across the country to discuss how leaders can enhance the quality of sport and physical activity in Canada. An international conference on furthering the principles of LTAD within the multiple sectors is also hosted by S4L. The biennial International Physical Literacy Conference (IPLC) brings these sectors together from around the world to discuss ways to advance knowledge, application and implementation of physical literacy theory and programming. The inaugural IPLC in 2013 hosted over 260 leaders, and by 2017 there were over 400 attendees. Furthermore, the number of countries represented has increased from 10 in 2015 to 24 in 2017.

The Coaching Association of Canada, HIGH FIVE and S4L have partnered to offer the Physical Literacy Instructor Program. This initiative gives front-line physical activity workers the tools they need to design and deliver quality programmes to enhance the development of physical literacy. The target demographic of the programme is recreation staff and management; the secondary targets are education staff, public health staff, and others responsible for the delivery of physical activity programmes. HIGH FIVE is Canada's quality standard for children's sport and recreation programmes; it is committed to assisting children ages 6 through 12 towards healthy development by working with programme leaders and parents/guardians.

An increasing number of Canadian scholars have been engaging in physical literacy-related scholarship in recent years (details of these publications can be found on the IPLA website, www.physical-literacy.org.uk). By way of their presence at national conferences or summits that focus upon physical literacy, their physical literacy-related presentations at these sorts of events, and their peer-reviewed publications, these Canadian scholars have been active participants in an emerging body of important scholarship. A recent review of these publications highlights these efforts (Robinson et al., 2018). Since 2009, Canadian scholars have contributed no fewer than 23 peer-reviewed physical literacy papers to the growing body of research. The majority of these contributions are conceptual in nature (13) – perhaps unsurprisingly, as we have seen physical literacy grow from its infancy in Canada in this time period. Research-based contributions are both qualitative (two) and quantitative (six) in nature, with an additional two publications reporting on the results of mixed-methods research. Found within a number of familiar high-impact journals, including *Quest, Journal of Teaching in Physical Education, Measurement in Physical Education and Exercise Science* and *Research Quarterly for Exercise and Sport*, many of these contributions have likely reached a large and far-reaching audience. Additionally, some of these contributions have been published within a Canadian 'practitioner-friendly' journal, *Physical & Health Education Journal*, allowing for easier access to local physical education teachers.

Physical literacy measurement/evaluation/assessment: Canadian contributions

A recent global scan of physical literacy revealed that Canada – compared to all other countries – has been especially active with respect to physical literacy assessments (Spengler and Cohen, 2015). Currently, there are three physical literacy assessment instruments that enjoy a somewhat privileged status within Canadian school communities (Robinson and Randall, 2017). These include PHE Canada's Passport for Life, CS4L's Physical Literacy Assessment for Youth (PLAY) and the Healthy Active Living and Obesity Research Group's (HALO) Canadian Assessment of Physical Literacy (CAPL).

Passport for Life (PHE Canada)

PHE Canada developed the educational support resource called Passport for Life (PFL) to support the awareness, assessment and advancement of physical literacy among physical education students and teachers (see http://passportforlife.ca/what-is-passport-for-life). Physical literacy is assessed through the online and in-person measurement of four components: active participation, living skills, fitness skills and movement skills. The PHE Canada tools are unique in that there are three separate sets of assessment instruments: one for grades 4–6, one for grades 7–9 and one for grades 10–12. PHE Canada is very clear in stating that PFL is not meant to be used as a report card grade, and that results are formative and meant to support improvement of an individual's physical literacy. PFL was recently validated for students in grades 3–6 and grades 7–9. Recent research has also enabled students to offer support for the measure along with recommendations for its use (Lodewyk and Mandigo, 2017).

PLAY (S4L)

Canada Sport for Life developed six tools intended to assess physical literacy. These assessment instruments are known as the Physical Literacy Assessment for Youth (PLAY) tools, and are meant to be used with individuals aged 7 and higher. *PLAYfun* is a comprehensive tool that assesses 18 movement skills. A shorter version of the *PLAYfun* assessment is the *PLAYbasic* tool, which assesses five movement skills. *PLAYfun* and *PLAYbasic* are meant to be used by someone with a background in movement, and require the assessor to physically observe a child complete a specific movement and score the movement performance. *PLAYcoach* and *PLAYparent* are questionnaire-type instruments whereby the coach or parent/guardian provides their perspective on the child's physical literacy. A child can self-assess his or her own physical literacy with the *PLAYself* questionnaire. *PLAYinventory* is a form that helps a parent/guardian or child track and record activity participation over a period of time.

Canadian Assessment of Physical Literacy (HALO/CAPL)

The Canadian Assessment of Physical Literacy for children and youth (CAPL; Healthy Active Living and Obesity Research Group, 2017) measures physical literacy in four domains: physical competence, daily behaviour, motivation and confidence, and knowledge and understanding. The rationale for measuring physical literacy using the CAPL is to identify areas of weakness so that interventions can be targeted, and ultimately more successful at improving physical literacy over time (Longmuir, 2013). The CAPL was recently used as part of the broader Royal Bank of Canada (RBC) Learn to Play Project – CAPL, which has now concluded testing on over 11,000 Canadian children. Results are now published in BMC Health 2018 (see Chapter 6 for references).

As beneficial as these tools may be, they are not without their faults. Most notably, all three models tend to focus heavily on the physical domain. For example, of the 100 points in HALO's instruments, 32 are awarded for physical competence, with another 32 points awarded for daily behaviour; the remaining 36 points are split between knowledge and understanding, and motivation and competence. Although all of the PLAY tools are scored out of 100, physical literacy *training* tends to focus on the physical domain, more specifically fundamental skills. Perhaps the focus on the physical domain may be due to the fact that it is the easiest category to measure objectively. Although the physical component is important, the importance and significance of motivation must not be overlooked. An individual (of any age) can score very well on all skill, fitness and knowledge tests, but if they are not motivated or have no desire to be active, their motor abilities and knowledge will be meaningless.

The three assessment tools all use the language of 'charting progress'; however, the progress is in relation to reaching a desired end (the 'achieving' or 'excelling' category or the 'acquired' or 'proficient' levels). The intended purpose of assigning a numerical score with an accompanying descriptor is so it can be used to gauge improvements. Although this can be motivating for some (oftentimes those who are already active), it must be recognised that this can be demotivating for many. Assessing physical literacy is not an easy task. Perhaps future instruments will be developed that more accurately capture the integrated, holistic essence of the concept, as well as capture the importance of motivation.

A consideration of (some) Canadian minorities and physical literacy

Several minority groups in Canada have been identified as needing targeted efforts for increased involvement in sport and physical activity, and therefore physical literacy development. These include indigenous peoples, women and girls, people with disabilities, and French-speaking Canadians.

Aboriginal peoples

In 2015, the Government of Canada, through the Truth and Reconciliation Commission of Canada, published 94 Calls to Action in an effort to address the negative impacts from actions taken in the past toward Aboriginal Peoples (Truth and Reconciliation Commission of Canada, 2015). Of the 94 Calls to Action, five are specifically related to sport and physical activity. It is recognised that aboriginal peoples present with a different set of experiences than many other Canadians. Namely, many migrate between cities and their reserves, posing challenges for athlete development. Furthermore, many face a disproportionate level of poverty, lower educational outcomes and health concerns – largely because of systemic racism. Layered with this is a different set of traditional and non-traditional values and beliefs. With this in mind, sport for aboriginal people may carry a different purpose, including that of building self-esteem and connectedness with community. For these reasons, a specific Aboriginal Long-Term Participant Development Pathway for sport was created (Sport for Life Society, 2016).

A two-stream model has been proposed for aboriginal athlete development based on the mainstream LTAD pathway (Sport for Life Society and Aboriginal Sport Circle, 2017). This model identifies the ways in which athletes can participate within aboriginal communities and mainstream communities, and where the opportunities for crossover exist. In conjunction with S4L, a resource aimed at aboriginal communities to engage in sport and physical activity was written (Sport for Life Society and Aboriginal Sport Circle, 2017). Through sharing the stories of aboriginal athletes, creating opportunities for participation and developing inclusive environments, the aim is to generate a sense of collaboration, education and acceptance using sport and physical activity. Importantly, this aboriginal model included considerable input from aboriginal leaders, and it includes a meaningful space for spirituality (see Figure 9.1), something that might eventually be considered by others who recognise the role that this might have in one's physical literacy journey (e.g. see Robinson, 2018). Such a purposeful physical literacy connection to spirituality (as well as to culture) embraces a monist and embodied sense of being. Indeed, this sort of indigenous holistic view of the interdependent and mutually enriching place of these four traditional teachings ought to (re) awaken others to the potential of physical literacy to contribute to living a whole and flourishing life. We would suppose that other indigenous groups (e.g. Maori, Aborigine) might also offer similar suggestions about the place and significance of spirituality and culture as they relate to physical literacy. All others, particularly settlers, would be well served to listen to and contemplate such perspectives when they are offered by indigenous peoples.

Canada's National Coaching Certification Program (NCCP) offers specific professional training for aboriginal and non-aboriginal coaches who work with aboriginal athletes. Learning objectives include: understanding the role of sport in aboriginal communities; understanding and positively influencing the community in which you coach; coaching the whole person; coaching beyond the physical to include the mental (intellectual and emotional), spiritual and cultural; responding to racism in sport; establishing a code of behaviour for your team that respects differences and addresses racism; and helping those you coach to make healthy lifestyle choices. Other long-term objectives include: imparting the wisdom of aboriginal culture in mainstream sport: increasing awareness of the aboriginal coaching modules (ACM); allowing coaches and communities the opportunities to embrace culturally sensitive practices to better meet the needs of aboriginal athletes; having coaches at all levels of sport use the ACM material; creating opportunities for dialogue at all levels of sport organisation to meet the needs of aboriginal athletes; and increasing the number of NCCP-certified aboriginal coaches (Coaching Association of Canada, 2017).

Women and girls

The Canadian Association for the Advancement of Women and Sport and Physical Activity (CAAWS), along with CS4L, published a document aimed at addressing the psychosocial factors that affect female participation in sport (CAAWS, 2012). Although women (and girls) represent more than 50% of the Canadian population, this group is grossly under-represented in sport at all levels of participation, and as coaches, officials and leaders. Furthermore, even from a young age, girls are less active than boys (Canadian Fitness and Lifestyle Research Institute, 2014), a trend that tracks forward into adulthood (Canadian Fitness and Lifestyle Research Institute, 2009b). The premise of the CAAWS/CS4L resource is to address the failure of conventional programming and the LTAD framework to adequately recognise gender differences. It highlights that equality is not synonymous with equity, where equity emphasises that needs, interests and experiences ought to be

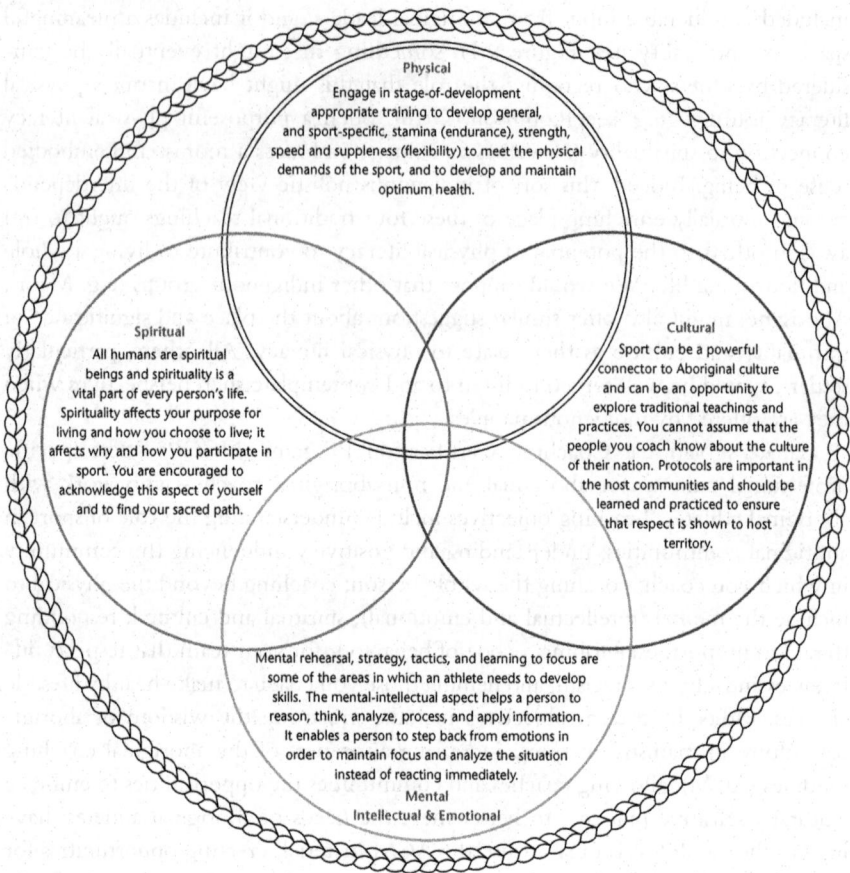

Physical

Engage in stage-of-development appropriate training to develop general, and sport-specific, stamina (endurance), strength, speed and suppleness (flexibility) to meet the physical demands of the sport, and to develop and maintain optimum health.

Spiritual

All humans are spiritual beings and spirituality is a vital part of every person's life. Spirituality affects your purpose for living and how you choose to live; it affects why and how you participate in sport. You are encouraged to acknowledge this aspect of yourself and to find your sacred path.

Cultural

Sport can be a powerful connector to Aboriginal culture and can be an opportunity to explore traditional teachings and practices. You cannot assume that the people you coach know about the culture of their nation. Protocols are important in the host communities and should be learned and practiced to ensure that respect is shown to host territory.

Mental rehearsal, strategy, tactics, and learning to focus are some of the areas in which an athlete needs to develop skills. The mental-intellectual aspect helps a person to reason, think, analyze, process, and apply information. It enables a person to step back from emotions in order to maintain focus and analyze the situation instead of reacting immediately.

Mental Intellectual & Emotional

FIGURE 9.1 The holistic model of physical literacy

Source: Created by Rick Brent for the Aboriginal Sport Circle (reproduced courtesy of Australian Aboriginal Sport Circle)

taken into account rather than simply providing an equal programme for a different group of participants.

Women and girls face barriers that other segments of the Canadian population may not face. Barriers prevent them from participating in sport and physical activity, limit skill development, and negatively impact overall development. These include: physical barriers (e.g. low physical fitness, low motor proficiency); psychological barriers (e.g. limited confidence in abilities or knowledge, low perceived behavioural control); time-based barriers (e.g. too much work or school, responsibilities for younger siblings, children or elderly parents); interpersonal barriers (e.g. low motivational support from family, partner or caregiver, lack of peer support); access and opportunity barriers (e.g. cost, access to appropriate equipment); and programming barriers (e.g. lack of choice and variety, no female-only opportunities) (CAAWS, 2012).

Due to some of the barriers listed above, many girls do not receive enough quality opportunities to develop both basic and advanced skills. These barriers can be addressed at all levels of the LTAD framework in sport, recreation and physical education. Beginning with the FUNdamentals, skills can be taught through fun and games, followed by basic and sport skills, all with the intent of encouraging young girls and women to continue participating and fostering the motivation to do so. Because of a potential lack of adequate instruction in the basic skills, adult women who wish to participate in sport may require basic skill development opportunities as well. Contrary to that, specialising at a young age contributes to a lack of basic movement skills, overuse injuries and early burnout/dropout. Early specialisation sports (e.g. gymnastics, figure skating, diving) tend to attract young female athletes due to their artistic and acrobatic characteristics and their social perception as appropriate for women and girls. Providing opportunities to transfer skills from one sport to another through exposure to a broad range of activities will help to foster overall physical literacy and encourage women and girls to be active for life.

Canadians with disabilities

All Canadians deserve the opportunity to be active. In an effort to provide athletes with disabilities the opportunity to participate in activity or sporting events at either a recreational or competitive level, S4L developed the LTAD model for athletes with disabilities titled *No Accidental Champions* (Higgs et al., 2011). The model mirrors the original LTAD with two additional changes. First is the recognition of additional or unique factors that must be considered when working with and delivering activity and sport programmes for athletes with disabilities. Second, the model contains two additional stages, namely the awareness stage and first contact stage. The awareness stage is meant to make not just the athlete aware of the potential opportunities, but parents/guardians, healthcare providers and the general public as well. The first contact stage stresses the importance of initial experiences being positive for the athlete. Positive initial experiences will increase the likelihood that athletes will remain engaged.

Another notable development in Canada in relation to physical literacy is the Abilities Centre. This is a charitable organisation in Whitby, Ontario committed to enhancing quality of life, health and well-being, and social inclusion for people of all ages, abilities and backgrounds. The Centre comprises a community hub, a research lab and an inclusion incubator. The success of the Centre lies in the development of programmes for diverse populations with varied needs through the lenses of inclusion and accessibility. Inclusion, from the Centre's perspective, means encouraging people of all abilities to engage in meaningful participation (see explanatory glossary) together in an environment that fosters a sense of belongingness and independence. The perspective of the Centre is that physical literacy is a lifetime journey that is unique to every person. This makes it naturally well-suited for people of all abilities, skills and interests. The holistic nature of physical literacy allows every person to demonstrate and reach their physical literacy potential in a variety of ways, regardless of physical capacity. By providing variations within activities, the Abilities Centre supports participation in anyone who is under-participating, who is lacking confidence and competence, or is starting the cycle of improved physical literacy. As the Abilities Centre continues to nationalise their physical literacy initiatives, they reinforce the notion that anyone, at any age, has the ability to pursue physical activity for life.

French-speaking Canadians

In 2011, discussions were held with the official language minority communities (OLMCs) and Sport Canada as part of the Canada Sport Policy renewal (Sport Canada, 2011). The province of Quebec presents as an interesting challenge for sport and recreation in that both minority French-speaking and minority English-speaking groups exist in different parts of the province. While both groups feel as though sport brings Canadians together, francophones see it as a way of strengthening ties to other francophones, while anglophones see it as a way to forge stronger ties with the francophone community (Sport Canada, 2011). A barrier to sport participation is accessing programmes in the official language of their choice. Francophones do not wish to have to limit themselves to English programmes; however, French-only programmes are not widely available, nor are French-speaking coaches and officials. Moreover, Quebec has seemingly refused to endorse/accept the CS4L/LTAD model for political reasons (Dowling and Washington, 2017).

Physical literacy in Canada: just how 'on track' are we?

Despite others, as well as ourselves, recognising that Canada has been one of the West's physical literacy leaders (e.g. see Mandigo et al., 2013; Spengler and Cohen, 2015), we oftentimes pause and wonder if Canada's perception of physical literacy (i.e. as it has been taken up within Canada's sport, recreation and education sectors) is the same physical literacy concept that Whitehead (2010) envisions. Is it aligned with Whitehead's intimated philosophical foundations (e.g. related to phenomenology, existentialism, embodiment and monism) and the IPLA's most recent definition?

We have concluded that despite the many positive changes that physical literacy has provided the sport, recreation and education sectors in Canada, we are still oftentimes off track with Whitehead (2010) and the IPLA's intentions. This is to say that although we do not oppose physical literacy's current and/ or potential influence within these sectors, we see that its uptake has been, at times, (over)simplified or misapplied. We are not alone in this opinion: some of our Canadian colleagues have taken on the challenge of critiquing local applications of physical literacy. The scholarly and often critical response is especially illuminating about specific shortcomings. Consider, for example, the following:

Lloyd and Smith (2006) suggested physical literacy's comparisons with language literacy perpetuate a dualist perspective; Jurbala (2015) suggested popular physical literacy assessment tasks 'lead to reductionist reverse engineering of the original concept' (p. 372); and McCaffery and Singleton (2013) suggested that physical education teachers' application of physical literacy can have injurious consequences upon students' sense of (in)competence. Herein, it is especially essential to acknowledge that none of these scholars are opposed to physical literacy. Rather, they too see dissonance between physical literacy's philosophical foundations and the consensus definition and its manifestations in contemporary practice. Critiquing our sectors' and institutions' applications of physical literacy should not be seen as an act of resistance against the concept. Rather, to us, it is an act of great concern and interest.

Clearly, there is more that physical literacy can offer these sectors and their institutions. It has been our observation that one of the greatest barriers to actualising 'true' physical literacy-informed sport, recreation or education has been what is perceived to be its seemingly abstruse and abstract philosophical foundations. We believe that it is because of these perceptions that many have seemingly adopted and/or introduced piecemeal and incomplete versions of physical literary, versions that sometimes address some of the most easily relatable parts of it. We believe that future efforts towards embracing physical literacy more fully within these sectors will require individuals and groups to take what may seem esoteric and make it more familiar. This will not be an easy task, though we believe it to be an essential one.

Acknowledgement

The authors of this chapter are grateful to the contributions made by Kim Nagan. She assisted the authors by doing background research, preliminary writing and editorial follow-up.

References

Balyi, I. (2001) Sport system building and long-term athlete development in British Columbia. *Coaches Report*, 8(1): 22–28.

Canadian Association for the Advancement of Women and Sport and Physical Activity (CAAWS) (2012) *Actively Engaging Women and Girls: Addressing the Psycho-Social Factors*. Available at: www.caaws.ca/ActivelyEngaging/documents/CAAWS_CS4L_Engaging_Women.pdf (accessed 12 March 2019).

Canadian Fitness and Lifestyle Research Institute (2009a) *2006–2007 Sport Monitor. Bulletin 8: Sport Participation in Canada*. Available at: www.cflri.ca/sites/default/files/node/365/files/CFLRISportMonitor-Bulletin8_English.pdf (accessed 12 March 2019).

Canadian Fitness and Lifestyle Research Institute (2009b) *Let's Get Active! Physical Activity in Canadian Communities: 2009 Physical Activity Monitor Facts and Figures. Bulletin 8: Sport Participation Rates of Canadian Adults*. Available at: www.cflri.ca/sites/default/files/node/128/files/PAM2009Bulletin8.pdf (accessed 12 March 2019).

Canadian Fitness and Lifestyle Research Institute (2013a) *Getting Kids Active: 2010–2011 Physical Activity Monitor Facts and Figures. Bulletin 6: Preferences for Types of Activities.* Available at: www.cflri.ca/sites/default/files/node/1194/files/CFLRI%20PAM%20 2010-2011_Bulletin%206%20EN.pdf (accessed 12 March 2019).

Canadian Fitness and Lifestyle Research Institute (2013b) *Getting Kids Active: 2010–2011 Physical Activity Monitor Facts and Figures. Bulletin 2: Nature of Children's Sport Participation.* Available at: www.cflri.ca/sites/default/files/node/1149/files/CFLRI%20PAM%20 2010-2011_Bulletin%202%20EN.pdf (accessed 12 March 2019).

Canadian Fitness and Lifestyle Research Institute (2013c) *Sport Participation in Canada: 2011–2012 Sport Monitor. Bulletin 8: Government Involvement in Sport.* Available at: www. cflri.ca/sites/default/files/node/1247/tables/CFLRI_Bulletin%208_2011-2012%20 Sport%20Monitor_EN.pdf (accessed 12 March 2019).

Canadian Fitness and Lifestyle Research Institute (2014) *Kids CAN PLAY! Encouraging Children to Be Active at Home, at School, and in Their Communities. Physical Activity Levels of Canadian Children and Youth.* Available at: www.cflri.ca/sites/default/files/node/1353/ files/Bulletin%201_CANPLAY%202011-2014_National.pdf (accessed 12 March 2019).

Canadian Fitness and Lifestyle Research Institute (2016a) *Municipal Opportunities for Physical Activity: 2015 Survey of Physical Activity Opportunities in Canadian Communities. Bulletin 7: Information for the Development of Physical Activity and Sport Programming.* Available at: www. cflri.ca/sites/default/files/node/1489/files/2015%20Municipalities%20Bulletin%207%20 Info%20for%20programming%20EN.pdf (accessed 12 March 2019).

Canadian Fitness and Lifestyle Research Institute (2016b) *Municipal Opportunities for Physical Activity: 2015 Survey of Physical Activity Opportunities in Canadian Communities. Bulletin 4: Provision of Informaiton on Physical Activity.* Available at: www.cflri.ca/sites/default/ files/node/1455/files/2015%20Municipalities%20Bulletin%204%20-%20Provision%20 of%20information%20EN.pdf (accessed 12 March 2019).

Canadian Fitness and Lifestyle Research Institute (2016c) *Encouraging Active Schools: 2015 Opportunities for Physical Activity at School Survey. Bulletin 1: School Policies Supporting Physical Activity and Sport.* Available at: www.cflri.ca/sites/default/files/node/1411/files/2015%20 Schools%20Bulletin%201%20-%20School%20policies.pdf (accessed 12 March 2019).

Canadian Fitness and Lifestyle Research Institute (2017) *Encouraging Active Schools: 2015 Opportunities for Physical Activity at School Survey. Bulletin 11: Barriers and Supports for Physical Activity within the School.* Available at: www.cflri.ca/sites/default/files/ node/1523/files/2015%20Schools%20Bulletin%2011%20Barriers%20and%20supports. pdf (accessed 12 March 2019).

Canadian Heritage (2002a) *Canadian Sport Policy 2002–2012.* Available at: http://sirc.ca/ sites/default/files/content/docs/pdf/2002-the_canadian_sport_policy.pdf (accessed 12 March 2019).

Canadian Heritage (2002b) *Canadian Sport Policy: Federal-Provincial/Territorial Priorities for Collaborative Action 2002–2005.* Available at: http://sirc.ca/sites/default/files/content/ docs/pdf/sp0092.pdf (accessed 12 March 2019).

Canadian Heritage (2007) *Canadian Sport Policy: Federal-Provincial/Territorial Priorities for Collaborative Action 2007–2012.* Available at: http://sirc.ca/sites/default/files/content/ docs/pdf/booklet-eng.pdf (accessed 12 March 2019).

Canadian Heritage (2010) *Interprovincial Sport and Recreation Council Evaluation of the Canadian Sport Policy: Final Report.* Available at: http://sirc.ca/sites/default/files/content/docs/ pdf/csp_evaluation_final_reporten.pdf (accessed 12 March 2019).

Canadian Heritage (2012) *Canada Sport Policy 2012.* Available at: http://sirc.ca/sites/ default/files/content/docs/pdf/csp2012_en.pdf (accessed 12 March 2019).

Canadian Heritage (2016) *Canadian Sport Policy 2012 Formative Evaluation and Thematic Review of Physical Literacy and LTAD: Final Report.* Available at: http://sirc.ca/sites/default/files/content/docs/CSP_documents/tsgi_pim_formeval_csp_themrev_final_report.pdf (accessed 12 March 2019).

Canadian Parks and Recreation Association and Canadian Sport for Life (2013) *Building Enhanced Collaboration between Recreation and Sport.* Available at: http://sportforlife.ca/portfolio-view/building-enhanced-collaboration-between-recreation-and-sport/ (accessed 12 March 2019).

Coaching Association of Canada (2017) *Aboriginal Coaching Modules.* Available at: www.coach.ca/aboriginal-coaching-modules-p158240 (accessed 12 March 2019).

Decorby, K., Halas, J., Dixon, S., Wintrup, L. and Janzen, H. (2005) Classroom teachers and the challenges of delivering quality physical education. *The Journal of Educational Research*, 98(4): 208–221.

Dowling, M. and Washington, M. (2017) Epistemic communities and knowledge-based professional networks in sport policy and governance: a case study of the Canadian Sport for Life leadership team. *Journal of Sport Management*, 31(2): 133–147.

Healthy Active Living and Obesity Research Group (2017) *Canadian Assessment of Physical Literacy: About.* Available at: www.capl-ecsfp.ca/about/ (accessed 12 March 2019).

Higgs, C. (2010) Physical literacy: two approaches, one concept. *Literacy*, 6(2): 127–138.

Higgs, C., Balyi, I., Way, R., Cardinal, C., Norris, S. and Bluechardt, M. (2008) *Developing Physical Literacy: A Guide for Parents of Children Ages 0 to 12.* Available at: http://sportforlife.ca/portfolio-view/developing-physical-literacy-a-guide-for-parents-of-children-ages-0-to-12/ (accessed 12 March 2019).

Higgs, C., Bluechardt, M., Balyi, I., Way, R., Jurbala, P. and Legg, D. (2011) *No Accidental Champions: Long-Term Athlete Development for Athletes with a Disability.* Available at: http://sportforlife.ca/wp-content/uploads/2016/06/NAC_ENGLISH_SCREEN_rev2013.pdf (accessed 12 March 2019).

Jurbala, P. (2015) What is physical literacy, really? *Quest*, 67(4): 367–383.

Kentel, J. and Dobson, T.M. (2007) Beyond myopic visions of education: revisiting movement literacy. *Physical Education and Sport Pedagogy*, 12(2): 145–162.

Lloyd, R.J. and Smith, S. (2006) Interactive flow in exercise pedagogy. *Quest*, 58(2): 222–241.

Lodewyk, K.R. and Mandigo, J.L. (2017) Early validation evidence of a Canadian practitioner-based assessment of physical literacy in physical education: Passport for Life. *Physical Educator*, 74(3): 441.

Longmuir, P.E. (2013) Understanding the physical literacy journey of children: the Canadian Assessment of Physical Literacy. *ICSSPE Bulletin*, 65: 277–283.

Lu, C. and De Lisio, A. (2017) Specifics for generalists: teaching elementary physical education. *International Electronic Journal of Elementary Education*, 1(3): 170–187.

Mandigo, J.L., Francis, N., Lodewyk, K. and Lopez, R. (2009) *Position Paper: Physical Literacy for Educators.* Ottawa: PHE Canada.

Mandigo, J.L., Harber, V., Higgs, C., Kriellaars, D. and Way, R. (2013) Physical literacy within the educational context in Canada. *ICSSPE Bulletin*, 65: 360–366.

McCaffery, M. and Singleton, E. (2013) Why are we doing this anyway? Physical literacy, monism, and perceived physical competence for Ontario's elementary students. *Physical & Health Education Journal*, 79(3): 6.

ParticipACTION, Sport for Life Society, Healthy Active Living and Obesity Research Group, Physical and Health Education Canada, Canadian Parks and Recreation Association, and Ontario Society of Physical Activity Promoters in Public Health (2015) *Canada's Physical Literacy Consensus Statement.* Available at: http://stage.participaction.com/sites/default/

files/downloads/Participaction-CanadianPhysicalLiteracy-Consensus_0.pdf (accessed 12 March 2019).

Physical and Health Education Canada (PHE Canada) (n.d.) *What Is the Relationship between Physical Education and Physical Literacy?* Available at: www.phecanada.ca/sites/default/files/Physical_Literacy_Brochure_2010.pdf (accessed 12 March 2019).

Robinson, D. (2018) Religion as an other(ed) identity within physical education: a scoping review of relevant literature and suggestions for practice and inquiry. *European Physical Education Review*, doi: 10.1177/1356336X17747860.

Robinson, D. and Randall, L. (2017) Marking physical literacy or missing the mark on physical literacy? A conceptual critique of Canada's physical literacy assessment instruments. *Measurement in Physical Education and Exercise Science*, 21(1): 40–55.

Robinson, D.B., Randall, L. and Sheehan, D. (2018) *Physical Literacy Scholarship within Canada: An Overview of Literature.* Available at: www.physical-literacy.org.uk/physical-literacy-scholarship-within-canada-an-overview-of-literature/ (accessed 12 March 2019).

Spengler, J.O. and Cohen, J. (2015) *Physical Literacy: A Global Environmental Scan.* Washington, DC: Aspen Institute Sports & Society Program.

Sport Canada (2011) *Summary Report, Canadian Sport Policy Renewal: Consultation with Official-Language Minority Communities.* Available at: http://sirc.ca/sites/default/files/content/docs/pdf/official-language.pdf (accessed 12 March 2019).

SportforLife Society (2016) *Aboriginal Long-Term Participant Development Pathway.* Available at: http://sportforlife.ca/portfolio-view/long-term-participant-development-pathway-1-1/ (accessed 12 March 2019).

Sport for Life Society and Aboriginal Sport Circle (2017) *Aboriginal Communities: Active for Life.* Available at: http://sportforlife.ca/wp-content/uploads/2017/06/Aboriginal-Communities-Active-For-Life-Web-Oct2017.pdf (accessed 12 March 2019).

Stanec, A.D. and Murray-Orr, A. (2011) Elementary generalists' perceptions of integrating physical literacy into their classrooms and collaborating with physical education specialists. *PHEnex Journal*, 3(1): 1–18.

Stoddart, A. and Humbert, L. (2017) Physical literacy is … ? What teachers really know. *PHEnex Journal*, 8(3): 1–18.

Truth and Reconciliation Commission of Canada (2015) *Truth and Reconciliation Commission of Canada: Calls to Action.* Available at: www.trc.ca/websites/trcinstitution/File/2015/Findings/Calls_to_Action_English2.pdf (accessed 12 March 2019).

Whitehead, M. (2010) Introduction. In M. Whitehead (ed.), *Physical Literacy throughout the Lifecourse.* New York: Routledge, pp. 3–9.

10

PERSPECTIVES ON PHYSICAL LITERACY IN CONTINENTAL EUROPE

Jeroen Koekoek, Niek Pot, Wytse Walinga and Ivo van Hilvoorde

Introduction

In this chapter we discuss physical literacy against the background of the history and ideologies that have shaped and founded the continental European context of physical education. We will address the question of why physical literacy can be considered a concept with strong European, continental roots (hereafter, generally referred to as Europe). We will argue that the philosophical and pedagogical foundation of physical literacy is strongly integrated within European thinking about education and physical education. We will further discuss the inherent tension between the ideological orientation and the factual situation in many European countries in which medical, biological and military orientations on physical activity have dominated.

Before going into detail about the integration of physical literacy in several European countries, we question the current worldwide popularity of the concept. Physical literacy provides a shared and integral framework for thinking about the cultural significance of movement behaviour, as opposed to the more instrumental and health-oriented perspectives on human movement. We will touch on this worldwide attraction against the background of a decreasing need to be physical active and also discuss some of the weaknesses of the concept, paradoxically due to its popularity and ease by which it is integrated, even within opposing frameworks. Furthermore, we will discuss the use of physical literacy in the sports and physical education context. The chapter will end with an overview of several European countries in which physical literacy has been more or less integrated.

European roots of physical literacy

Why do we need physical education? Why do we need to educate youngsters to be able to enjoy movement and sport? Why do we value physical literacy, and what does it mean to be physically literate? Many different answers can be found to these perennial questions. In order to understand the current attraction of physical literacy, we need to stress the origin of physical education as a typically nineteenth-century phenomenon, in the context of a renewed attention to the healthy body as a response to urbanisation, secularisation and industrialisation.

The nineteenth century provided a fertile scientific and medical soil in which a general interest in physical culture could be cultivated. Sedentary lifestyles stimulated a concern for 'physical compensation', which fostered discourses on degeneracy and prevention (van Hilvoorde, 2008: 1307). European institutes for physical education (PE) were dominated by pedagogical and medical thinking, and were often characterised by their resistance to sport and an overly strong focus on the body-object and competition. Physical education in many European countries is highly influenced by German (J.C. Gutsmuths, 1759–1839; F.L. Jahn, 1778–1852; A. Spiess, 1810–1858), Swedish (P.H. Ling, 1776–1839) and Austrian (K. Gaulhofer, 1885–1941; M. Streicher, 1891–1985) systems of physical education. The explicit use of gymnastics for the powers of military defence also played an important role in many European countries (van Hilvoorde, 2008).

During the 1920s and 1930s, a more 'relational paradigm' emerged that was adopted by a broad group of scientists and philosophers. This paradigm was highly influenced by 'personalist thinking' and shared a critical stance towards Cartesian notions of the human being. Important representatives of this movement were German thinkers such as Arnold Gehlen and Helmuth Plessner and the French philosopher Maurice Merleau-Ponty (1908–1961). Characteristic of these thinkers was their ability to bridge scientific gaps between biology, physiology, psychology and philosophy (Dekkers, 1995). They considered the human being as a unity and strongly opposed mechanistic explanations of human behaviour. The body should not be understood as a machine to be trained and disciplined. Instead, the body should be considered, following Merleau-Ponty, as 'active as a preconscious disposition of our personal existence' (Dekkers, 1995: 24). Entire generations of PE teachers were trained from the 1960s onwards not to use the notion of 'physical education' (because of its dualistic connotation), but rather to favour the more personalistic concept of 'movement education'. In several European countries, this paradigm aided in transforming physical education from a medically and physiological-oriented practice towards a more pedagogical-oriented, educational practice. In the words of one of the main advocates of this development in the Netherlands, bodies are not trained or educated, but pupils are instead being taught to move and play (van Hilvoorde et al., 2010). Objectives of PE were formulated in terms of the realisation of personal movement competencies and of the developments of the identity of the youngsters. This point will be further explained in the section about physical education.

Under the influence of strong neo-positivistic tendencies in the social sciences, the importance of the phenomenological approach lost ground in the 1960s and 1970s. Hermeneutical and phenomenological research in the field of sport and PE was marginalized, and empirical and experimental research became dominant. This 'scientisation of physical education' started to dominate the more pedagogical and phenomenological paradigm.

Interesting, but largely beyond the scope of this chapter, is the explanation for the current popularity of physical literacy. This widespread use of physical literacy does not stand alone, but can be explained in the context of a broader revival of 'personalistic' thinking and value-based and phenomenological approaches within educational science. This change of view arose from several partly opposing developments. Before elaborating more on the content and implications of European concepts of physical literacy, we mention three of these developments:

1. There is a growing resistance, both within education as well as science, to reduce educational systems to 'evidence-based education' or the measurement of outcomes (cf. Biesta, 2015). In relation to physical education, this means a critical position towards the reduction of the values and importance of physical education, just in terms of quantifiable outcomes, for example by measuring fundamental movement skills (Pot et al., 2017). Ironically, or some would say its weakness, is the fact that physical literacy is itself being adopted by propagators of a more reductional science. This situation has arisen because those adopting this view have little or no understanding of the philosophical underpinning of the concept (cf. Barnett et al., 2016).

2. The growing dominance of (digital) technology in our society plays a paradoxical role. On the one hand, it facilitates new kinds of measurements of the body, which nurtures ideologies such as the *quantified self* (e.g. Lupton, 2015). Many of these developments are in conflict with the foundations of physical literacy. However, these kinds of reductions of embodiment to the monitoring of specific parameters can engender support for physical literacy in instigating a renewed focus on meaningful and autonomous movement behaviour. When teachers experience that certain measurable outcomes do not reflect the value of their daily work, this could stimulate their wish to revitalise a discourse that is more in line with the educational and pedagogical reality of teaching. There is a clear need for a language that also deals with uncertain outcomes, without implicating that this uncertainty is a proxy for lack of quality. Physical literacy offers a broader vocabulary for framing the importance and values of physical activity and PE than more limited concepts, such as fitness or 'physical activity', do.

3. There is a growing European interest in 'personal learning', stimulated by the propagation of the so-called twenty-first-century skills (e.g. Voogt and Roblin, 2012). These skills, such as creativity, exploration, communication, discovery and problem-solving, better fit an accent on movement education in which the personal goals and self-regulating skills are of more importance than the fulfilment of standardised tests or fitness criteria. Physical literacy pays more attention to the enjoyment of movements and stresses the importance of creativity. The notion of a personal journey towards a 'sport identity' conflicts with a strong focus on general goals or generalised levels of FMS (see Chapter 17). Being physically literate should be considered inherent to human flourishing, instead of being a state of possessing a fixed set of (motor) skills. To be physically

literate is, however, more than just a process or personal journey. It can also be considered a value or goal in itself, to be(come) physically literate. The criteria for this mode of literacy are at the same time highly dependent on the context, living circumstances and motivation.

Physical literacy in sport

As physical literacy originated from a pedagogical and philosophical background, school and physical education is the most obvious context to see it being applied. For instance, in Malta, the Netherlands, Norway, the Czech Republic and Denmark, physical literacy is mainly used in the educational sector. However, the concept also attracts some attention from the world of sport. In most European countries, this can at least partly be explained by the popularity of the long-term athlete development (LTAD) model (Balyi, 2004). This model is used by many European sport federations as a guideline for talent development.

Within the LTAD model, the first three stages are often summarised as 'physical literacy'. However, when taking a closer look at these stages (Active Start, FUNdamentals and Learning to Train), it could be argued that these stages reflect an emphasis on movement skill acquisition. Often a 'building block' metaphor has been used in this respect (Abbott et al., 2002; Balyi, 2004; NOC*NSF, 2011). This means that it is conceived that teaching children certain (fundamental) movement skills (building blocks) will lead to more refined movement patterns later in life. Although this is a contested idea (Pot et al., 2017), this reinforces the interpretation of physical literacy as (the learning of) mere movement skills (Pot and van Hilvoorde, 2013), and leads to translation of physical literacy in terms of 'motor alphabet', 'movement ABCs' or 'physical grounding'.

For instance, in the Netherlands and Denmark, physical literacy is starting to be used as an overarching concept that stimulates intersectoral ways of working, such as common goal-setting of the sport, physical education and health sectors. On the other hand, the Norwegian sport sector is considered to be conservative in its views, and physical literacy is not expected to become a central topic. What can be concluded is that physical literacy is hitherto an educational concept in Europe, and other sectors, such as the sport sector, are only beginning to pick up on the term. Because of the relative novelty of the concept in these sectors, changes in policy and practice are not expected in the short term. The ways in which physical literacy are part of the educational context is described in the next paragraph. We will start with a description of how the concept relates to the educational practice in the Netherlands. After that, we will focus on the similarities and differences compared to other European countries regarding the implementation of the concept in practice.

Physical literacy in Dutch physical education

In the Netherlands, the backgrounds of physical literacy are most represented – but not equal to – the way the standards of physical education (PE) are structured.

In this paragraph, we will discuss practical implications of the conceptual approach in Dutch PE as an example of the European orientations towards physical education and the role of physical literacy. In 2017, the concept of physical literacy received considerable attention in physical education in the Netherlands (Steenbergen, 2017). In spite of the fact that physical literacy itself is not explicitly part of the Dutch standards, there seems to be a large resemblance in the philosophical groundings between physical literacy and the Dutch standards of PE (Mooij et al., 2004). As explained in the first part of this chapter, one physical education teacher education (PETE) faculty and a university of human movement sciences share a history of approaching human movement behaviour grounded in existential phenomenological philosophy. This had a major influence on the Dutch standards of physical education in several ways. This was most visible in the appellation transition from 'physical education' to 'human movement education', which was suggested by Gordijn (1961), as an attempt to delete rudimentary attitudes that were based on dualistic approaches. Of course, one could say that in the end, it is not how we name the approach, but how we act according to it. Nevertheless, the discussion initiated a new stimulus to consider a major shift in thinking about physical education in the Netherlands: education is not only about educating or training the physical part, but rather about the meaningful relations a human being encounters while moving. Human movement is about the interaction between the mover and the environment, and should be taught in ways that articulate and understand that significance. Learning to interact is present from birth (and even before). From that moment on, the direction of the development of the human depends on personal, physical, social and cultural constraints.

The curriculum implications

The pertinent shift in thinking about the undividable and embodied human being – which is fundamentally different from the more dualistic paradigm of 'training the physical' (cf. Tamboer, 1992) – influenced the forming of the Dutch curriculum to a practical and meaningful approach (ten Brinke et al., 2007). For example, in the Dutch standards, the aim is preparing a learner to be part of the (cultural) movement environment. This goal was further developed in four key concepts in which learners could be educated. Besides the responsibility towards *health* questions, movement education in the Netherlands primarily focuses on teaching children how to 'arrange movement activities, improve movement activities and value movement activities' (ten Brinke et al., 2007: 30). There seems to be a shared thought that PE is not only an instrumental way of building competencies through the acquisition of skills. A broader development is stressed by focusing on other types of goals, such as increasing skilled competence (and perceived competence), performance, health, enjoyment, and maintaining relationships (i.e. social contact) with the aim of a life-long commitment to be involved in movement activities (ten Brinke et al., 2007).

The first mentioned aspect of Dutch PE standards, *arranging movement activities*, points to the aim of teaching children the aspects of interpersonal constraints in movement activity. In line with social constructivism (Rovegno and Dolly, 2006), children are introduced to different forms of organised movement that necessitate collaboration with others (Koekoek and Knoppers, 2015). This collaboration is not an isolated goal that is reached through movement education, but rather an essential part of human movement activity. How children tune in to each other, arrange different settings of activities, get acquainted to different forms of organisations, and choose their positions and roles in different group dynamic phases is part of the teacher's focus and guidance in PE at school.

The second aspect of the Dutch standards, *improving movement activities*, is part of an ongoing discussion and needs some explanation. The key element is how movement skills are defined. Under influence of the current assessment culture (i.e. the tendency to value what we can measure instead of measuring what we value), there is an increased attention for measuring fundamental movement skills. Without denying the importance of a solid foundation for children, we hesitate to embrace this culture. Starting from a relational approach, it is of great importance to further discuss the interpretation of skilled behaviour and the effects of its assessment. From our perspective, the metaphor to learning language offers a sufficient analogy to discuss the two approaches towards education of movement activities (Jurbala, 2015; Pot et al., 2017). To avoid the simplification of the metaphor, Jurbala (2015) warns not to interpret the metaphor 'physical literacy' only in a parallel to learning to read and write, but rather to linguistic lingual communication. In other words, the question is whether we approach the learning process content as separate building blocks towards an uncertain future, or attempt to find meaningful relations that are tailored to the ability of the learner in which the meaning of the activity is prominently present. This suggestion is reminiscent of the Dutch discussion about assessing 'isolated' skills or more holistically following children's embodied interaction with the world. From our perspective, learning to move is comparable to learning to communicate. Thus, learning to move is not the same as the building of separate blocks that in the future will accumulate towards a successful participation in movement activities. Just like learning to communicate, a child is interacting with his or her environment from day one, and, in line with that, learning to move needs guidance from the start in order to become even more meaningful.

Teachers should always try to implement this meaning-making, instead of teaching the children meaningless tricks or isolated skills that perhaps lead to future (unknown) success. In addition, the ability of individuals to choose their preferred environment in which to be active and successful, tailored to their current abilities and interests, might be just as, and perhaps even more, important than the acquisition of a set of fundamental skills. The role of fundamental movement skills, and the increasing call for assessing these skills, is a much-debated topic in the Netherlands, and this debate resembles the discussion about physical literacy and fundamental movement skills (Pot et al., 2017). Given the fact that the concept of physical literacy, as introduced by Whitehead (2001), is a holistic approach to human movement that describes participation throughout life, it seems almost logical to presume that motor skills of humans in their earlier years are related to the activity levels throughout life. However, there is very little, and if any poor, evidence that motor skill abilities are related to being active for life. Research that has attempted to show the correlation between the two have encountered methodological difficulties (Giblin et al., 2014).

Knowing that there seems no necessary relationship begs the question regarding what kind of skills should be assessed in PE. Rather than narrowing this to isolated fundamental movement skills that are easy to assess, we aim for development in activities based on their core meaning. In the late 1980s, a categorisation of motor activities for PE was developed at the physical education teacher education (PETE) institutes, and is still in use in the Dutch national curriculum standards. Similar to a categorisation of game activities (e.g. teaching games for understanding's net and wall, target, invasion and tag games; see Bunker and Thorpe, 1986), a group of PE teachers at the PETE university tried to cluster activities on criteria of so-called *core problems*. A core problem represents the meaning of the activity that is independent of the different executional forms or levels. The *core problem* approach uses a description of activities that are globally described in a sense that the activity is stripped down to the essential meaning. The categorisation of activities was used to define learning tracks. A learning track is a group of activities that share the same core problem (e.g. balance activities, target games) structured in a sequence from introductory to complex. Children work in various age groups that match their development. For example, the core problem (aim) of volleyball is to place the playing object in the opponents' field while the opponents are trying to prevent this. Although this is done with specific techniques in the sport context, a (modified) game of volleyball with catch rules shares the same core challenge. Indeed, badminton and tennis share these characteristics, and therefore belong to the same cluster of activities.

Designing activities while retaining the core problem by stripping overly complex techniques and rules is key to providing learners a meaningful and rich learning environment (Koekoek et al., 2014). Stripping these sport-like activities to the core meaning also allows teachers to design similar games that retain the core meaning but are tailored to the abilities of the learner. If the activities a teacher offers throughout the years are built in complexity, the teachers will create designs of so-called 'learning tracks' (ten Brinke et al., 2007). Based on analysis of activities, the Dutch curriculum distinguishes categories such as jumping and balancing in gymnastics but also jumping, running and throwing in athletics. Different meaning is attributed to these activities. Jumping in athletics, for example, shares the core problem of *citius, altius, fortius* (i.e. faster, higher, stronger), but differs in those activities where height is problematised compared to those where distance is problematised. Jumping in gymnastics, on the other hand, shares the same core of using a surface to get airborne and postponing landing, which drastically changes the approach towards the learning of this type of jumping. This is a good example of how meaning-making matters to the behaviour. Ways of executing various movements in terms of prescribed 'techniques' are only addressed when they serve to solve the core problem of an activity. Structuring the categories in terms of complexity has resulted in the development of progressive practices and resulted in 12 learning tracks that are now used in Dutch PE in primary school. For example, the global learning track 'scoring games' (alongside tag games, aiming and rally games) is divided into three central themes: (1) keeper games; (2) possession games; and (3) small-sided modified invasion games. The keeper games share the same core problem of placing the playing object in the goal while the opponent is trying to prevent this. Various games that build in complexity are suggested for various age groups (such as penalty games). The possession games share the same core meaning of keeping possession of the ball while the opponent wants to take over the possession of the ball. Examples of activities are pass and intercept games, rondo, and end zone ball. The modified invasion games all share the same core meaning of passing the opponent in attempting to score while the opponent wants to prevent this, and vice versa. Modified (small-sided) invasion games are clustered in this theme.

Finally, the third aspect of Dutch movement education is focused on *the valuing of movement activities*. Through reflection, children are introduced to components of personal involvement in activities such as personal preferences, responsibility, fair play, authenticity or motivation (ten Brinke et al., 2007). The central theme in this part of physical education is about the experience of individual learners (e.g. by questioning the students about how they perceived the PE lessons). This approach leads to reflective questions regarding their perceived abilities but also their preferences. It can be questioned whether or not children should choose their own preferred activity that fits their needs. Therefore, it is necessary to explore the extent to which they are influenced by their peers. For example, are they able to choose with whom they want to play and learn in groups or teams? In addition, what culture of play would be appropriate in that PE setting (e.g. competition, recreation, show)? But also, do they have the ability to estimate the opportunities for active lifestyle in their personal environment? This third goal of Dutch PE also seems to be the least developed. Related to physical literacy, valuing movement activity might, however, be a crucial aspect of PE.

The situation of Dutch physical education as we have described in this section is used as an example of European orientations towards physical education and the role of physical literacy. In addition, the aforementioned existential phenomenological philosophy on PE and its implications for the curriculum can be considered as a starting point for developing future directions, and also for questioning the role of physical literacy in Europe. The Dutch PE context has shown that education should be meaningful and always related to personal developments and goals. Therefore, in the European practice, there might be some key issues to address. For example:

1. How do we protect a broad perspective of physical literacy and PE in a time where measuring details of human movement challenges the implications of a holistic approach?
2. Can we further develop the *valuing of movement activities* within the PE context?

European similarities and differences

The central purpose of this section is to provide insight into the current status of several European countries in respect of how they are developing the physical literacy concept. To gain this information, some scholars and policymakers who were seen as committed to physical literacy received a questionnaire. Most of these individuals are currently actively advocating physical literacy in their country. In order to obtain information about the development of physical literacy in their particular country, they were asked to respond to a series of questions.

Main findings of the physical literacy questionnaire

The questionnaire consisted of 19 questions and explored the status of physical literacy. Six responses were received from continental Europe: Malta, the Czech Republic, Denmark, Norway, Portugal and the Netherlands. In order to give an overview of the initiatives of each country on physical literacy, a few central elements were used to highlight their current status. The following elements contribute to the picture of physical literacy for each country, which will be discussed below: (1) the initial reason to develop the physical literacy concept; (2) the way each country disseminates physical literacy; (3) the sector(s) involved in this process; (4) the impact of physical literacy in several sectors; (5) the opportunities for spreading and developing the concept; (6) perceived barriers to promote physical literacy; and (7) the issues that need to be addressed for adoption of physical literacy.

The most important reason for interest in physical literacy in many countries in continental Europe is the search for a new concept that is related to sport and physical activity. In each country, different starting points were used, but they all considered physical literacy as an important and promising concept. The arguments for exploring physical literacy consisted of expanding the understanding of the definition of physical literacy (by not only focusing on competence or physical activity), linking physical literacy to other concepts (such as LTAD), or searching for the legitimisation of current initiatives (i.e. from a health and physical activity perspective).

In all countries, the universities are particularly responsible for disseminating the concept. In addition, there is a tendency to establish project groups (with both policymakers and scholars) or work to secure a degree of governmental influence (the Czech Republic). In Denmark, the National School Sport Association is closely involved in the dissemination of national physical education and sport objectives. Because the universities are particularly involved in disseminating the concept of physical literacy, several articles and chapters are published in national journals and books relevant to the context of physical education, physical activity and sport. Furthermore, seminars and symposia were organised (Malta, the Czech Republic, the Netherlands). A few countries developed courses (Malta, the Czech Republic) and presentations on a university level. In the Netherlands, the status of physical literacy has been explored in a national research project. The findings of this project have resulted in a document setting out a few scenarios to further develop the concept (Steenbergen, 2017).

This publication pays attention to physical literacy in relation to new trends, interdisciplinary collaboration, and new perspectives on sport and physical activity for all ages. One of the results is that a group of scholars from 10 different institutes developed a White Paper that aimed to identify how people can be stimulated for lifelong participation in physical activity and what physical literacy may contribute to this intention (Steenbergen et al., 2018).

Differences between countries were found regarding the impact of the physical literacy concept in several sectors. In the Czech Republic, the physical literacy concept has been discussed in several university discussion groups. More specifically, a few research studies have been conducted that thoroughly explored the value of the concept for the country (Vašíčková, 2016). Quantitative and qualitative studies were conducted in order to explore what physical literacy meant for the Czech environment. These studies focused on awareness among students and PE teachers, for example, by investigating students' motivations to be physically active, their knowledge about health and physical activity, and their attitudes towards PE lessons were mentioned as entry variables to physical literacy. In Malta, several lectures were given for early childhood educators. In Denmark (and in a similar way for Norway), physical literacy in school has been developed by researchers of a PETE university because the term physical literacy is closely related to the Danish understanding of PE and sport. Physical literacy in the Netherlands has been explored only in the educational sector (university level), although other sectors also showed their interest, as illustrated by the White Paper written and signed by 10 different institutes (Steenbergen et al., 2018). Furthermore, in one university in the Netherlands, several critical perspectives were discussed on the use of FMS within physical literacy concepts (Pot et al., 2017).

The researchers and policymakers from the countries who participated in the questionnaire also reflected on both the opportunities of physical literacy as potentially a valuable concept but also stressed the limitations of the concept. For example, Norway noted the potential of physical literacy in order to find alternatives for the physical activity discourse in their country. In Denmark, physical literacy contributed to the Danish school reform from 2014 that promotes physical activity of 45 minutes for all children on a daily basis. This example shows how physical literacy has an important influence on the school curriculum. In Malta also, a new curriculum has been implemented (2012) and new PE learning outcomes were determined (2015). Physical literacy in the Czech Republic and the Netherlands have not yet influenced the (PE) school curriculum. In these countries, (funded) projects and conferences dealing with physical literacy were organised in order to explore how the concept could be a valuable approach for schools and children. All countries faced similar barriers when addressing the concept. For example, because of the prevailing culture (e.g. different focus or other priorities), the introduction of new concepts was limited. In the Netherlands, physical literacy was seen as a theoretical approach, with relatively little attention given to the practical consequences. In Denmark, no specific barriers were found, but the term physical literacy was not so much perceived as an innovative concept. Norway reported a significant lack of understanding of the term literacy, specifically because of the lack of an appropriate Norwegian word that accurately represents its meaning. This is also a struggle in the Netherlands, on account of the somewhat dualistic connotations of the concept.

The countries formulated several issues that need to be addressed in order to adopt the physical literacy concept. The most important issue for all countries is the promotion of the concept to key stakeholders with the aim of understanding the nature of physical literacy. Furthermore, sedentary lifestyles and physical inactivity (e.g. Denmark, the Czech Republic, the Netherlands) were seen as decisive developments. In Norway, physical literacy is mainly used for the justification of PE and physical activity as meaning-making processes. The Czech Republic reported the tendency of significant dropout from compulsory PE as an important issue.

Conclusions

It is delicate to discuss a complex concept such as physical literacy in a generic way, based upon general continental European traditions of PE. It is no problem to stress the common philosophical ground of physical literacy within European, continental philosophy, in particular in the phenomenological and personalistic tradition. When looking in more detail, we do, however, see an enormous variety of understandings and practical translations of physical literacy in different European countries.

In this chapter, we have first used the situation in the Netherlands as a case to understand what the implementation of physical literacy could mean for sport or for the curriculum. The understanding and implementation of the concept in several European countries shows a wide variety of understanding and uses. This variety illustrates both the power and potential of physical literacy, as well as its pitfall. When there is no clear and common understanding, this could lead to diffusion, miscommunication, and use of the concept by sectors with interests other than those that the main stakeholders have in mind. A possible way to develop such common understanding is where people from key national organisations or institutes work together on the concept and establish close links with the International Physical Literacy Association (IPLA). In most of the European countries that responded to our questionnaire, the concept has been introduced and investigated by (sport and movement) universities that focused on sport and human movement, as well as faculties for physical education teacher education. It also appeared that the educational context in most countries is the leading context and often the starting point in which physical literacy has been developed. It is a misunderstanding that for developing the concept in a particular country, all national leading (governmental) institutes, sport organisations or universities should be directly involved. It is recommended to first bring together those institutes that have a decisive influence in the national educational policies and curriculum reformations. Obviously, in a second tranche, it would be valuable to invite other important stakeholders.

One of the main findings from our exploration among different European countries is that researchers and policymakers use physical literacy to legitimise their national initiatives for purposes that are not always doing justice to the content of the concept. For example, commonly, it is the prevailing culture to establish research projects that are based on general health problems (e.g. obesity, sedentary behaviours), and therefore the focus is often on a single pillar of the concept (i.e. competence, confidence or motivation). Assessing, monitoring and improving motor skill behaviour are often taken for granted without including important contextual influences (e.g. the social impact of school, sports club, neighbourhood, parents, etc.).

However, we also see an increasing tendency to shift this paradigm by describing physical literacy as a broad, more holistic perspective (e.g. in the Czech Republic and the Netherlands). Lifelong participation in sport and physical activity should not be used as a decisive reason for isolating the 'physical part' of our existence from other domains ('mental', 'social', 'environmental'). Broad interpretations of physical literacy can be useful for collaboration and provide an impulse for new research and policy with contributions from a variety of stakeholders.

Acknowledgement

We would like to thank all the colleagues from different continental European countries who helped us by completing the questionnaire. Their insights were a valuable contribution to this chapter.

References

Abbott, A., Collins, D., Martindale, R.J. and Sowerby, K. (2002) *Talent Identification and Development: An Academic Review*. Edinburgh, UK: Sport Scotland.

Balyi, I. (2004) *Long-Term Athlete Development: Trainability in Childhood and Adolescence. Windows of Opportunity, Optimal Trainability*. Victoria: National Coaching Institute British Columbia & Advanced Training and Performance.

Barnett, L., Stodden, D., Cohen, K.E., Smith, J.J., Lubans, D.R., Lenoir, M., ... Morgan, P.J. (2016) Fundamental movement skills: an important focus. *Journal of Teaching in Physical Education*, 35(3): 219–225.

Biesta, G.J.J. (2015) *Good Education in an Age of Measurement: Ethics, Politics, Democracy*. Boulder, CO: Paradigm.

Bunker, B. and Thorpe, R. (1986) The curriculum model. In R. Thorpe, D. Bunker and L. Almond (eds), *Rethinking Games Teaching*. Loughborough, UK: University of Technology, Department of Physical Education and Sports Science, pp. 7–10.

Dekkers, W.J. (1995) FJJ Buytendijk's concept of an anthropological physiology. *Theoretical Medicine*, 16(1): 15–39.

Giblin, S., Collins, D. and Button, C. (2014) Physical literacy: importance, assessment and future directions. *Sports Medicine*, 44(9): 1177–1184.

Gordijn, C.C.F. (1961) *Bewegingsonderwijs [Movement Education]*. Baarn: Bosch & Keuning.

Jurbala, P. (2015) What is physical literacy, really? *Quest*, 67(4): 367–383.

Koekoek, J. and Knoppers, A. (2015) The role of perceptions of friendships and peers in learning skills in physical education. *Physical Education and Sport Pedagogy*, 20(3): 231–249.

Koekoek, J., Dokman, I. and Walinga, W. (2014) *Sportspelen* [*Sportgames*]. The Hague: Boom Lemma.

Lupton, D. (2015) Data assemblages, sentient schools and digitised health and physical education (response to Gard). *Sport, Education and Society*, 20(1): 122–132.

Mooij, C., van Berkel, M. and Hazelebach, C. (2004) *Basisdocument bewegingsonderwijs. Leerlijnen, tussendoelen en methodisch didactische uitwerkingen* [*Basic Document for Physical Education: Learning Categories, Goals and Methodical and Didactic Descriptions*]. Zeist: Jan Luiting Fonds.

NOC*NSF (2011) *Meerjaren Opleidingsprogramma* [*Multiyear Educational Program*]. Available at: www.nocnsf.nl/cms/showpage.aspx?id=7642 (accessed 12 March 2019).

Pot, N. and van Hilvoorde, I. (2013) A critical consideration of the use of physical literacy in the Netherlands. *ICSSPE Bulletin*, 65: 313–320.

Pot, N., van Hilvoorde, I., Afonso, J., Koekoek, J. and Almond, L. (2017) Meaningful movement behaviour involves more than the learning of fundamental movement skills. *International Sports Studies*, 39(2): 5–20.

Rovegno, I. and Dolly, J.P. (2006) Constructivist perspectives on learning. In D. Kirk, D. Macdonald and M. O'Sullivan (eds), *The Handbook of Physical Education*. London: Sage, pp. 242–261.

Steenbergen, J. (2017) *Physical Literacy – verkenning naar het wat, wie en hoe* [*Physical Literacy: Explorative Study of the What, Who and How*]. Nijmegen: Kennispraktijk.

Steenbergen, J., Van Hilvoorde, I., De Vries, S., Mombarg, R., Barendse, P., De Martelaer, K., Savelsbergh, G., Van der Poel, H., Lucassen, J. and Brouwer, B. (2018) '*Physical Literacy*'; *bouwstenen voor een leven lang bewegen van jong tot oud* [*Physical Literacy: Building Blocks for Lifelong Participation from Early Years to Older Age*]. Ede: Kenniscentrum Sport.

Tamboer, J.W.I. (1992) Sport and motor actions. *Journal of the Philosophy of Sport*, 19(1): 31–45.

Ten Brinke, G., Brouwer, B., Houthoff, D., Massink, M., Mooij, C., van Mossel, G., Swinkels, E. and Zonnenberg, A. (2007) *Basisdocument bewegingsonderwijs voor de onderbouw in het voortgezet onderwijs* [*Basic Document for Physical Education in the First Two Years of Secondary School*]. Zeist: Jan Luiting Fonds.

van Hilvoorde, I. (2008) Fitness: the early (Dutch) roots of a modern industry. *The International Journal of the History of Sport*, 25(10): 1306–1325.

van Hilvoorde, I., Vorstenbosch, J. and Devisch, I. (2010) Philosophy of sport in Belgium and the Netherlands: history and characteristics. *Journal of the Philosophy of Sport*, 37(2): 225–236.

Vašíčková, J. (2016) *Physical Literacy in the Czech Republic*. Olomouc: Palacký University Olomouc.

Voogt, J. and Roblin, N.P. (2012) A comparative analysis of international frameworks for 21st century competences: implications for national curriculum policies. *Journal of Curriculum Studies*, 44(3): 299–321.

Whitehead, M. (2001) The concept of physical literacy. *European Journal of Physical Education*, 6(2), 127–138.

11

PHYSICAL LITERACY IN INDIA

Pankaj Markandey and Nigel Green

Introduction

In 2015, Shri Pullela Gopichand was coaching badminton to a 12-year-old girl at a summer camp (Shri is used in India before the name of a highly respected person). He threw a shuttle to her, which she failed to catch. He asked her to catch the shuttle again from a throw, but she could not do it even after a few more attempts. When leaving the court, the girl went over to Shri Gopichand and asked him, 'Can you teach me how to catch?' He was stunned by the question and considered why it was that a young girl who was developing her badminton expertise at an academy could not perform the simple skill of catching. Shri Gopichand reflected on his early childhood experiences and felt that his interactions with the natural environments allowed him to develop simple skills that he then nurtured through more specific sporting activities. He wondered whether children today were not getting adequate opportunities for playing in a range of varied environments, and therefore were not developing the skills and experience that are essential to future participation in physical activities. Shri Gopichand then talked to friends from within his coaching community and realised that young children were not developing the fundamental skills that the coaches believe are needed as a base for engagement in physical activity in later life.

In January 2016, Shri Gopichand met with two individuals who were exploring answers to similar questions on their own and trying to positively influence the sports ecosystem in the country – Pankaj Markandey and Amit Malik. They were concerned that the rising obesity and diabetes levels would have a significant impact on their nation, and believed that the population as a whole should be engaged in more physical activity as a form of prevention in relation to these problems. They also acknowledged that a country with a population of 1.3 billion should be more successful in international competition. By chance, they discussed these issues with Shri Gopichand, and all agreed that the 'philosophy of excellence' was a focus throughout the world in relation to sport. However, in order to attain excellence, there needs to be a high level of participation within a country and there is a need to go beyond medals. Unfortunately, for many, their experiences in sport were not positive and there was a high dropout rate, with many participants not continuing to engage in physical activity. The other issue they considered in relation to sport is the not uncommon incidence of exclusion, with many potential participants being excluded as they 'did not make the grade'. These issues were a concern to the group, and they all agreed that they should do something to improve the health, fitness, engagement and success of the Indian nation. They wanted to make a difference, and collectively they agreed to try to find solutions.

Becoming aware of physical literacy

Shri Gopichand, being a highly regarded coach having won the All England badminton singles title in 2001, was held in extremely high regard within the country. Following his victory in the All England Championship, he set up an academy in Hyderabad, which has since produced many successful badminton players. His links, from an international perspective, brought him into regular contact with a fellow Indian who was the Canadian national badminton coach. Discussing the problem of young children developing basic physical skills and the issues of long-term athlete development with the coach, Shri Gopichand was introduced to Canada Sport for Life (CS4L). CS4L is an organisation with significant experience in long-term athlete development. Following a discussion with CS4L, it was agreed that they would run a session for sports coaches in India to share their experience of developing young children as athletes. The state of Andhra Pradesh was an enthusiastic partner in this project. This Indian state has a population of around 53 million people and is based in the south of the country. The workshop was run by members of CS4L over seven days, and was perceived by the coaches to be successful. During the coaching session, Shri Gopichand became aware of the term 'physical literacy', as it was mentioned by the CS4L team. Shri Gopichand immediately found the concept interesting and wanted to learn more about physical literacy, so he created a team and tasked them to search the globe for more information about the concept.

Even prior to this workshop in January 2016, Shri Gopichand had a video conference in January 2016 with Margaret Whitehead, the president of the International Physical Literacy Association (IPLA), which was facilitated by his colleagues. The short 30-minute conversation with the president led to his self-exploration and connection with physical literacy. The team, working under the Gopichand Foundation umbrella, was committed to taking up this cause in India, and consisted of committed individuals from a variety of professional backgrounds. The team located links to physical literacy in Australia, Canada and New Zealand, and eventually found the IPLA, which is based in the UK. Initial discussions with the president of the IPLA made the team realise that the concept of physical literacy could be the focus they were looking for. The more they researched the concept, the more they wanted to know, and by talking to the president of the IPLA they were provided with a much more profound introduction to the concept – so much so that the group decided that it not only linked to their country's philosophy, but it was a concept that should underpin their work.

Indian culture

Indian culture has a rich history in art, music and physical activities, which have allowed the population to engage in pursuits of self-exploration. Yoga originated in ancient India thousands of years ago. The word 'yoga' derives from the Sanskrit (ancient Indian language) word 'yug', meaning to yoke or unite. Though many people think of yoga as physical practices that foster physical health, the deeper purpose of yoga practice is spiritual, intended to help unite the individual soul with universal consciousness. The holistic developmental nature of yoga was seen by the Gopichand Foundation team to provide clarity in relation to physical literacy and its monist/holistic philosophy. The focus of self-exploration through physical pursuits, experienced holistically, as opposed to being framed by the dualist philosophical approach of the Western world, where in some circumstances the mind and body are seen as separate entities, resonated with the group as being aligned to Indian culture. The philosophies of highly regarded Indian academics such as Shri Aurobindo, Shri Swami Vivekananda and Shri Rabindranath Tagore concur with the importance of an emphasis on self-exploration through physical pursuits (see notes at the end of the chapter). Many similar terms such as physical culture have been used in Indian literature, where the concept of spirituality is internalised by the Indian society. The many gurus in India guide individuals on a path of mind, body and soul evolution, acknowledging that this is a holistic experience. This approach resonates with the monist nature of physical literacy.

Sport

From a sporting point of view, the team believed that they had tended to look only at the outcomes, and not the process involved in sport. Helping everyone reach their potential was only significant in relation to successful performance in competition. Although self-excellence is a key focus in the sports ecosystem, the contrast to physical literacy is distinct. Sport often tends to have extrinsic motivation and a focus on self-excellence, whereas physical literacy has a focus of encouraging each individual towards self-development and intrinsic motivation, where the engagement in physical activity is valued in itself rather than for the success in competition. In this context, the team in India found a synergy between the roots of the concept of physical literacy and Indian culture.

The Indian nation is going through a transition period where there is an aspiration for an increased appreciation and recognition of its own culture, beliefs and practices. The modern-day influences of technology are having an impact from both a positive and negative point of view. Technology has the potential to enhance the quality of life, but there is also a concern that with the advent of newer aspirations and technology, the population is losing out on their physical literacy development. The team felt that children in particular are either spending a great deal of time studying or interacting with IT toys such as computers, tablets, television and mobile phones. In addition, many adults are not engaging in physical activity, and if this epidemic is not corrected now, it has the potential to create a generation who will suffer from the side effects of physical illiteracy (see explanatory glossary). It was perceived that this would be very costly for the nation, as it would have a significant impact on the country's resources, with rising healthcare cost, loss of productivity, and severe risk to the holistic health and well-being of the nation.

Physical education

Through increasing their understanding of physical literacy as a concept, the team came to appreciate how the key ingredients of physical literacy aligned closely with the local beliefs, arts and dance forms. However, away from physical education and sports, the Indian education system as a whole was also going through a transformation stage. Concepts such as experiential learning, inclusive education and engagement-driven learning were being introduced into schools. The holistic development of an individual was at the heart of these developments, and therefore the team felt that it would be totally appropriate for physical literacy, as a philosophy, to be the guiding light in the transformation in the whole education system.

Examples of this development can be found in the Heritage Xperiential Learning School in Gurgaon (see http://heritagexperiential.org/), where the learning community now allows each child to be free to grow towards the realisation of his or her highest human potential through a harmonious integration of spirit, heart, mind and body. The Indian National Curriculum Framework (2005) was also a step in the right direction, with a focus on making learning a joyful experience. The goal was to provide an education system that focused on a child-centred approach, irrespective of caste, creed, religion and gender. This inclusive focus on each individual's progressive journey has significant links with the physical literacy concept.

With a desire to make something happen, the Gopichand Foundation team were keen to start to plan a large-scale development within the state of Andhra Pradesh. By attracting funding from the government, the team looked at potential future possibilities. They believed that physical literacy could be the focus they were looking for, and as such they wanted this concept to be central to their plans. They realised that in order to improve an individual's engagement in physical activity, they needed to ensure that experiences from a young age were positive and varied. The team felt that schools could play a significant role here, so their initial target was schoolteachers. However, they were also aware of the need, as with any initiative, for research. To realise this goal, the foundation of a university of physical literacy became an aim in their long-term plans. This institution could combine the training of teachers with research into the concept.

Preparing teachers

As in many countries in the world, training for general primary-level teachers in physical education is very limited, and this is certainly the case in India. Provision of facilities is also an issue, but the team felt they had to start somewhere, and training teachers would provide a stimulus. With 62,000 schools in Andhra Pradesh, initial thoughts were of using a cascade method to share an understanding of physical literacy, and so an initial event for teachers was planned. This was in their holiday time, but with payment. This event was held at the Acharya Nagarjuna University, Vijayawada, Andhra Pradesh. As the team already had links with CS4L, the aims of which were to create cross-sectoral partnerships between sport, education, recreation and health, while aligning community, provincial, and national sport and physical activity programming, they decided to invite them to run a teachers' workshop. As planning for this event went ahead, so further discussions with the IPLA were taking place and the Gopichand Foundation team were becoming more aware of the philosophical depth and complexity of physical literacy. They agreed that they needed to deepen their understanding of the concept if it was to be a focus for their initiative, and as a result the team invited two members of the IPLA from Liverpool John Moores University in the UK to work with them during the teacher training event. Dialogue with the IPLA members stimulated further discussion concerning the creation of a university for physical literacy, a programme of action research, doctoral research programmes, and training for teachers on a larger scale. All were agreed as valuable and possible future developments. Six hundred teachers attended the nine-day workshop in Acharya Nagarjuna University, run by nine coaches from CS4L. The task was enormous, with language issues and very large classes. However, the workshop was well received by the teachers.

Working to establish support to develop physical literacy

Discussions with the IPLA during the workshop revealed the depth and significance of physical literacy as a concept, and the Gopichand Foundation Team were keen to share this with government representatives. At incredibly short notice, opportunities for the IPLA team to share the concept of physical literacy with education government ministers were provided and well received. This gave the Gopichand Foundation team the confidence to meet with the Chief Minister of Andhra Pradesh, where suggestions to use physical literacy to promote physical activity in the state were well received and acknowledged as a potential mission for the government in the future. Physical literacy was being considered as a focus for the government to increase participation of its population in physical activity, to improve the holistic health of the state, and in the long term potentially to produce athletes of international status.

The Gopichand Foundation team had been talking to different states who were ready to embrace the concept of physical literacy. The team believed that the physical literacy concept was closely allied to a range of national government initiatives. Shri Gopichand's support allowed the team to gain access to a significant number of state chief ministers, sports ministers and other bureaucrats. All these individuals acknowledged and appreciated the concept once it had been explained to them by the team. Shri Gopichand even had a unique opportunity to present physical literacy to the honourable Prime Minister of India, who acknowledged the importance of the concept.

The team also organised a workshop, promoted by the Directorate of Education from Delhi, entitled 'Physical Literacy and Sports for All Delhi Citizens'. The Chief Minister of Delhi and celebrated Olympians were in attendance, along with 200 coaches/teachers/sports administrators. This workshop allowed the concept of physical literacy to be shared with the coaches and dignitaries. Once again, it was considered to be a very successful event, with the delegates recognising the potential for physical literacy to become a key focus for the government in promoting physical activity in schools and local communities.

Promoting physical literacy

The Gopichand Foundation team continued to focus their energy on promoting physical literacy across the country. The route chosen by the team focused on working with physical education teachers and coaches initially, through training courses, and then via creating a wider structure that would also facilitate impact in the community.

The team continue to advocate the concept at all levels, including central and state government, and Shri Gopichand has consistently promoted physical literacy in all of his many public engagements. Interest in the concept has progressed slowly, with more positive action being forthcoming in some states, such as Andhra Pradesh and Gujarat. Talks with the Andhra Pradesh government led to Andhra Pradesh introducing one hour of physical literacy a day in all schools from June 2016. This was to be provided by all schools and would take place at the end of the day. A lack of specific resources to support the teachers and limited opportunities to share this concept with such a diverse population has meant that the impact of this initiative has been limited. However, further work by the team has resulted in developments within the government of Andhra Pradesh. The Commissioner of the School of Education for Andhra Pradesh produced guidelines for the state. Within the document G.O.M.S. 35 (2017), they set out their plan to implement a physical literacy policy framework, with the intention to introduce physical literacy into all schools for the academic year 2017–2018. One of the key goals of the policy was to shift the focus of physical literacy from being an extracurricular activity to a curricular activity. This document suggested the aspects of physical literacy were a range of activities and concerns, including:

1. body awareness and yoga;
2. movement skills;
3. rhythmic movements/group activities;
4. fun, creativity, leisure and recreation;
5. multi-environment exposure;
6. organised sports;
7. regional sports; and
8. expressions/performance arts.

The proposals included recommendations for the inclusion of continuous professional development and training for PE teachers and class teachers. This would include the design of an appropriate infrastructure for physical activity in schools, assessment of students, use of technology, effective monitoring and community engagement. In addition, setting up a resource institute of physical literacy (RIPL) would allow certain schools to become centres of excellence, which would then cascade materials and support developments in local schools. It was agreed that there would be a time allocation of at least six one-hour periods a week of physical literacy and yoga in every school that was designated as a centre of excellence. Also of significance was point III.12 in G.O.M.S. 35 (2017), which suggested that the school of education would allocate 5% of their budget for this initiative. These points clearly indicate a determination to introduce physical literacy as a key element in school life, which is fully supported by the government.

As part of the implementation plan, the school of education stated their intention to reach out to teachers, parents and other stakeholders from an advocacy point of view, and to provide an infrastructure that supported teachers with lesson plans and assessment tools. There appeared to be a clear recognition of the need to inform and educate the community of the concept of physical literacy and the benefits of it being a focus in both schools and the community. The commitment related to a five-year time frame and a phased development of facilities, infrastructure, equipment and training. This clearly demonstrated an obligation to enhancing the quality of physical education experiences and community opportunities. The RIPL structure was planned to enable a cascading of knowledge, resources and experience that would further support this initiative. Initiatives to attract sponsorship/funding from local donors would also aid the advancement of provision.

Physical literacy in the community

The importance of engaging communities has not been lost in this initiative, and the promotion of village-level activities that are inclusive was seen as key to the success of this project. Physical literacy champions within each community were tasked to further support and promote the importance of culturally relevant activities for all of the community. Significantly, there is also an intention to liaise with the medical, health and sports departments to increase the depth and breadth of the impact of this initiative. As yet, there has been no formal indication of the success of this implementation plan. However, there have been other developments that supported the notion of a state looking to develop the physical literacy of its population.

While the team were advocating physical literacy at national and state levels, their efforts had mainly been related to the education system. They realised the lifelong notion of the concept was also important, and therefore decided to attempt a community activation project at a city level. Shri Gopichand connected with and motivated more passionate enthusiastic people. Together, these people formed a team that worked on initiating 'physical literacy days' designed to celebrate participation in physical activity. Every Sunday, in Hyderabad initially (but similar programmes have since been established elsewhere, such as Delhi, Gurgaon and Vijayawada), a 'physical literacy day' was organised. The blueprint for these days was shared with all local administrators as a means of ensuring support for the initiative. The plan included the closure of one road, of around 200 metres in length and 20 metres in width, so that varied physical literacy days could be engaged in by the local population on a Sunday. Initially, a trial run was undertaken with a small set of 100 people from all age groups. In that trial run, various awareness campaigns related to physical literacy were provided for the participants and related to a range of varied activities (records of these events can be seen at www.facebook.com/pldays/).

The response to this initiative was exceptional. From all age groups, the first week saw more than 1,000 attendees. Week on week, different forms of dance, art, culture and physical activities were showcased and enjoyed by the local community. Participants from schools, colleges, local non-governmental organisations, hospitals and other parts of the community attended, and this allowed a wide range of the population to enjoy the events and the opportunity for physical activity that was provided. There were many requests to conduct similar events at other places, but limitations with regard to planning teams meant that this was too much of a challenge at this early stage. Programmes were designed in such a way that all age groups and genders could participate and enjoy the activities. This concept of community activation made the team believe that physical literacy community activation would really complement physical literacy within schools, and this could lay the foundation for a more physically literate nation.

The physical literacy initiative continues to benefit greatly from the involvement of Shri Gopichand. He is involved at the highest level with regard to Olympic and Commonwealth competition, and is in demand to speak at prominent events. He always manages to mention physical literacy and is a very influential supporter of the concept. The advocacy of the 'physical literacy' concept is very close to his heart. He passionately talks about the prominence of alphabet literacy and numeric literacy, and goes on to suggest that physical literacy should be equally important. As a nation, Shri Gopichand perceives that individuals do not engage in physical activity as much as they did in the past. He sees an increased need to see physical literacy as an integral part of education and throughout the lifecourse of an individual. This is required not only to broaden the base of the number of people playing sport, but also to foster the happiness and well-being of the society at large.

Status of physical education teachers, training and resources

Of significance in India, and related to the initiative, was the realisation that the status of PE teachers was an issue in moving physical literacy forward in education. PE teachers have quite a low status in India due to more importance being attached to the core education subjects such as maths and science. A very low ratio of PE teachers to students, given large class sizes, linked to varied availability of facilities, impacted on the quality of what could be achieved within PE lessons. Climatic conditions also impact significantly, with the diverse weather – from very hot to very cold, or very rainy to very windy. While similar weather conditions may be experienced in other countries, the lack of indoor facilities can limit impact.

One of the smaller interventions that the Gopichand Foundation team suggested was to motivate the PE teachers by changing the name of PE teachers to physical literacy teachers, as this could raise the status of teachers and of physical activity, while emphasising the focus on holistic development. Education departments are recognising the need for active and thriving PE (physical literacy) teachers in schools, and are becoming more accepting of the importance of physical literacy as a key focus.

It has been acknowledged by the Gopichand Foundation team that there is a need to impact on the training of teachers at teacher training colleges. Many colleges are unaware of the concept, and traditionally the teaching of physical education has been very didactic. However, the team are keen to have an impact here by developing programmes that look more widely at pedagogy that can be adopted by teacher training colleges to support the PE teachers of the future. This idea is still in the early stages, but projects have been undertaken where a full day of training teachers has been provided. However, since the college education system is governed by a separate ministry in the country, this development may take time to implement.

Discussions more recently have been in relation to the provision of resources to support teachers that link to their training needs. While the philosophy is holistic and readily accepted, it is the contextual implementation that needs solutions. Individuals need to understand how they can operationalise physical literacy in their schools and communities, and what resources can support them in this quest. The scale of work is considerable, with around 70,000 schools in the state of Andhra Pradesh and similar numbers in other states. Many schools only have one teacher and very limited facilities. Generally, private schools have better facilities than state schools, and these private schools also have more funding for teacher training and the development of resources. The team recognise the need to develop materials that can educate the nation in relation to the concept and also train the teachers and coaches so that they can provide opportunities for people to develop their physical literacy.

Traditional cultural games

The acknowledgement that traditional cultural games should be a significant part of any development was seen as critical, as it is important to promote heritage activities and establish a link to the many sports played in India. In more recent times, traditional sports have had a resurgence in India. One example has been the success of kabaddi, where a league has developed a significant following, even though kabaddi is not an Olympic sport. Local mass participation has allowed this cultural activity to thrive and provide opportunities for many people to engage in physical activity.

The way forward

'The more we know, we realise that there is more we do not know' is a phrase used by the Gopichand Foundation team to explain where they were at the start and where they are now. India does not have one key agency driving the physical literacy knowledge and research dissemination in India. However, what it does have is a team who are committed to 'physical literacy and sports excellence', led by Shri Gopichand. This team is advocating that physical literacy, in its purest form, should influence the policymakers so that opportunities are created for all individuals to be motivated to engage in physical activity for life. There are many teachers and coaches working in their own micro-environment who are ready and able to foster physical literacy among children. However, a significant mindset shift is required in India if it is to embrace the physical literacy philosophy among various sectors and stakeholders. There is a strong need to:

- include native content;
- present and promote native knowledge;
- influence education structures;
- influence policymakers and practitioners to embrace physical literacy as a concept;
- increase awareness levels across the general population about the concept; and
- provide the necessary tools and resources for practitioners that can help them provide opportunities for others to engage in physical activity in appropriate environments.

The team have taken a path towards physical literacy, with a clear remit to thread the concept through all aspects of life in India, but more specifically through education and sport. While they work on developing opportunities and implement activities, they learn, improve, revise and modify as the need arises. However, the passion for driving the physical literacy concept through all aspects of life in India and the significant progress that has been made in only a few years are remarkable, given the size of the country. Achievements have been made through education and political integration, and physical literacy is starting to make an impact in and on the nation.

Notes on Indian philosophers named in the text

Aurobindo, Shri Aurobindo was an Indian philosopher, yogi, guru, poet and nationalist (https://en.wikipedia.org/wiki/Sri_Aurobindo).

Tagore, R. Shri Rabindranath Tagore, sobriquet Gurudev, was a Bengali polymath from the Indian subcontinent, a poet, musician and artist (https://en.wikipedia.org/wiki/Rabindranath_Tagore).

Vivekananda, S. Shri Swami Vivekananda was an Indian Hindu monk, a chief disciple of the nineteenth-century Indian mystic Ramakrishna (https://en.wikipedia.org/wiki/Swami_Vivekananda).

References

G.O.M.S. 35 (2017) *Andhra Pradesh Government Order for Implementation of Physical Literacy.* Available at: www.schools360.in/implementation-physical-literacy-andhra-pradesh-schools-2017-18-guidelines-go-ms-35/

Indian National Curriculum Framework (2005) *National Council of Research and Training in India.* Available at: https://en.wikipedia.org/wiki/National_Curriculum_Framework_(NCF2005) (accessed 13 March 2019).

12

AOTEAROA/NEW ZEALAND'S PHYSICAL LITERACY JOURNEY

Karen Laurie

Introduction

The 'physical literacy journey' of Aotearoa/New Zealand is still in its formative and foundation years; however, the path has been set and our trip is well under way! Like an individual's physical literacy journey, the pathway has not necessarily been a linear one. Along the way, there have been highs and lows, successes, challenges and learning, and this will continue as we work towards embedding the understanding, principles and practices associated with the concept, and ensure its relevance and meaning to the people of Aotearoa/New Zealand.

Where have we come from?

The initial awareness concerning the terminology of 'physical literacy' came through several channels and was met with mixed reactions. Sport New Zealand (Sport NZ), as the crown agency responsible for oversight and leadership of the sport and recreation sector in New Zealand, was in the process of developing a new 'community sport' strategy through 2013 to 2014. The establishment and implementation of this strategy has been the key driver of physical literacy's profile within New Zealand. That strategy is to enrich and inspire New Zealanders through participating in community sport, achieving this by ensuring quality experiences that grow people's confidence, competence and motivation for a lifelong love of physical activity. The focus of the strategy is young people aged 5–18.

Sport NZ is a crown agent established under the Sport and Recreation New Zealand Act 2002 (New Zealand Government, 2002) to 'promote, encourage and support physical recreation and sport in New Zealand'. Its functions broadly cover investment, promotion of participation, support for capability development in the sport and recreation sector, and the provision of policy advice. Sport NZ is part of the Sport NZ Group, which is made up of High Performance Sport New Zealand (HPSNZ), a wholly owned subsidiary that delivers Sport NZ's high-performance outcomes, and Sport NZ, which is responsible for community sport. Together, the teams form the Sport NZ Group, whose role is to lead, enable and invest in delivering a world-leading system whose purpose is to 'enrich lives and inspire a nation through sport and active recreation' (Sport NZ, 2015a). 'Community sport' within New Zealand has a wide definition, and includes play, active and outdoor recreation, and competitive sport taking place through clubs, schools and events at a local, regional and national level. It aligns to a broad physically active concept, and does not include passive recreation such as gardening. It also does not include elite and international competition, which is the focus area of HPSNZ.

The backdrop for the creation of this community sport strategy was a realisation that 'things are changing' and we needed to act. New Zealand historically has been a country with high rates of physical activity participation by both young people and adults, and an enviable record of winning on the world stage. An active playful childhood was viewed as the norm, with sport and recreation being an integral part of the Kiwi lifestyle. Our environment, Maori cultural history, and pioneering spirit have all played a significant role in developing our 'Kiwi psyche', reflected in the idea that 'sport is in our DNA'. This wonderful active heritage in essence reflected a population where the customary lifestyle naturally developed and progressed an individual's physical literacy without specifically naming it as such. While this was certainly viewed as something to celebrate, there was also a recognition that it was, and still is, under threat from societal changes, the changing face of New Zealand, and global trends towards inactivity.

Research

Research and work delving more thoroughly into understanding New Zealanders' participation in sport and physical activity were undertaken by Sport NZ, with a focus on identifying issues and elements – both negative and positive – that were systematic drivers impacting on the quality and quantity of sport and physical activity, particularly for young people. Sport NZ had, and continues to have, a specific focus in understanding the world of young people, as we strongly believe that the early sporting and physical activity experiences of children and young people are crucial in their future lifelong involvement in being active.

In 2011, Sport NZ undertook the most significant piece of research into young New Zealanders' participation in sport and recreation in more than 10 years. The New Zealand 2011 Young People's Survey (Sport NZ, 2012) was a school-based survey of over 17,000 young New Zealanders (5–18 years old). The scale of the survey allowed exploration into how sport and recreation fit into the lives of young people of different ages and backgrounds. It provided a voice for young people to talk about physical activity in their lives. Overall, while results were fairly positive and New Zealand had relatively good participation rates, there were also indications from this survey, and others, of issues that, if not addressed, would undermine young people's participation in physical activity, sport and recreation.

Other influential information was gathered from a project called the School Sport Futures Project (SSFP), which Sport NZ established in 2014 to better understand issues and long-standing concerns about the quality and quantity of physical activity, physical education (PE) and sport available to young people in New Zealand within the school setting. The project aimed to develop a series of solutions to the challenges identified within the school setting. This was not a top-down approach, but one that was built from the ground up. Sport NZ took an iterative, collaborative approach (i.e. all analysis and documentation was undertaken with stakeholders who critically analysed the issues, workshopped and commented on each other's views).

In undertaking this review process, we asked many questions and talked to people who work in various fields. We heard about a range of experiences, from Māori, Pasifika, Asian, European New Zealanders, immigrants, people with disabilities, different socio-economic groups, people in remote areas, and people in built-up urban environments.

We identified that we were essentially at a 'tipping point'. Simply trusting that our sporting and outdoor culture would continue through into future generations was perhaps naïve and unlikely to address the changes, trends, opportunities and challenges we would face now and into the future. We needed a 'reality check' that the way people want to be active and engage in sport was changing. Inaction on issues that seemed in the 'too hard basket' could undermine the strengths we had built over past decades, and there was a strong awareness we needed to do something concrete to address the very real perception that if we did not act now, our sporting culture, and all the benefits it provides to New Zealand and New Zealanders, could be lost. Once gone, it is just about impossible to get back.

The international context

Internationally, other nations were, and still are, struggling with a tidal wave of physical inactivity and increasing sedentary behaviour. This is a global problem, and one from which we recognised we were not immune. With this understanding, Sport NZ continued to actively investigate practices and trends both nationally and internationally.

The concepts and growing international momentum associated with the concept of physical literacy as it was being expressed through the work of the International Physical Literacy Association (IPLA), as 'a disposition to capitalize on the human embodied capability, wherein the individual has the motivation, confidence, physical competence, knowledge and understanding to value and take responsibility for engagement in physical activities for life' (Whitehead, 2010: 11), aligned and resonated with what we were aiming to achieve around enriching and inspiring New Zealanders though sport and physical activity.

Key elements such as the following were not new ideas in New Zealand:

- understanding the interplay of the human domains in sporting participation;
- viewing 'sport' in its broadest sense; and
- encouraging lifelong participation because of the wider holistic value it plays in people's lives.

Our previous New Zealand Community Sport Strategy and Young People's Plan (2010–2015) already encouraged a broader holistic view of sport, and identified the many benefits of sport participation, including improving social connectedness, educational value, health and well-being, and personal and social development.

Promotion of adopting a holistic approach to understanding and delivering sport and physical activity experiences had long been a component and feature of our system, policies and programmes (programmes such as Active Movement, Active Schools and He Oranga Poutama, to name a few). There was a sense that aligning with an international consensus and taking firm overt action to shine a brighter light on these messages could be achieved by focusing on and expressly using the concept and terminology of physical literacy.

There was a view that the opportunity to both learn and contribute within a larger worldwide united community could certainly strengthen and develop our capability to deliver on our aims, messages and ideas.

The New Zealand context

These messages and ideas had developed in response to New Zealand culture, with its strong bicultural roots, which has long promoted a monist perspective in the understanding of our people.

Maori health expert and research professor Mason Durie developed the Te Whare Tapa Whā model (Durie, 1994) that is utilised across a variety of sectors (health, education and justice). Te Whare Tapa Whā encapsulates a Maori view of health and wellness, and has four dimensions: *taha wairua* (spiritual health), *taha hinengaro* (mental health), *taha tinana* (physical health) and *taha whānau* (family health). Different parts of a *wharenui* (meeting house) represent each of these dimensions.

Similarly, this model and the concept of well-being, or *Hauora* (Ministry of Education, 2014), underpins our national health and physical education (HPE) curriculum, and encourages a holistic approach in this learning area, where the focus is on the well-being of the students themselves, of other people, and of society through learning in health-related and movement contexts. We asked ourselves, 'Could the promotion of a similar model that specifically targeted fostering lifelong meaningful engagement in physical activity, and considered how physical activity contributed to holistic well-being, provide a platform from a community sport perspective to enable us to explore ways of working that would help to draw links and clarify roles and responsibilities?'

A strategic step forward

This culmination of five years of learning, new evidence and scanning good practice at home and abroad led to the development of our current Community Sport Strategy (2015–2020) (Sport NZ, 2015a), which stressed the need for a system that was 'participant-focused', and identified three interrelated approaches that would work together to deliver this. These approaches were based on the concepts of physical literacy, locally led development, and use of evidence-based data and insights. This reflected the awareness of a need for a stronger information base for investment and planning, more cross-government engagement and collaboration, and a strong focus on a system-led, participant-centred approach that acknowledges the need to understand and get closer to the participant. The strategy looks to preserve and build off existing strengths, and, where necessary, develop alternative options to ensure the needs of all New Zealanders are recognised and met. The strategy was designed to invite innovation and ongoing learning practices, thus challenging conventional thinking on the delivery of sport and active recreation, focusing on what participants want rather than simply following traditional provision.

This reflected a change in focus from 'development for sport' to 'development through sport'. While both relate to encouraging sport participation, development for sport generally focuses on progression-oriented actions and outcomes to grow the sport itself, and nurturing talent to encourage elite-level success. Development through sport is concerned with the use of sport to achieve wider individual and societal development goals. It relies on participation, but for different reasons, with sport existing as a vehicle through which desirable behaviours can be encouraged, positive messages can be transmitted and social connections made. It highlights the breadth of the agenda to which sport may contribute, and is increasingly becoming the underpinning philosophy shaping the work of Sport NZ.

The wider sporting sector and partners

Across other sectors within New Zealand, namely education, our sporting partners and, to a lesser extent, the health sector, awareness of physical literacy was also growing, but it was predominantly linked to the work and ideas being developed with a focus on fundamental movement skills and basic sport skills. It would be fair to say there was a combination of excitement and apprehension from the various agencies and organisations involved in our community sport sector. Most apprehension came from misunderstandings of physical literacy and assumptions based on how this was being utilised in other countries. From a more traditional sport perspective, this concept either appeared to induce confusion as to the inclusion of the term 'literacy' or was interpreted as 'more of the same', as the understanding referred specifically to targeting the early primary years and involved a mastery of fundamental movement skills and basic sport skills. New Zealand had a very strong and successful delivery network around basic skill learning, and arguably had a more holistic approach to the development of these sport foundations than was evident in newer activities around the globe that were being promoted under the heading of physical literacy.

Within the education sector, awareness of the concept came through international research and connections. The education sector had a mix of both positive responses and a dislike for the use of the word 'literacy', as well as some concern over its promotion at the expense of physical education. Specifically, the critique that came from the educational sector was connected to three themes. First, there were questions that arose concerning the name physical literacy and the translation of the name. Many higher educators in New Zealand challenged the use of 'physical activity' instead of movement, and additionally wanted to know more about the use of the term literacy. Second, there was a question asked about whether physical literacy accounted for the social element of learning, and whether physical literacy could essentially be seen to be promoting healthism. This was also linked to debate concerning whether physical literacy would be able to be used critically and authentically in New Zealand, considering its Eurocentric origins. Third, there was concern and questions raised around the idea of 'monitoring' or 'assessing' of physical literacy through separating components of the experience (such as the affective, cognitive or physical). This gave the impression that a measurement of different elements of physical literacy would end up reinforcing a dualistic perspective, and not necessarily achieving the monist philosophical intent it sought to achieve. There were clear links between this concern and prior understandings of physical literacy that had come from international sources that seemed to prioritise fundamental movement skills. This certainly did cause some challenges initially!

Sport NZ's physical literacy approach

Fairly early in this journey was the understanding and commitment from Sport NZ, as the lead agency and driving force, towards the power of collaboration and partnerships if we were to gain any traction and momentum in embedding a focus on enhancing a person's physical literacy, rather than a concern with participation numbers and sport organisational growth. A commitment based on collaboration aimed to explore the possibilities of how lifelong physical literacy could develop within a New Zealand context. Once again, we reflected, 'Could physical literacy in fact be an umbrella concept to potentially unify sectors and enhance positive outcome for participants?'

To begin the dive into answering this, Sport NZ invited a wide and broad range of experts to come together to formulate how we would begin the groundswell necessary. This initially took the form of focus groups and shared workshops. This further emphasised the mixture of both positive excitement, questions and confusion through to more negative resistance to the terminology of physical literacy that existed because of its inclusion in our policy and strategy documentation.

The outcome of this work reflected the intent of being truly collaborative in contextualising physical literacy. It rapidly changed the initial plan concerning the creation of a physical literacy 'framework' to the notion of further building capability around physical literacy being expressed as an 'approach' that highlighted developing ownership by those directly involved. A very early New Zealand contextual component was the addition of a spiritual component in considering the holistic nature of our people.

This interactive process with partners and the wider sector led to the creation of the Sport NZ Physical Literacy Approach document (Sport NZ, 2016a). This was a leading policy document to support system building. An academic philosophical backdrop of physical literacy was needed to be operationalised into functional practice-based support, and this process was the start of that journey. This document could be used as a base to begin to delve into understanding our participants in a broader, more holistic way, and reinforce our commitment to viewing physical literacy as a lifelong commitment.

This policy document outlines the rationale behind Sport NZ's focus on physical literacy based on the belief that understanding and embracing a physical literacy approach would lead to more people being more active, more often throughout their lives, regardless of age, gender, ability, socio-economic group or culture. The document shared our vision and intent of using the concept of physical literacy, and its associated holistic approach, to enhance a shared understanding and add value to the provision and support of quality experiences across the many different partners and providers within New Zealand.

As socialisation and use of this policy progressed, again together with our partners, further clarification of the approach was developed. It was agreed that a physical literacy approach is one that:

- supports physical activity experiences that respond to the holistic nature of people;
- recognises the effect that sport and physical activity have across all elements of well-being;
- encourages people to value and take responsibility to be physically active for life;
- considers the different needs and reasons people choose to participate in physical activity at different life stages; and
- recognises the importance of play and quality physical education in ongoing sport and physical activity participation.

While Sport NZ's strategy had a focus on 5- to 18-year-olds, the working group was committed to ensuring the concept of physical literacy was understood to be a lifelong journey, and as such identified five broad life stages to frame the initial consideration of individuals' holistic needs. These life stages were identified as:

- babies and toddlers;
- children;
- young adults;
- adults; and
- seniors.

The approach then looked at each life stage and outlined a 'starting point' of initial needs and considerations across the domains the working party had ascertained. This was a very long and well-discussed process as it was acknowledged that trying to consider and identify factors of a dimension in isolation was possibly at odds with the underlying holistic framework. It was also identified that there were needs that are common across all life stages, such as:

- the chance to be playful, creative and have fun;
- physical opportunities that match individual physical ability;
- the chance to grow and develop at an approriate pace;
- a safe physical environment;
- a safe emotional environment where an individual is welcomed, respected, accepted and could be themselves; and
- the support and love of friends, family and whanau.

Where are we currently? Sport NZ and our partners

With a strategy, policy and investment commitment to enhancing the physical literacy of New Zealanders (particularly young people) in place, we needed to concentrate on operationalising this, and really bringing it to life. Due to its initial mixed reception and learnings from its integration into other countries, a significant piece of the work that Sport NZ has carried out in the past three years, since the adoption of the strategy, has been advocating and ensuring a shared and consistent understanding exists concerning physical literacy. This has been coupled with an acknowledgement of the need for various organisations and communities to have the flexibility to contextualise how it may 'look' within their setting, which builds and supports taking a locally led approach.

Understanding the crucial importance of the education setting in fostering physical literacy and the concerns surrounding replacement of PE with sport, the national subject association for PE, Physical Education New Zealand (PENZ), was invited from the beginning to work collaboratively with Sport NZ. The intent of this was to increase both the sporting and education sectors' understanding of the concept and terminology. This also reinforced a key emphasis for both parties in ensuring quality PE in schools is strongly advocated, and not wholly replaced by sport.

Together, Sport NZ and PENZ undertook a national tour holding a series of 'Introduction to Physical Literacy' workshops and training forums in each region across New Zealand. These were open to any organisations or individuals who wished to attend, and focused on:

- understanding physical literacy;
- unpacking the Sport NZ Physical Literacy Approach document; and
- collaborating and developing co-constructed partnerships exploring how this approach could add value to our work.

Dispelling myths and fairy tales associated with physical literacy

These workshops were a key first step in dispelling 'myths and fairy tales', and began the process of linking into a broader range of organisations that could be involved. Attendance included health-based organisations, councils and local government, with other national government agencies and private companies, along with the sport and education sector representation. There seemed to be an appetite for a unified message.

A development from this awareness campaign was the creation of a New Zealand physical literacy advocacy group, whose role is to champion and advocate physical literacy across the sector, and be the key network tasked with developing the tools, support, training and feedback mechanisms required across the range of settings within our New Zealand community sport system. Membership of this group was predominantly individuals who were early adopters of the concept and strong advocates of the approach. Representation was from several organisations, including our key partners – national sporting organisations, regional sporting trusts, PENZ, and youth development organisations. Additional members are constantly being added to this network as partners and providers adopt more overt practices aligned to enhancing physical literacy, and we envisage these members will continue to join from more varied settings than we have had to date.

The physical literacy advocacy group has had a concentration on professional development and capability-building opportunities, including all completing the IPLA level 1 foundation physical literacy learning programme. The aim of this group is to widen members' expertise and capacity concerning physical literacy to support Sport NZ's overall focus of creating quality experiences that enable young people to develop the broader skills and competencies needed to encourage a lifelong love of being physically active. We have focused on understanding and building systems to ensure this quality is consistent across all physical activity experiences within the different settings of home, school, clubs and community.

Quality indicators

Consideration of the importance of 'quality' in progressing an individual's physical literacy led to the development of a set of 'quality indicators' (Sport NZ, 2016b) These are not a means of measurement; rather, they are an initial series of descriptors and statements that Sport NZ believes should all be addressed. The support, opportunities and experiences provided via attention to these quality indicators should make a positive contribution to fostering an individual's physical literacy. These descriptors enable us to have conversations with people at all levels of the system to co-construct the way in which we support ongoing lifelong participation. Rather than a checklist to complete, these descriptors are better viewed as guides to ensure we are on the right track. The indicators consider:

1. *quality experiences* that are fun, positive, inclusive, valued and challenging that meet the aspirations and needs of young people;
2. *quality support* provided by people who are motivating, knowledgeable, principled, committed and encouraging; and
3. *quality opportunities* that are consistent, safe, minimise barriers, are accessible, and meet young people's abilities and aspirations.

These indicators are shaping the work we are undertaking with our key partners, in particular national sporting organisations and regional sports trusts, and we are now well under way in being able to answer those physical literacy questions around 'how' and 'what does it look like'.

Physical literacy is adding weight and strength to quality player-centred coaching programmes and parent awareness campaigns, and ensuring our grass-roots sporting system still emphasises the simple message that 'kids play sports for the fun of it, and they are more likely to stay playing when they enjoy it'.

While we still have much work to do, and it is still early days, there is a sense that our question of whether using the concept and terminology of physical literacy to shine a brighter light and advance our messages is starting to show some positive developments across our sporting system.

The power of play

A significant development within Sport NZ has been recognising and advocating the importance of play in laying the foundations of an individual's physical literacy journey. In November 2017, Sport NZ released a set of Play Principles (Sport NZ, 2017a) that recognise, and can be used to protect, the right of young New Zealanders to play. The principles clearly articulate the concept of intrinsic motivation and self-determination, with no additional justification of outcome required other than just participation itself. They aim to support and guide our communities around the value of joy and fun in movement, and its vital role in the well-being and ongoing choices concerning physical activity involvement. Sport NZ works in partnership with a number of local government territorial authorities and has established a network of play champions across these organisations. Their role is linked to the broader physical literacy advocacy group; however, it also taps into an additional partner network and is very focused on promoting and enabling play as a specific key area within a physical literacy approach.

Physical literacy and the education setting

Like many countries, New Zealand has experienced a blurring of the lines between physical education and sport, which has had the potential to impact negatively on the development of a lifelong love of movement and activity. This lack of clarity concerning roles and responsibilities is the result of a range of impacting factors, many of which were identified by the Sport NZ School Sports Futures Review project (Sport NZ, 2015c). Some of these were associated with the commercialisation and talent focus sometimes evident within sport and, in part, due to the lack of quality teacher training and professional development, regarding physical education (Petrie, 2008). While there is a great deal of variation across different schools and regions, in many cases primary school teachers have become increasingly reliant on or even replaced by external sport providers delivering sport instead of PE. The sport sector's understanding of PE is often limited, and typically their delivery is simply sport. Adding to this problem is the situation that the primary education sector often lacks the understanding of how to utilise sports effectively as a context of PE, and how to use sporting providers in a support role to enhance learning and teaching.

First, there was a need to reassure and emphasise to the education sector that physical literacy in New Zealand would not be used as a form of curriculum, programme or a replacement for PE. This was an essential step, and indicated the acknowledgement by both Sport NZ and PENZ that if the New Zealand HPE curriculum is being taught effectively in schools, then this would inevitably lead towards the outcome of progressing physical literacy.

This would mean nothing further would need to change within the curriculum design. However, it was also widely recognised that continued support and education is required in primary and secondary schools to deliver this curriculum effectively. This was more so for the primary sector, as HPE is just one of eight curriculum areas taught by generalist teachers.

The New Zealand HPE curriculum has a strong focus on the well-being of the students. When taught well, it is reflective of all four of its underlying strands (*Hauora*, attitudes, socio-ecological perspective and health promotion). These strands are all crucial enablers of an individual's development and progression of physical literacy, and as a result there was no need to argue for one or the other.

Schools, however, offer far more opportunities for the progression of physical literacy than just curriculum PE. Sport NZ has a long history of supporting schools and these wider opportunities, which we will continue with. Sport NZ invests in and leads many school community initiatives that now more overtly prioritise the outcome of supporting individuals' physical literacy, which we believe will provide greater and more consistent quality, and are more responsive to children and young people's needs.

Physical literacy and wider community settings

Another question we had asked was whether physical literacy could contribute to unify wider sectors and support our partnership at a cross-government level. Once again, we are in early days, but we are beginning to see some evidence of how this is emerging. The recently published Ministry of Health physical activity guidelines for under fives, *Sit Less, Move More, Sleep Well* (Ministry of Health, 2017), reflect the development of this partnership. The physical activity component of this guide has more of an emphasis on active play and holistic development than the fundamental movement skill development focus of the previous guidelines. We have a long history of collaboration with the health sector, and our continuing move towards broader holistic outcomes engendered through sport, physical literacy and a well-being focus will enable us to align more closely with their agenda. This wider focus has enabled additional opportunities, such as supporting a recent project of Oranga Tamariki (Ministry for Children) concerning connecting children in care to their communities. As we continue to further progress the embedding of our Community Sport Strategy and its three interrelated approaches, concentration and outcomes based around this wider value of sport is an area that will continue to develop.

Where is our journey heading?

Three years into our five-year strategy, physical literacy is now a cornerstone of our approach to delivering community sport and recreation for New Zealanders, and has progressed notably in terms of its acceptance and appreciation of its social relevance in New Zealand. The strategy is beginning to generate evidence and tangible examples of how physical literacy is being woven into the work in which we and our partners are involved. The growth and expansion of the physical literacy group and the reciprocal learning network that has been created has facilitated productive reflection and valuable partnerships. In addition, this network has played a significant role in creating links between philosophy and practice.

The major initiative Sport NZ developed and led from 2015, which is underpinned by supporting young people's physical literacy, is now beginning to provide evidence and examples to deepen our learning and inform our current work and future opportunities.

Known as 'Play.sport' (Sport NZ, 2017b), this initiative takes a strengths-based community-led methodology, which works across schools and communities, and draws from the collective expertise of all partners involved. Play.sport is about creating quality and engaging physical activity experiences (play, physical education, sport and active recreation) that encourage lifelong value and participation in physical activity.

The increasing focus on unpacking the 'value' that physical activity and movement can bring to individuals and communities, in terms of wider well-being outcomes, is further cementing the role that physical literacy is playing in the work of Sport NZ and in those with whom we partner.

Next steps

As we begin to consider and shape our new strategy, which will take effect from 2020, developing and supporting the physical literacy journeys of individuals is becoming a predominant aspect. The strong focus from our government concerning the well-being of young people and a collaborative cross-government focus on intergenerational well-being is adding additional reinforcement to this commitment.

There have been considerable efforts to contextualise physical literacy with respect to New Zealand's unique culture, history, and its people. As we continue to learn and develop our thinking, principles and practices, these discussions and research opportunities should continue.

At the same time, the growth globally of the importance of physical literacy has meant that the opportunity for greater collaboration across countries has been enhanced. Sport NZ has worked closely with Sport Wales and the Australian Sports Commission, and will continue to advance the potential this wider network can bring. Ongoing collaboration with the IPLA remains a focus for our organisation moving forwards.

Unpacking yet retaining the philosophical origins of physical literacy while simplifying and articulating these into valuable practical outcomes is a process we will continue to progress. We know we cannot expect people to get the most out of their sport and physical activity experiences if we are not considering their physical, social, emotional, cognitive and spiritual needs. We cannot expect to develop a lifelong love of being active if our thinking and resultant activity predominantly has a focus on physical competency (or a narrow objective of sporting success).

Unpacking how a system can support individuals to determine their own priorities and decisions to take responsibility for an active lifestyle must be understood and addressed. We as a national body will have justified expectancy around demonstrating the return on investment concerning a focus on physical literacy. Like so many countries globally, we are experimenting and grappling with aspects such as evaluation of our approach, tracking individuals' progress and understanding our impact, and this provides both challenge and exciting opportunity.

The future

Sport NZ aims to sustain the positive momentum that has been created, and lead the New Zealand sports and active recreation sector in taking the next step in the evolution of community sport as we both continue our work within the current strategy and develop the work that will result from the next strategic period. There is a validation and an appetite to continue to further evolve our emphasis relating to well-being. The answers to our questions and evidence to support the rationale concerning the inclusion and promotion of physical literacy will continue to accumulate and will inform the ongoing journey. We look forward to the upcoming twists, turns and prospects it will undoubtedly provide.

References

Durie, M. (1994) *Whaiora, Maori Health Development*. Auckland: Oxford University Press.

Ministry of Education (2014) *Health and Physical Education in the New Zealand Curriculum*. Wellington: Learning Media.

Ministry of Health (2017) *Sit Less, Move More, Sleep Well: Active Play Guidelines for Under-Fives*. Wellington: Ministry of Health.

New Zealand Government (2002) *Sport and Recreation New Zealand Act 2002.* Available at: www.legislation.govt.nz/act/public/2002/0038/latest/whole.html (accessed 13 March 2019).

Petrie, K. (2008) Physical education in primary schools: holding onto the past or heading for a different future. *Journal of Physical Education New Zealand,* 41(3): 67–80.

Sport NZ (2012) *Sport and Recreation in the Lives of Young New Zealanders.* Wellington: Sport NZ.

Sport NZ (2015a) *Community Sport Strategy.* Available at: www.sportnz.org.nz/about-us/our-publications/our-strategies/community-sport-strategy/ (accessed 13 March 2019).

Sport NZ (2015b) *Group Strategic Plan.* Available at: www.sportnz.org.nz/about-us/our-publications/our-strategies/sport-nz-group-strategic-plan-2015-2020/ (accessed 13 March 2019).

Sport NZ (2015c) *School Sports Futures Review.* Available at: www.sportnz.org.nz/assets/Uploads/attachments/managing-sport/young-people/School-Sport-Futures-Project-Final-Report.pdf (accessed 13 March 2019).

Sport NZ (2016a) *Physical Literacy Approach.* Available at: www.sportnz.org.nz/about-us/who-we-are/what-were-working-towards/physical-literacy-approach/ (accessed 13 March 2019).

Sport NZ (2016b) *Quality Indicators.* Available at: www.sportnz.org.nz/assets/Uploads/Young-People-Quality-Indicators-FINAL.pdf (accessed 13 March 2019).

Sport NZ (2017a) *Play Principles.* Available at: www.sportnz.org.nz/assets/Uploads/attachments/Sport-New-Zealand-Play-Principles-Nov-2017.pdf (accessed 13 March 2019).

Sport NZ (2017b) *Play.sport Evaluation* Available at: www.sportnz.org.nz/site-search/?q=play.sport&action_search=Search (accessed 13 March 2019).

Whitehead, M.E. (ed.) (2010) *Physical Literacy throughout the Lifecourse.* London: Routledge.

13

PHYSICAL AND FOOD LITERACY

A holistic approach to public health in Scotland

*Chris Topping, Jo Kopela, Isla Gibson
and Sandy Whitelaw*

Introduction

Contrary to everyday understanding, 'literacy' is clearly so much more than intellectual development and acquisition of information and skills. When appreciated as fundamental to our self-efficacy, confidence, empowerment, understanding and meaning, literacy becomes a profound way of experiencing life and the world around us. From a health and well-being systems perspective, it therefore offers a different way of considering health and health improvement. Literacy affords the opportunity to move away from our long-standing affinity with cognitive development and presumed behaviour change strategies that overlook the fundamental role of the social and emotional context in shaping people's health (Vidgen, 2016). In Dumfries and Galloway (D&G), *physical and food literacy* (PFL) is being explored and developed in a way that could significantly impact on the lives of individuals, communities and the environment to enhance the quality of life.

This chapter describes the processes undertaken to define the theory of physical literacy and start to move it into practice, ultimately 'operationalising' the concept (Chen, 2015). We start by describing work undertaken within the remit of the region's *physical activity strategic partnership*, The Physical Activity Alliance (PAA). This formed a starting point for conceptual work that sought to broaden a literacy focus, creating a wider systematic notion of PFL. We then describe a series of 'engagement sessions' conducted with health and well-being professionals in order to test this concept. We conclude by reflecting on the potential for PFL to act as a common ethos in addressing the complexities of healthy diet and active living.

Background

There has been significant long-term investment in healthy diet and active living-related work internationally, nationally and locally within D&G. However, some argue that this has been reactive, based on delivering isolated projects with variable levels of strategic coordination (WHO, 2018). These projects have also, more often than not, been oriented towards fostering propositional knowledge and personal skills for behaviour change (Morris et al., 2016).

Relatively less attention has been paid to social, psychological, cultural and environmental influences (Kelly et al., 2017a). Current work is more likely to focus on deficits, with the consequence of those who cannot cook or who are not physically active tending to be blamed for lacking in knowledge or motivation. Rhodes and Kates (2015) also point out that approaches tend to emphasise cognitive rather than affective determination.

As such, levels of overweight and obesity and physical inactivity in the D&G region are still high: 69.5% of adults (aged 16+) are overweight or obese (Scottish Government, 2015a); 27.5% of children are overweight or obese, while 18.8% are at a level of overweight or obesity that may warrant referral to child healthy weight services (Information Services Division, 2016); and 22% of schoolchildren (Currie et al., 2015) and 60% of adults (Scottish Government, 2015a) meet Chief Medical Officer recommendations for physical activity (Department of Health, 2011).

D&G's strategic approach to the implementation of a long-term athlete development approach (Balyi, 2001) has been supportive of a fundamental movement skills (FMS) approach to improve activity levels (Okely et al., 2001). FMS was seen as valuable, in theory teaching skills in early years that provide a foundation for activity. It was also felt that it was something that could be conveniently 'packaged' as a resource and utilised easily by professionals. While still having some merit, those within NHS D&G acknowledged the potential limitations of FMS as an effective basis of lifelong physical activity (Edwards et al., 2017). There was a belief that in and of itself, it lacked the sophistication of a physical literacy approach (Barnett et al., 2016). It follows that the development of lifelong physical activity fails to consider social, emotional and environmental influences within our communities (Almond, 2014; Chen, 2015; Cairney et al., 2016) and is unlikely to be achieved in isolation from approaches that provide knowledge, foster motivation and create environments that are supportive of physical activity (Edwards et al., 2017). This resulted in a reorientation towards a more holistic approach and the practical application of physical literacy arising from Whitehead's (2010) physical literacy definition (Lundvall, 2015).

Whitehead (2010) believes that the primary reason for inactivity is a lack of motivation, often a consequence of previous negative physical activity experiences that impact self-confidence and interest in an active lifestyle (Whitehead, 2010; Chen, 2015). Qualitative research undertaken in D&G in 2017 with active/inactive young people found that while learning and mastering new skills were associated with enhanced enjoyment, social (e.g. promoting enjoyment through the social element), emotional influences (e.g. enjoyment through variety) and physical environment (e.g. location and accessibility) were more prominent (Kelly et al., 2017b). These findings are supported by wider research into physical activity correlates and determinates. For example, Bauman et al. (2012) highlight the association between physical activity and individual factors, including 'self-efficacy'/'motivation', while Biddle et al. (2011) highlight 'motivation' in addition to 'behaviour correlates' such as 'previous physical activity' and 'environmental correlates', including 'access to facilities'.

First steps towards physical literacy

From these initial steps, the cross-sector partnership D&G PAA agreed in 2014 to a series of principles that would support the group's policy and practice, including, for example, the commitment to collaborative working, taking a lifecourse approach, tackling health inequalities, building capacity, and, of most significance to this chapter, *adopting a physical literacy approach* as a common theoretical base. The breadth of this group (representation from various NHS, local government and third-sector agencies) was an important basis in increasing awareness and building understanding of physical literacy via dialogue and shared understanding and a holistic culture (Dudley et al., 2017).

This common knowledge and understanding was seen as a basis for enhancing the effectiveness of localised interventions across different sectors and settings (Davis et al., 2015), and the partnership recognised that this approach had potential to contribute positively to the achievement of the various physical activity outcomes contained within the Scottish Government national framework (Scottish Government, 2015b).

A significant strength of the physical literacy approach, and what attracted the partnership in the first instance, was the perceived academic rigor and theoretical foundations upon which it is based (IPLA, 2017a). However, while this *theoretical* discourse on physical literacy and physical activity promotion is generally rich (e.g. Sallis et al., 2016), a dearth of implementation-oriented insights was noted – members feeling unclear about *how to apply* this approach in the 'real world'.

It was therefore apparent that if the approach was to be progressed, work to build cross-sector consensus, understanding and commitment to action was required. The PAA then contacted the International Physical Literacy Association (IPLA), who had developed a physical literacy introductory course. The course had various aims: to foster an understanding and appreciation of the concept of physical literacy; to encourage individuals to reflect on their own physical literacy journey (phenomenology); and to empower participants to appreciate and then adopt the notion of choosing physical literacy for life (IPLA, 2017a).

The PAA then commissioned the IPLA to deliver a modified version of their introductory training course to explore the potential of the approach to improve local physical activity. The partnership was also interested in testing the concept within a setting with professionals/practitioners and community members. If physical literacy was to be enacted, an assessment of its accessibility and relevance was deemed critical. At this time, two partnership primary schools in the west of the region were working with NHS D&G to develop themselves as 'healthy school communities'.

The Scottish Government's education strategy, Curriculum for Excellence, promotes learning through health and well-being in ways that develop confidence and understanding in order to develop mental, emotional, social and physical well-being (Scottish Government, 2008).

In this context, engagement with parents, pupils, staff and relevant partners had identified healthy diet and physical activity as priorities for this community. The partnership head teacher was therefore interested in the potential of physical literacy, and discussions began on the process of considering healthy diet from a similar perspective. It was agreed to deliver bespoke physical literacy training sessions in April 2016 (details summarised in Table 13.1). Each session introduced physical literacy as an inclusive and holistic approach encompassing equally the physical (e.g. movement patterns), cognitive (e.g. knowledge) and affective (e.g. motivation) domains of 'human nature' within our environments (IPLA, 2017a, 2017b).

Insights were collected during the sessions. Generally, participants engaged well with the concept. However, many questions remained as to how to translate the theory into grounded practice – how to make this 'real'. In addition, the rich dialogue that emerged throughout these training events highlighted the complexities of approaching general health improvement through single 'topic' issues such as healthy diet and physical activity. Follow-up conversations, particularly with the school staff and partners, shifted the focus onto literacy as a *social* practice, and the importance of focusing on *strengths* rather than *deficits*. In summary, the training emphasised (Green et al., 2016):

- the importance of recognising and respecting both individual and community starting points, and capability to make progress within the physical, affective and cognitive domains;
- that barriers may restrict individual and community abilities to engage and the necessity to look at how structural and attitudinal barriers can be overcome;
- that the status quo should be challenged and positive action should coordinate the growth of opportunities within a community; and
- that coordinated strategies within communities that are effectively communicated and promoted need to be developed.

Extending the concept to physical and food literacy

From this base, the next phase of the work centred on more conceptual matters and with respect to two lines: a specific extension of the physical aspect of the concept to include food, and thereafter reflection on the broad orientation of this 'topic-based' approach with a general health improvement perspective. First, the three major public health priorities in D&G at this time were overweight and obesity, physical inactivity, and mental health and well-being. Taking a systems approach, a 'test of change' process was initiated to investigate the potential impact of the wider influence on individual and community health behaviours taking a PFL approach, underpinned by improving mental health and well-being.

TABLE 13.1 D&G physical literacy training, April 2016

Venue	Target audience	Information
Dumfries	Policymakers across physical activity settings (e.g. education, health, sport, environment)	A three-hour course based on the philosophy and concept of physical literacy that will be undertaken with policymakers who are keen to develop a strategy for education, leisure and travel
Wigtown Primary School	School staff and key partners	Continued processional development for primary school staff plus some key stakeholders; associated secondary school to be invited
Wigtown Primary School	Parents, sport/activity coaches and community groups	A 60-minute course for parents, coaches and community
Kirkcowan Primary School	Parents, sport/activity coaches and community groups	A 60-minute course for parents, coaches and community
Kirkcowan Primary School	School staff and key partners	A two-hour follow-up course that develops thinking from school staff and key partner sessions into action plan

We believed that there was a lessened desire for 'isolated' single-topic approaches, and that a more integrated orientation had the potential to be a more powerful long-term approach. Particularly, some professionals appear to require an expansion beyond current topic-based work towards more generic healthcare approaches.

Second, in the context of a 'systems' approach to public health that is congruous with the ethos underpinning physical literacy, 'the richer the interactions with the environment, the greater one will understand their human potential' (Whitehead, 2007: 285). This systems approach seeks to redress the potentially isolated and disjointed nature of many aspects of current health improvement initiatives and interventions (Green, 2006; WHO, 2018). Therefore, it is suggested here that focusing on a single domain of a system is unlikely to bring about deep and sustained change. Rather, systematic approaches attempt to understand the varied 'determinants' of health issues and consider the various levels at which health improvement can be achieved (Henderson, 2017). With specific respect to the focus of this chapter, various 'ecological' models have been proposed within public health generally (Green, 2006). This has provided a foundation for expressions in a number of topic areas, including physical activity (Giles-Corti et al., 2005) and overweight and obesity (Ohri-Vachaspati et al., 2015), wherein changes in culture, environment, organisational behaviour and marketing, as well as change in group, family and individual behaviours, are stressed.

Bringing these ecological principles and PFL together, the following can be seen as a potential model of such interaction (see Figure 13.1). Crucially, the contextual or environmental element of ecological models is seen as significant in relation to the individual motivation, confidence, physical competence, and knowledge and understanding. This conceptual model has been beneficial in demonstrating to practitioners the equal and balanced importance of each domain on an individual's potential engagement in physical activity and healthy diet choices. The model also illustrates possible harmful consequences of removing one or more domains in terms of the likelihood of positive engagement – recognising that responses will be unique to the individual's physical and food literacy journey.

Further unpacking shows that the dynamics that shape the attainment of *food* literacy have the potential to be seen as highly congruous with those associated with *physical* literacy; that is, both are influenced by the same affective, physical and cognitive domains, resulting in attaining the motivation, confidence, competence, knowledge and understanding that leads to the empowerment and the responsibility for healthy eating and engagement in physical activity, respectively. The relationship between these two literacies and their contribution to improved health and well-being via promoting lifelong engagement in physical activity and healthy eating is shown in Figure 13.2, which highlights the need for appropriate domains to be addressed while demonstrating environmental influences on behaviour. The benefits of including these domains, and the problems arising from lack of attention to some or all of the domains, are identified. The figure also shows that where domains are addressed, there is potential for positive engagement and the development of the capacity to take responsibility, throughout life, for active participation and healthy eating.

We believe that an amalgamated PFL concept potentially offers an inclusive approach that focuses on building the potential every individual has to be physically active and responsible for their diet quality throughout their lives.

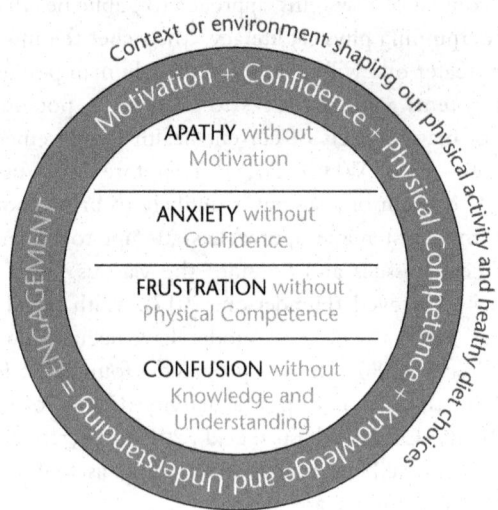

FIGURE 13.1 Holistic concept designed to promote lifelong engagement in PFL

Source: Courtesy of E. Durden Myers, adapted from Durden-Myers (2017)

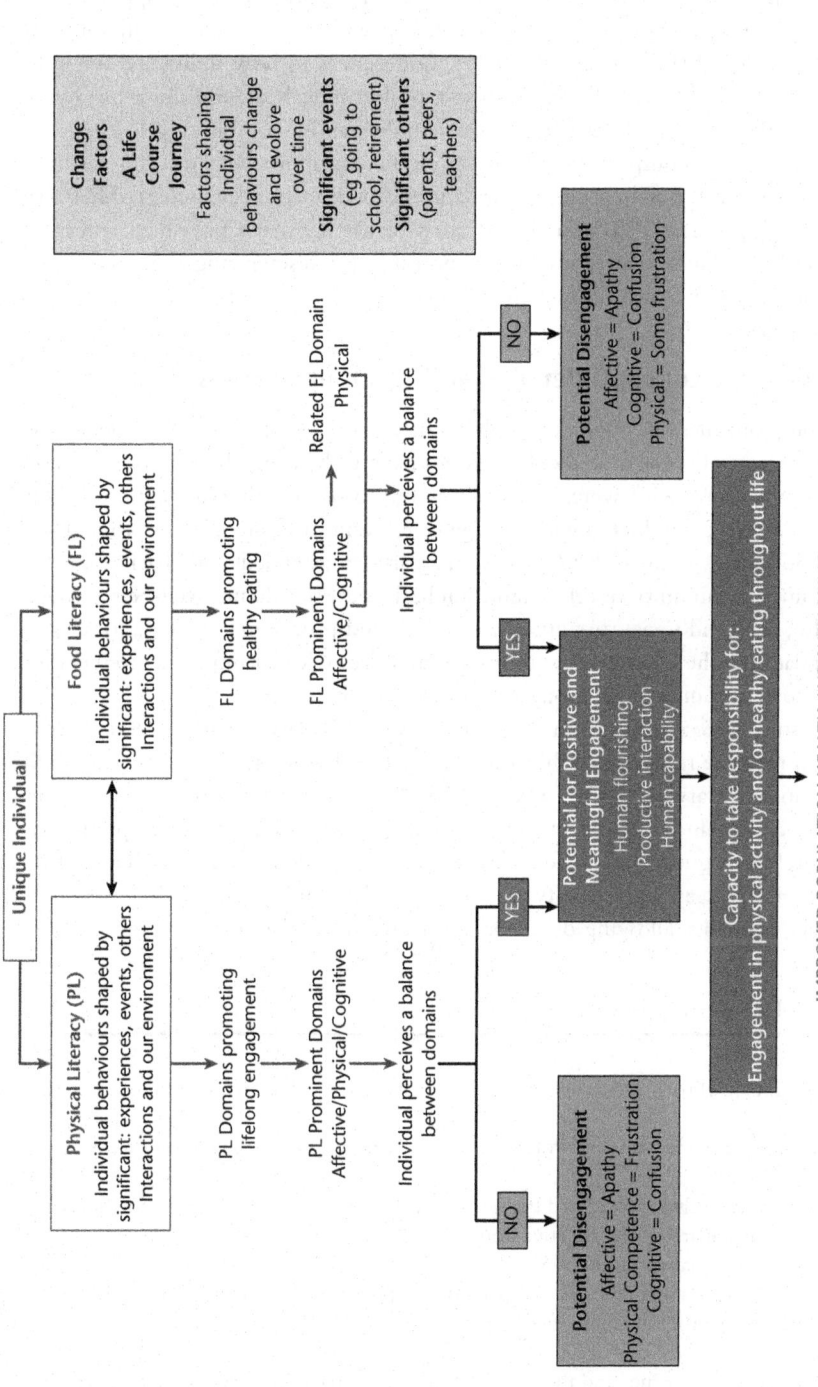

FIGURE 13.2 A model showing the relationship between physical and food literacies

Important to the public health perspective, the approach can be applied across the lifecourse, regardless of ability level, and will be experienced differently by each individual (Edwards et al., 2017). Differences in how individuals view the world are related to phenomenology, a philosophical underpinning of physical literacy (Edwards et al., 2017). A greater understanding of individual experiences related to PFL complement wider public health approaches towards changing behaviours (e.g. person-centred care and motivational interviewing). Therefore, wider adoption of PFL as a shared cross-sector approach provides a means to tackle long-standing determinates responsible for disengaging individuals from physical activity and healthy eating choices.

Testing the concept: detailed engagement sessions

Throughout these developmental phases, it was recognised that if the concept was to be ultimately operationalised, it would have to be accessible and have congruence with those who were potentially going to use it. 'Engagement workshops' were therefore conducted with a range of relevant professionals from the region's four localities in early 2017. Thirty-six partners attended with backgrounds in teaching, community development, public health, health and well-being, mental health, care and social support, active travel, and professionals from a local sports foundation. The workshops comprised a mixture of leader input and presentation, anecdotal accounts, small group tasks, and open discussions.

A student researcher from the University of Glasgow was deployed to capture the immediate reactions to the concept and to subsequently assess its accessibility and utility (Harwell, 2003). The methodology chosen for this was a post-event focus group and a short qualitative questionnaire. This form of preliminary research is aligned with a 'formative' approach, and relatedly 'concept testing'. This provides an opportunity to assess whether target groups understand and accept concepts, allowing developers to learn to translate complex messages in a

TABLE 13.2 Key themes

Need for PFL
- A number of participants felt that the concept did not offer anything unique to their practice.
- Comments were made by professionals that characteristics of the concept were 'backwards'.
- In contrast, others recognised the need for new approaches and saw the potential in PFL, particularly in the affective domain.

Barriers to concept advancement
- Included issues surrounding the terminology, perceived lack of tangibility, and concerns over the breadth of concept.

Ideal prerequisites for concept advancement
- Included partnerships and the need for multidisciplinary conversations, resources, time and staff.

---

way that will be accepted by target groups and to fix any issues that arise in the developmental process (Parvanta et al., 2011). Key themes from the research , also explored by Gibson et al. (2019), are shown in Table 13.2.

In this context, and in positive terms, the majority of participants recognised that new ways of looking at healthy diet and physical activity were needed, and supported the potentially inclusive nature of a PFL approach. These participants felt that more holistic ways of working that go beyond the limits of traditional approaches may be more successful in reaching target groups. Concerns were expressed, however, in two main respects: either the concept was *not unique enough*, or it was felt that some of its characteristics were outdated (e.g. the reduction-ist tendencies of specific *food* and *physical* domains are contrary to contemporary broad-based holistic principles). A number of participants felt that the concept was not distinctive enough to offer any alternative to their current practice. Although the engagement sessions asked participants to reflect on whether their practice did indeed access all three of the discussed domains (cognitive, affective and behav-ioural/physical), some participants were certain that these principles were already in the scope of their practice, and thus could not see the uniqueness of this con-cept. Additionally, other participants likened the breaking down of the concept into discrete categories as being similar to an outdated division between mental and physical health. It was felt that introducing such a concept with this division was harmful to progression in this area.

Concerns over the meaning of 'literacy' were also raised. Despite a definition being given at the start of the sessions, many believed it to remain unnecessarily com-plicated – simple Google searches had highlighted some very complex definitions and theory. Parent feedback from the IPLA workshops also highlighted that some were concerned by the connotations with reading. It was felt that if, as professionals, they could not capture its meaning easily, it would be unlikely for the concept to be transferable to a lay audience. One participant particularly felt that the use of the term 'literacy' may be problematic, stating that it 'undermines illiterate people and makes them seem less valuable'. That is, by using the word 'literacy' in relation to healthy diet and physical activity, we are creating another area where individuals can potentially have a 'deficit' (i.e. be '*il*literate) (see explanatory glossary).

Another anxiety centred on the tangibility of the concept. Despite the discussion in the session being introductory and developmental, allowing participants to gain incremental insights into the concept, it was clear that the professionals wished to *immediately* understand how it might work pragmatically within their current prac-tice. Participants felt that if they were to consider taking the approach forward, they would need more tangible examples, particularly of how it would fit within their local circumstances. These positions are very much congruent with a perspective that professionals can be 'application-minded', with tangibility being a significant factor when judging the appropriateness of any approach (Yelon et al., 2004).

The scope of the concept was also considered problematic. Many participants stated that the sole focus on healthy diet and physical activity was considered too narrow for their increasingly multifaceted remit. In more operational terms, a combination of complex theory and lack of tangibility were considered prohibitive in attracting or appealing to internal/external grant funders (or other resource allocation) for physical literacy, even when outcomes are within health and well-being. Many of those who supported the 'essence' of the concept, particularly centred around the 'affective' domain, which many have pointed to having the potential to deliver positive change (e.g. see Rhodes et al., 2009; Morris et al., 2016). Finally, some participants asked for the approach to be extended towards a broader 'health literacy'. Despite voicing these concerns, participants discussed a range of factors that would make the transition to a PFL approach more accessible – framed as 'prerequisites' that would be particularly advantageous if established in the early stages of planning and delivery. Participants cited a series of factors that were considered necessary, specifically:

- community participation;
- partnerships;
- multidisciplinary conversations;
- organisational support; and
- basic funding and resources.

Participants specifically praised the multidisciplinary conversation generated in these engagement sessions for allowing them to share good examples of practice and increase their knowledge of other local services. They felt that having professionals from a wide range of backgrounds 'enabled a different type of conversation', with one participant claiming, 'It opened up my way of thinking'.

In summary, a number of themes were highlighted in this work that were broadly congruous with the emergent 'research questions related to physical literacy' that have recently been highlighted by Longmuir and Tremblay (2016). In particular, in relation to their set domains, we have similar interests in understanding how we might 'enhance' and 'monitor' physical literacy, and these suggest a series of positive 'next steps' that will be undertaken over the next few years. This will involve further work to operationalise the concept and to test its utility as a

TABLE 13.3 Physical literacy: navigating challenges in D&G

Factor	Challenge(s)	Navigation
Leadership/ ownership	Comprehension Capacity Developing networks	Policy alignment Uniqueness Training Evidence
Operationalising Language Holistic approach	Tangible Accessible Focus on 'person-centred approach'	Context-specific examples/resources User-friendly Partnerships Transferable The 'affective'

common ethos in bringing about cultural change. This change will require collective decision-making processes that shape investments in healthy diet and active living work. These are summarised in Table 13.3.

Planning the way ahead

D&G has set out four key next steps that aim to navigate the challenges set out in Table 13.3:

1. PFL as a strategic priority – *leadership and ownership, holistic.*
2. Operationalising PFL – *operationalising, language, holistic.*
3. Building PFL workforce capacity – *operationalising, language, holistic.*
4. Maintaining current measures of PFL in practice – *operationalising, holistic.*

1. PFL as a strategic priority

In the context of Longmuir and Tremblay's (2016) desire to understand, 'how to most effectively support progress on the physical literacy journey' (p. 32), the PAA was asked by public sector senior leaders in D&G (e.g. Chief Executives of Council and NHS) to identify the evidence-based interventions that would be expected to lead to a cultural shift in the percentage of the D&G population participating in physical activity to recommended levels. Twenty-one recommendations aiming to increase population levels of physical activity by 5% in over five years were identified by the PAA from review of current practice, expert testimonial and research.

Recommendations were categorised into five categories recognising the varied types of action required to deliver population-level change. These included the retention and expansion of current successful projects and changes to policy, including budget realignment and transformational change actions requiring system-wide leadership to implement. A fifth category entitled underpinning is an action core in the implementation of all other recommendations. The development of a D&G PFL framework that underpins the promotion and delivery of physical activity has been agreed across sectors and settings. Recommendation no. 21 identifies a need to create a PFL framework. This framework should be prioritised across all physical activity interventions. Recommendations have been approved by local public sector senior leaders, and formal reporting mechanisms and implementation plans are in progress.

2. Operationalising PFL

Again in relation to Longmuir and Tremblay's (2016) aim of enhancing, 'our understanding of the approaches, settings, and intervention content most likely to promote and support the physical literacy journey' (p. 33), Public Health in D&G are planning to partner the University of Glasgow to undertake further research to identify how and if a PFL approach can be implemented as a multi-agency and cross-sector policy approach in D&G. Qualitative research with PFL practitioners will explore:

- current practice in relation to PFL (successful, unsuccessful, best practice, etc.);
- links to policies, plans and everyday interactions;
- relevance to practice – usability and feasibility (language, resources, etc.);
- factors critical to adaptability, longevityd an uptake across sectors and settings (holistic); and
- opportunities for PFL collaborations.

3. Building PFL workforce capacity

Longmuir and Tremblay (2016) suggest a need for a 'greater knowledge of ... factors that characterize successful interventions' (p. 32), and, in line with Kohl et al.'s (2012) recognition of the significance of 'workforce capacity' and 'strategic leadership', the PAA has focused on these concepts in the context of physical literacy. Partnerships crossing sectors/settings will be essential, as well as training and implementation approaches. D&G will progress a two-pronged approach to training led by Public Health. First, continuing delivery of a locally developed and free PFL training session. This two-hour workshop introduces PFL as an approach, and aims to bring together varied partners to discuss and reflect on opportunities within their personal and professional practice to promote PFL. Second, the IPLA foundation certificated course that introduces physical literacy with consideration to the individual's journey across life (3.5 hours). This is delivered at no cost to maximise uptake.

The next step is to develop a PFL early years training course in collaboration with local partners from the health, education and sport sectors, with an academic research component provided by the University of Glasgow. Training will be designed to enhance the knowledge, skills, confidence and motivation of practitioners to deliver and apply a physical and food literacy approach across their teaching and learning experiences/environments. Research will aim to develop understanding on how practitioners can embed FPL into their practice, with the hope that tangible examples to progress concept operationalising and uptake will be identified.

4. Maintaining current measures of PL in practice

Finally, Longmuir and Tremblay (2016) place monitoring and evaluation at the heart of their critical research questions related to physical literacy, and work in D&G has very much conformed to this assertion. In November 2017, D&G Council, in partnership with NHS D&G, administered the annual survey of school physical activity in school pupils aged 11–17 years (NHS Dumfries and Galloway and Dumfries and Galloway Council, 2018). This survey aims to report the number

TABLE 13.4 Physical literacy measure (scale and domain measured)

Item	Domain measured
I want to take part in physical activity	Motivation
I feel confident to take part in lots of different physical activities	Confidence
I am good at different physical activities	Physical competence
I know why physical activity is good for me	Knowledge and understanding
I enjoy the places I go for physical activity	Environment

of school pupils meeting recommended levels of physical activity over the previous seven days (60+ minutes of health-enhancing physical activity daily). This figure is a key performance measure of physical activity levels in D&G.

If PL is to become an underpinning approach, there is a need to understand how physically literate children and young people perceive themselves to be in order to chart future progress. A PL measure of this nature could prove a more informative and holistic means to understand the complex nature of physical activity engagement for each individual (Silva et al., 2017), while providing a baseline for future assessment rather than the current classification of being 'active' or 'inactive'. Embedding physical literacy offers a new and potentially important approach to raising levels of physical activity in D&G. To demonstrate this potential, the PAA agreed to the inclusion of physical literacy as a survey item in an annual population survey of school pupils in D&G. The survey aimed to develop an understanding of the contribution each physical literacy domain has on school pupils' decisions to be physically active. This insight offers potential to improve the effectiveness of physical activity behaviour change interventions.

A five-item measure was included in the 2017 D&G Schools Physical Activity Survey, one for each physical literacy domain developed by the IPLA/ Department for Culture, Media and Sport (Green et al., 2017), plus the environment domain developed by Public Health D&G (see Table 13.4). Questions related to the pupils' current perception of each domain rather than an actual measure of each aspect. Each item was scored on a Likert scale from 0 (not like me) to 10 (very like me). The survey was administered to pupils in primary seven (11 years), secondary one (12–13 years), secondary three (14–15 years) and secondary five (16–17 years) only.

Two stages of statistical analysis were conducted (Topping et al., 2018):

1. The correlation between pairs of physical literacy items was assessed using the Pearson correlation coefficient.
2. Generalised linear models were used to assess the relationship between the outcome variables for each physical literacy item, and the summed scores (four items excluding 'environment' and five items) – and the following predictor variables:

    a.   Year group
    b.   Gender
    c.   Number of days pupils reported being physically active to guidelines in the past week (60+ plus minutes of health-enhancing activity):

        i.   0–2 days = inactive
       ii.   3–6 days = some activity
      iii.   7 days = meets guideline

Just under 3,000 survey responses were received ($n = 2,851$), with all PL items completed. There was a positive correlation ($0.53 \leq r \leq 0.80$) between all pairs of PL domains, the strongest being between the first three items (motivation, confidence and physical competence). Interestingly, the locally added environment item had a higher correlation with the first three than the 'why is it good for me' item did. Key findings from pupil responses are summarised below, and were statistically significant unless stated ($p < 0.05$):

- Pupils who were less physically active had lower physical literacy scores across all five domains and domains combined.
- Girls perceived confidence and physical competence was lower than boys. Domains combined found girls had lower perceived physical literacy.
- With the exception of knowledge and understanding, perceived physical literacy scores decreased as year group age increased.

Positive correlations were reported between all physical literacy domains. This is important as physical literacy gives equal weighting to each domain, recognising that they interconnect/intertwine to shape behaviours (IPLA, 2018). Scores by gender, year group and activity level provide insight into where resources should be invested to support and empower children and young people to be active now and in the future.

Research carried out in D&G in 2017 into why 13- to 25-year-olds did not engage in physical activity emphasised the importance of 'organisational delivery of physical literacy training to key physical activity partners emphasising equally the physical, social, affective domains and how they are influenced by competency' (Kelly et al., 2017).

Public Health also developed and tested a new primary schools' physical activity and sport event evaluation form in Autumn 2018 considering the domains of physical literacy. The aim was to better understand experiences of school-aged children in order to ensure that future events could enhance engagement, experiences and environments of participants. Event feedback is collected from teachers (e.g. the extent to which pupils enjoyed or not taking part) and pupils via hands-up responses for speed (e.g. 'I enjoyed/did not enjoy taking part'). The form uses adapted questions and scales from the 2017 D&G School Physical Activity Survey – the aim being that events that positively engage and provide meaningful experiences for children.

Conclusion

This chapter has looked at how a PFL ethos has been developed conceptually and practically in one specific area, particularly concerned with its possible intangibility, and therefore how it might be reflected in real-world circumstances. We conclude by reflecting on the wider possibilities of such an interaction. The steps we have taken to develop and test an approach that focuses on physical literacy, and potentially builds towards a more holistic concept, including food literacy, clearly shows promise. By realistically and critically exploring the possible operationalisation of the concept, we have discovered a series of pragmatic issues that require further attention. First, there were views that practitioners and the public found the concepts complex, elusive and therefore, in applied terms, potentially unworkable. As such, there is a need to further 'operationalise' the concept into relatively accessible and tangible guidance that can be expressed in practice-based contexts. Likewise, in a systematic context, the relationship between a topic-specific orientation to literacy and wider holistic *health* literacy needs further exploration. Finally, testing whether the values contained within a PFL ethos can act to bind together various partners in the healthy diet and physical activity domain should be explored.

The publication of a series of recent policy documents from the Scottish Government (2018a, 2018b, 2018c) offers significant opportunity to include PFL as part of any national and local implementation approach. Scottish Government (2018b) is particularly supportive of a PL approach, stating, 'we will develop the physical confidence and competence of children and young people' (p. 22).

Work progressed in D&G and described in this chapter will provide a starting point from which to challenge current approaches, create new partnerships, and influence future policy and planning decisions. However, further progress will be restricted unless the practical application of PFL can be clearly and simply articulated to policymakers, practitioners and communities. Simply put, answers to the following three questions are necessary if PFL is to become a widely accepted approach:

- How can practitioners, services and communities deliver or incorporate PFL into everyday practice (tangible examples)?
- How can health and well-being changes (e.g. individual/community level) be measured as a result of implementing a PFL approach?
- Is there a service or health economic benefit of implementing a PFL approach?

In relation to the issues of operationalisation and the generic-specific relationship, we are currently undertaking more work to establish how PFL might be expressed pragmatically. The region is also trialling the possibility of deploying the concept as a cultural resource across the healthy diet and physical activity communities. In this latter context, there is little doubt that one of the main drivers that informs the current debate on the most appropriate public health approach to healthy eating and active living is the need to recognise *complexity*. The aforementioned strategy ambitions to improve diet, activity and healthy weight states that 'a broad range of interventions is needed because factors contributing to overweight and obesity are *complex*' (Scottish Government, 2017: 5, emphasis added). What flows from this is the significance of a *systems-based* orientation that draws on 'holistic' principles (Green, 2006). This has been expressed in a host of 'ecological' public health models – both generally (Todnem By, 2005) or in relation to specific areas of interest, such as healthy diet and active living (e.g. Giles-Corti and Donovan, 2002; Sallis et al., 2006). In relatively *structural* and *tangible* terms, these tend to map out the determinants of a healthy diet and active living, and then go on to propose possible actions and partnerships that flow from this analysis – resulting in a *system* of coordinated actions. Alongside this specific healthy eating and physical activity orientation, the general nature of any systems change also tends to lead with a *structural* emphasis – success will be achieved if we can just get the 'right' policies or organisational structures.

However, some dispute this assumption, suggesting the need for a common change *culture* to precede any structural adjustments across the range of perspectives and partners; for example, Glasby (2016) believes that 'although much less dramatic than creating new structures, focusing on organisational and professional culture is crucial – and we neglect this at our peril' (p. 2). This results in little effort being made to examine the potentially varied professional and community roles and perspectives that inform the nature of 'problems', 'determinants' and the 'solutions' that flow from this analysis in the healthy diet and active living field (Hamlin, 1998). In this sense, 'culture' would be considered to a be a collective set of deep and sometimes implicit and unconscious assumptions, values, beliefs, and perceptions of the world views that provide a 'lens' through which actions are identified and implemented (Improvement and Development Agency, 2004). Unsurprisingly, in complex, multidisciplinary areas, these can often be conflicting. The culture-based approach to change would address these tensions directly and suggest that consensus and progress can be fostered by a process of 'enculturation' – an active and conscious attempt to 'nurture a culture' (Improvement and Development Agency, 2004).

We believe the inclusive nature of a PFL approach that encompasses a wide range of perspectives and health behaviour change models is highly suited to these requirements of developing a holistic and community-led systems change (Dudley et al., 2017). At all levels, it offers the potential to provide stakeholders with an overview of the key domains of healthy diet and physical activity (cognitive/ knowing, affective/feeling, behavioural and physical/doing, and environmental/ context) that will inform investments and a requirement to address *all* domains – particularly the affective element, which commonly appears in policy directions but is rarely articulated in practice.

Postscript

This chapter is a slightly shortened version of the full paper. The full version can be found at: http://eprints.gla.ac.uk/.

References

Almond, L. (2014) Serious flaws in an FMS interpretation of physical literacy. *Science and Sports*, 29: 60–62.

Balyi, I. (2001) *Sport System Building and Long-Term Athlete Development in British Columbia.* Canada: SportsMedBC.

Barnett, L., Stodden, D., Cohen, K., Smith, J., Lubans, D., Lenoir, M., Iivonen, S., Miller, A., Laukkanen, A., Dudley, D., Lander, N., Brown, H. and Morgan, P. (2016) Fundamental movement skills: an important focus. *Journal of Teaching in Physical Education*, 35(3): 219–225.

Bauman, A.E. Reis, R.S. Sallis, J.F., Wells, J.C., Loos, R.J. and Martin, B.W. (2012) Correlates of physical activity: why are some people physically active and others not? *The Lancet*, 380(9838): 258–271.

Biddle, J.H., Atkin, A.J., Cavill, N. and Foster, C. (2011) Correlates of physical activity in youth: a review of quantitative systematic reviews. *International Review of Sport and Exercise Psychology*, 4(1): 25–49.

Cairney, J., Bedard, C., Dudley, D. and Kriellaars, D. (2016) Towards a physical literacy framework to guide the design, implementation and evaluation of early childhood movement-based interventions targeting cognitive development. *Annals of Sport Medicine and Research*, 3(4): 1073–1078.

Chen, A. (2015) Operationalizing physical literacy for learners: embodying the motivation to move. *Journal of Sport and Health Science*, 4: 125–131.

Currie, C., Van der Sluijs, W., Whitehead, R., Currie, D., Rhodes, G., Neville, F. and Inchley, J. (2015) *Health Behaviour in School-Aged Children: Dumfries and Galloway Report 2014*. St Andrews: University of St Andrews, Child and Adolescent Health Research Unit (CAHRU).

Davis, R., Campbell, R., Hildona, Z., Hobbsa, L. and Michiea, S. (2015) Theories of behaviour and behaviour change across the social and behavioural sciences: a scoping review. *Health Psychology*, 9(3): 323–344.

Department of Health (2011) *Start Active, Stay Active: A Report on Physical Activity for Health from the Four Home Countries' Chief Medical Officers*. London: Department of Health.

Dudley, D., Cairney, J., Wainwright, N., Kriellaars, D. and Mitchell, D. (2017) Critical considerations for physical literacy policy in public health, recreation, sport, and education agencies. *Quest*, 69: 1–17.

Durden-Myers, E. (2017) *Physical Literacy and Human Flourishing*. International Physical Literacy Conference, Toronto, Canada, April 2017.

Edwards, L.C., Bryant, A.S., Keegan, R.J., Morgan, K. and Jones, A.M. (2017) Definitions, foundations and associations of physical literacy: a systematic review. *Sports Medicine*, 47(1): 113–126.

Gibson, I., Whitelaw, S., Topping, C. and Kopela, J. (2019) Food and physical literacy: exploring an obesity prevention approach using formative research. *Health Education Journal*. https://doi.org/10.1177/0017896919029775

Giles-Corti, B. and Donovan, R. (2002) The relative influence of individual, social and physical environment determinants of physical activity. *Social Science & Medicine*, 54: 1793–1812.

Giles-Corti, B., Timperio, A., Bull, F. and Pikora, T. (2005) Understanding physical activity environmental correlates: increased specificity for ecological models. *Exercise and Sport Sciences Reviews*, 33(4): 175–181.

Glasby, J. (2016) If integration is the answer, what was the question? What next for English health and social care partnerships? *International Journal of Integrated Care*, 16(4): 1–3.

Green, L. (2006) Public health asks of systems science: to advance our evidence-based practice, can you help us get more practice-based evidence? *American Journal of Public Health*, 96(3): 406–409.

Green, N., Sprake A., Topping, C. and Kopela, J. (2016) Physical literacy – from concept to action: the International Physical Literacy Association guiding Dumfries and Galloway Scotland. *Physical Education Matters*, 11: 64–67.

Green, N., Whitehead, M., Foweather, L., Swaithes, W., Shakespeare, J., Cale, L., Stratton, G., Myers, L., Shearer, C., Goss, H., Morley, D., Holding, L., Thornton-Bousfield, K. and Roberts, W. (on behalf of the Department for Culture, Media and Sport) (2017) *Sport England: Children's Survey Physical Literacy KPI Development*.

Hamlin, C. (1998) *Public Health and Social Justice in the Age of Chadwick: Britain, 1800–1854*. Cambridge: Cambridge University Press.

Harwell, S. (2003) *Teacher Professional Development: It's Not an Event, It's a Process*. Available at: www.cord.org/uploadedfiles/HarwellPaper.pdf (accessed 8 November 2018).

Henderson, E. (2017) *Children, Obesity, and the Future*. Available at: https://blog.oup.com/2017/07/children-obesity-future/ (accessed 8 November 2018).

Improvement and Development Agency (2004) *Making Partnership Work Better in the Culture and Sport Sector: Successful Partnership Working – A Simple Guide to Improving How Your Partnership Works*. London: Improvement and Development Agency.

Information Services Division (2016) *Primary 1 Body Mass Index (BMI) Statistics Scotland School Year 2014/15*. Available at: www.isdscotland.org/Health-Topics/Child-Health/Publications/2016-02-16/2016-02-16-P1-BMI-Statistics-Publication-2014-15-Report.pdf (accessed 22 October 2017).

International Physical Literacy Association (IPLA) (2017a) *International Physical Literacy Association Conference: Physical Literacy and Holistic Health – June 2017*.

International Physical Literacy Association (IPLA) (2017b) *IPLA Foundation Course: Physical Literacy Professional Development*. Available at: www.physical-literacy.org.uk/ipla-foundation-course/ (accessed 13 March 2019).

International Physical Literacy Association Conference (2018) *Physical Literacy? It's Simple*. Available at: www.physical-literacy.org.uk/physical-literacy-simple/ (accessed 8 November 2018).

Kelly, P., McAdam, C. and Turner, K. (2017a) *Best Investments for Physical Activity in Dumfries and Galloway*. Edinburgh, UK: Edinburgh University Press.

Kelly, P., Reid, K. and Williamson, C. (2017b) *Insight Project: Improving Engagement of Young People with Physical Activity Services and Provision in Dumfries and Galloway*. Edinburgh, UK: Edinburgh University Press.

Kohl, H.W., Craig, C.L., Lambert, E.V., Inoue, S., Alkandari, J.R., Leetongin, M.D. and Kahlmeiier, S. (2012) The pandemic of physical inactivity: global action for public health. *Lancet*, 380(9838): 294–305.

Longmuir, P. and Tremblay, M. (2016) Top 10 research questions related to physical literacy. *Research Quarterly for Exercise and Sport*, 87(1): 28–35.

Lundvall, S. (2015) Physical literacy in the field of physical education: a challenge and a possibility. *Journal of Sport and Health Science*, 41: 113–118.

Morris, B., Lawton, R., McEachan, R., Hurling, R. and Conner, M. (2016) Changing self-reported physical activity using different types of affectively and cognitively framed health messages, in a student population. *Psychology Health and Medicine*, 21(2): 1–10.

NHS Dumfries and Galloway and Dumfries and Galloway Council (2018) *Dumfries and Galloway School Physical Activity Survey 2017*. Dumfries, UK: NHS Dumfries and Galloway.

Ohri-Vachaspati, P., DeLia, D., DeWeese, R., Crespo, N., Todd, M. and Yedidia, M. (2015) The relative contribution of layers of the social ecological model to childhood obesity. *Public Health Nutrition*, 18(11): 2055–2066.

Okely, A., Booth, M. and Patterson, J. (2001) Relationship of physical activity to fundamental movement skills among adolescents. *Medicine and Science in Sports and Exercise*, 33(11): 1899–1904.

Parvanta, C., Nelson, D., Parvanta, S. and Harner, R. (2011) *Essentials of Public Health Communication*. London: Jones & Bartlett Learning.

Rhodes, R. and Kates, A. (2015) Can the affective response to exercise predict future motives and physical activity behavior? A systematic review of published evidence. *Annals of Behavioral Medicine*, 49(5): 715–731.

Rhodes, R., Fiala, B. and Conner, M. (2009) A review and meta-analysis of affective judgments and physical activity in adult populations. *Annals of Behavioral Medicine*, 38(3): 180–204.

Sallis J., Cervero, R. Ascher, W., Henderson, K., Kraft, K. and Kerr, J. (2006) An ecological approach to creating active living communities. *Annual Review of Public Health*, 27: 297–322.

Sallis, J., Bull, F., Guthold, R., Heath, G., Inoue, S., Kelly, P., Oyeyemi, A., Perez, L., Richards, J. and Hallal, P. (2016) Progress in physical activity over the Olympic quadrennium. *The Lancet*, 388: 1325–1336.

Scottish Government (2008) *Health and Wellbeing across Learning: Responsibilities of All – Experiences and Outcomes*. Available at: www.education.gov.scot/Documents/hwb-across-learning-eo.pdf (accessed 22 October 2017).

Scottish Government (2015a) *Scottish Health Survey: 2015 Health Board Results*. Edinburgh, UK: Scottish Government.

Scottish Government (2015b) *Active Scotland Outcomes Framework*. Available at: www.gov.scot/About/Performance/scotPerforms/partnerstories/Outcomes-Framework (accessed 13 March 2019).

Scottish Government (2017) *A Healthier Future: Actions and Ambitions on Diet, Activity, and Healthy Weight – Consultation*. Edinburgh, UK: Scottish Government.

Scottish Government (2018a) *A Healthier Future: Scotland's Diet and Obesity Delivery Plan*. Edinburgh, UK: Scottish Government.

Scottish Government (2018b) *A More Active Scotland: Scotland's Physical Activity Delivery Plan*. Edinburgh, UK: Scottish Government.

Scottish Government (2018c) *Framework for the Prevention, Early Detection and Early Intervention of Type 2 Diabetes*. Edinburgh, UK: Scottish Government.

Silva, K.S., Garcia, L.T.G., Rabacow, F. and Sa, T.H. (2017) Physical activity as part of daily living: moving beyond quantitative recommendations. *Preventive Medicine*, 96: 160–162.

Todnem By, R. (2005) Organisational change management: a critical review. *Journal of Change Management*, 5(4): 369–380.

Topping, C., Brodie, S., Henry, C. and Whitelaw, S. (2018) *Measuring Physical Literacy in School Pupils: Developing a Critical Understanding of Physical Activity Behaviours in Children and Young People*. Available at: www.physical-literacy.org.uk/product/ipla-conference-2018-physical-literacy-coaching-community-education/ (accessed 13 November 2018).

Vidgen, H. (2016) *Food Literacy: Key Concepts for Health and Education*. London: Routledge.

Whitehead, M. (2007) Physical literacy: philosophical considerations in relation to developing a sense of self, universality and propositional knowledge. *Sport, Ethics and Philosophy*, 1(3): 281–299.

Whitehead, M. (2010) *Physical Literacy throughout the Lifecourse*. London: Routledge.

World Health Organization (WHO) (2018) *Global Action Plan on Physical Activity 2018–2030: More Active People for a Healthier World*. Geneva: WHO.

Yelon, S., Sheppard, L. and Sleight, D. (2004) Intention to transfer: how do autonomous professionals become motivated to use new ideas. *Performance Improvement Quarterly*, 17(2): 82–103.

14

PHYSICAL LITERACY IN THE UNITED STATES

E. Paul Roetert

Introduction

The construct of physical literacy was brought to the forefront in the 1990s by Margaret Whitehead with renewed interest and focus, in the United States as well as other countries (Whitehead, 1990). Since then, there has been significant activity, discussion and debate, as well as exchange and review of information regarding the value and position of the construct within different sectors of society. This chapter focuses on the progress made to date related to physical literacy in the United States, mostly notably in the sectors of education and sport, as progress in those two sectors has been the most evident. In addition, some specific examples of organisations that are active and successful in promoting and implementing physical literacy concepts will be highlighted.

Background

Like many other countries, the United States faces significant challenges dealing with increases in obesity rates as well as overall physical inactivity of its population. In fact, recent research highlighting the health effects of overweight and obesity in 195 countries over 25 years and published in the *New England Journal of Medicine* showed that among the world's 20 most populous countries, the United States had the highest level of childhood obesity, at 12.7% (GBD 2015 Obesity Collaborators, 2017). In addition, data from the Centers for Disease Control and Prevention (CDC, 2017) indicated that only one in five adults and one in five high school students fully met physical activity guidelines for aerobic and muscle-strengthening activities. The bottom line is that too few Americans get the recommended amount of physical activity. Inadequate levels of physical activity are associated with shorter lifespans, lower overall quality of mental and physical health,

When the United States was founded, there was much debate over the role of the federal government vs. states' rights. This conflict continues to this day. The U.S. Department of Education, for example, cannot mandate that every school in the United States teach physical literacy; it is up to each state and depending on the state, each school district. This decentralized system makes it challenging to reach every child in the U.S. with the concept of physical literacy. In addition, there is often an assumption that if a concept or a program is announced on a federal level, the states will easily adopt the concept or program on the local level. This does not happen automatically and can be especially difficult if there are no incentives or financial support.

FIGURE 14.1 Federalist system of states' rights

increases in annual healthcare costs, and many other overall health and wellness-related issues. This is a multifaceted problem, including health education issues such as proper nutrition habits, and continues to be addressed by a number of different researchers and organisations with moderate success. Additional challenges include a decline in physical education offerings, focus on early sport specialisation often leading to early dropout, and a greater focus on elite sports benefiting mostly the better athletes and/or early maturing children. For a variety of reasons, as will be expounded on in this chapter as well as other chapters in this book, physical literacy can play a major role in helping to solve the challenges listed above and provide a framework for learning the competencies necessary for lifelong physical activity. In fact, the confidence, desire and enjoyment for the lifelong pursuit of physical activity provide key components of physical literacy that should be addressed. With the appropriate help and support from national and state governments (see Figure 14.1), as well as key organisations and associations, who also need to embrace and support the concept, our country as a whole, as well as individuals, can develop the motivation, confidence, physical competence, and knowledge and understanding to value and take responsibility for engagement in physical activities for life (Whitehead, 2013). As this definition indicates, embracing physical literacy will help address obesity and inactivity challenges, but just as important, it will allow individuals to reap the benefits from the enjoyment of participating in physical activities for the full lifespan.

Introduction of physical literacy

Although the term physical literacy is not new to the United States (references in the academic literature can be found for over 80 years), a renewed focus can be traced for the past couple of decades. Physical literacy efforts in countries such as

Australia, Canada and England paved the way for the United States to consider ways to adopt the concept of physical literacy in our academic and educational institutions, as well as sports, recreation and other physical activity-related organisations. This led to early efforts by key national governing bodies (NGBs) of sport, with the assistance of the United States Olympic Committee (USOC) through coaching education programmes, specifically focused on alignment with long-term athletic development (LTAD) programmes. In the education field, the Society of Health and Physical Educators (SHAPE America), the national association for health and physical education in the United States, revised their K–12 physical education national standards, culminating in the incorporation of the term physical literacy (SHAPE America, 2014). Although the USOC and SHAPE America worked independently on their efforts, both included physical literacy-related components in their review of literature, discussions and actions starting at the beginning of this century. The Aspen Institute's (2015) Project Play Physical Literacy Report was the first major collaborative effort at developing ideas on how to introduce and implement physical literacy in the United States. The report provided a model, strategic plan and call to action for physical literacy in the United States. This effort and report addressed the importance of reaching multiple audiences and provided concrete recommendations for practitioners. Therefore, to encourage broad adoption, the Aspen Institute encouraged embracing the following cross-sector simple, useful definition: *physical literacy is the ability, confidence and desire to be physically active for life.* The authors of the report recognised that the pursuit of physical literacy does not end at age 12 (and should certainly be developed beyond that age); however, the main focus of the effort was on creating conditions encouraging habits of health and fitness for life for youth by that age. The recommendations of the report have spurred interest and activity among several organisations and sectors of society. Despite this significant early progress, the United States faces a number of challenges as physical literacy is still considered to be in its infancy. In fact, the greatest activity as well as progress has been in both the education and sport sectors. This chapter therefore highlights key successes, identifies some of the remaining challenges, and offers suggestions to increase the adoption and implementation of physical literacy in the United States in those specific sectors.

Education

As is the case with many other sectors, physical literacy is still very much in its infancy in the United States as it relates to education. A major obstacle to its adoption is the fact that our schools and school districts do not follow a federal curriculum. The closest we have come to a standardised system is the Common Core (www.corestandards.org), which is a set of math and English language standards developed by the National Governor's Association and adopted by 42 states and the District of Columbia, but this system has been controversial in the past few years. Many leaders (both Republican and Democrat) believe that local control may be the best way to ensure each state and district can develop an education system that serves their own students' unique needs. This has led to many non-profit organisations developing standards in fields such as science, art and world languages. In the large majority of states, these standards are adopted for most subject areas, but the adoption of curriculum to fulfil those standards is left up to the individual school districts.

Physical education

Despite the challenges listed above, SHAPE America has made significant strides in introducing and moving physical literacy forward through the inclusion in the national standards, communication with their constituency and dissemination at conferences. In the case of physical education, 50 out of 51 (including Washington, DC) states have adopted state standards that align with SHAPE America's national standards (see Figure 14.2). Since SHAPE America has identified physical literacy as the goal or outcome of physical education, workshops and webinars based on the national standards and grade-level outcomes for physical educators with specific assessment and communication strategies have been provided through both cognitive and psychomotor engagement. Webinars are available live and in recorded format for physical and health educators, sport coaches, and physical education teacher education (PETE) professionals. In discussions with faculty, PETE programmes continue to show interest in embracing physical literacy. The next challenge for SHAPE America regarding the standards is to complete the development of a programme called PE Metrics, a physical education assessment tool to evaluate student achievement of the standards, and therefore inherently physical literacy. This project is currently in progress.

Standard 1 — The physically literate individual demonstrates competency in a variety of motor skills and movement patterns.

Standard 2 — The physically literate individual applies knowledge of concepts, principles, strategies and tactics related to movement and performance.

Standard 3 — The physically literate individual demonstrates the knowledge and skills to achieve and maintain a health-enhancing level of physical activity and fitness.

Standard 4 — The physically literate individual exhibits responsible personal and social behavior that respects self and others.

Standard 5 — The physically literate individual recognizes the value of physical activity for health, enjoyment, challenge, self-expression and/or social interaction.

FIGURE 14.2 SHAPE America's national standards

From a policy perspective, SHAPE America has also assumed the lead in the physical education sector with the support of Voices for Healthy Kids, an initiative of the American Heart Association and the Robert Wood Johnson Foundation (SHAPE America, 2016). Since implementing physical literacy-related projects on the federal level in the United States is an enormous task, targeting key influential states would seem to be a way to ignite the physical literacy movement in the United States. If the above-named organisations are successful in a few states, it will be easier to convince other states to emulate the example of the physical literacy pioneer states. Support by governors does carry some weight in the form of governors' councils or programmes run by the executive office, but to provide sustainability at the state level, policy and legislation must be passed. State legislatures could be campaigned using the Voices for Healthy Kids model in a coordinated approach. The importance of allowing for adaptation at the state and local level is key in achieving widespread success or adoption. In addition, the physical literacy community needs to develop arguments that explain how adopting physical literacy standards in a state would help the governor's priorities. For example, promoting physical literacy could help reduce childhood obesity as well as overall physical inactivity, and over time reduce healthcare costs. Another related topic would be to evaluate the plans states submit for the Every Student Succeeds Act (ESSA), a bipartisan measure focused on a long-standing commitment to equal opportunity for all students. These plans indicate that a majority of states have selected 'chronic absenteeism' as their overall goal, and therefore SHAPE America can help to support our physical literacy efforts by attaching wellness benefits with overarching educational benefits (e.g. we know that healthier, fitter kids come to school more often). A similar way of thinking can and should be carried forward to the adult population. Clearly, a physically fit population is a potential asset for attracting new business to each governor's state. This type of approach can help in showing how the concept of physical literacy can improve the fiscal health of their states. Since funding for school districts around the country continues to be a challenge, and many do not have the resources to develop new curricula, convincing governors as well as state and local school leaders could provide the momentum needed to take the next steps in adopting physical literacy to a greater extent.

Military

Teaching physical literacy in our schools can ultimately help our national security in the future as well. People in the United States have a high esteem for the military, and with terrorist threats looming, Americans want to make sure we have strong military members. Only about 1% of Americans volunteer to serve in our armed forces, yet spending in the military is one of the largest portions of our federal budget. The biggest asset the US military has is its people. But like the rest of the United States, the military is seeing challenges with recruitment. Nearly one in four young adults are not eligible for the military because of obesity, and 1 in every 13 current troops are overweight. In fact, each year, the military discharges over 1,200 first-term enlistees because of weight problems. The military must then recruit and train their replacements at a cost of $50,000 for each man or woman, thus spending more than $60 million a year (NCPPA, 2017). Physical literacy leaders may want to research if there are military installations in the states where they have targeted governors to help further convince key leaders in each state that physical literacy is important for our safety and security. There are national organisations such as Mission Readiness (www.strongnation. org/missionreadiness) that have retired military leaders willing to speak about the importance of nutrition and physical activity in our schools. As Richard R. Jeffries, Rear Admiral, U.S. Navy (Retired) and former Medical Officer of the U.S. Marine Corps, said, 'If we don't take steps now to build a strong, healthy foundation for our young people, then it will not just be our military that pays the price – our nation as a whole will suffer also' (Trust for America's Health and Robert Wood Johnson Foundation, 2017: 13).

Research

Most of the research related to physical literacy in the United States thus far has focused on philosophical and promotional articles explaining the benefits of the concept (Roetert and Jefferies, 2014; Hastie and Wallhead, 2015; Roetert and Couturier MacDonald, 2015) or questioning if, and/or commenting on, how physical literacy is truly different from physical education or physical activity (Lounsbery and McKenzie, 2015; Corbin, 2016; Roetert, 2016). For example, changing the term from 'physically educated person' to 'physically literate individual' in the national standards met with some resistance either for philosophical reasons or the concern that a new term might cause confusion for the end user. However, taking a different view, and as has been explained in several follow-up articles in the United States, physical literacy as a lifelong journey provides the framework to update the definition of a physically educated person, and at the same time provides parallel language to other subjects in schools such as health literacy and math literacy (Castelli et al., 2015; Ennis, 2015; Lundvall, 2015; Roetert et al., 2017a). Among other groups, SHAPE America and the American College of Sports Medicine (ACSM) could play a major role stimulating and promoting research related to physical literacy. As a starting point, researchers have started encouraging different sectors of society, such as the sports medicine sector (Roetert et al., 2018), in addressing and embracing physical literacy. In addition, more research, such as a recent article highlighting the health, fitness and physical activity sectors with a focus on the older population, is needed to help promote physical literacy for the full lifespan (Roetert and Ortega, 2019). Measuring the benefits of the nationwide implementation of the national standards, enacting on successful models across schools, highlighting positive policy changes, and addressing new and different sectors of society are additional examples of potential future areas of research.

Sport

Unlike most developed countries in the world, the United States does not have a Ministry of Sport to develop national athletic priorities. Without a ministry, we also lack funding to promote sports concepts in the United States. The closest entity we have in the United States to a Ministry of Sport is the United States Olympic Committee (USOC). The Ted Stevens Olympic and Amateur Sports Act designated the USOC as the coordinating body for all athletic activity for international competitions, and they were also assigned the role of promoting and supporting physical fitness and public participation in athletic activities. Also, unlike other countries, the USOC does not receive federal funding, and relies on private donations and sponsors to implement its programming. With the pressure to bring home gold medals at every Olympic Games, the USOC does not have the resources to promote physical literacy in the United States on its own. Having stated that, the leadership of the USOC clearly understands the importance of promoting sport for the masses, and among other projects has most recently focused on long-term athlete development (LTAD), as well as addressing the concern of kids dropping out of sports at young ages (by age 12, there is typically a large drop-off in participation). The national governing bodies (NGBs) of sport, such as U.S. Swimming and U.S. Hockey, have been supportive of physical literacy as well, but their main goal is also to recruit and train champions, not educate the entire US population on physical literacy.

Progress at the national level

Fortunately, significant progress is being made in not only the awareness of physical literacy, but also the implementation of specific projects and programmes. Since the initial introduction of both the LTAD and physical literacy concepts by the USOC coaching education department and several NGBs at the beginning of this century, programmes were developed mainly based on the work of the Canadian Sport for Life programme (CS4L). The United States has since adopted its own version of the LTAD programme, which in the United States is now known as the American Development Model (ADM). The model focuses not just on Olympic and Paralympic success, but also utilises long-term athlete development concepts to promote sustained physical activity and participation in sport. These concepts have been tailored to create a framework for developing American youth through sport. The USOC and its NGBs have developed the following five key athlete development principles, which are in line with the concept of physical literacy and allow youth to utilise sport as a path towards an active and healthy lifestyle, and create opportunities for athletes to maximise their full potential:

1. Universal access to create opportunity for all athletes.
2. Developmentally appropriate activities that emphasise motor and foundational skills.

3. Multi-sport participation.
4. Fun, engaging and progressively challenging atmosphere.
5. Quality coaching at all age levels.

The ADM also features a physical literacy training component that is likely to grow and improve motor skill development of athletes at all ages. In 2017, the USOC formed a committee of experts from multi-sport organisations to study early sport specialisation concerns and dropout rates in youth sports. The mission statement for this committee was 'to increase youth sport participation and physical literacy education through improving collaboration with USOC partner and member organizations' (USOC Youth Sport Working Group, 2017). As listed above, providing universal access to create opportunity for all athletes was a key goal. An example of this group's work is an article prepared by a subgroup of this committee for *Olympic Coach* magazine focused on 'physical literacy for all'. The article highlights that:

> Just as it is important for the general population to continue to participate in sports and general physical activities throughout a person's full lifespan, it is also important for athletes with disabilities to explore and learn a full range of sports and recreation, so they can enjoy a healthy lifestyle alongside their family and friends.
>
> *(Roetert et al., 2017b: 12)*

Further, the article challenges coaches to consider if there are specific ways in which they can integrate children with disabilities within group lessons or training sessions, and better ways in which coaches could modify their teaching and coaching techniques. It concludes with the recommendation that coaches need to continue to look for ways to integrate athletes with and without disabilities to enhance both the coaches' growth and knowledge, but also that of the athletes themselves. Many of the NGBs provided input on the overall work of this youth sport participation committee. In addition to seeking alignment with the ADM, the focus will be on supporting the Aspen Institute's (2015) Project Play suggested strategies.

National governing bodies of sport

Due to size, financial challenges and individual differences, each NGB implements components that work best for their sport. Some NGBs have shown clear successes in the implementation of physical literacy components to their programmes. For example, U.S. Ski & Snowboard helped with the development of the initial ADM programme based on their Nordic skiing efforts, USA Track & Field introduced a run/jump/throw programme to help youth learn sport and movement through track-and-field-related activities, the United States Tennis Association has launched Net Generation by bringing together a national community of parents, coaches, players, teachers and volunteers through a variety of programmes, teaching and learning tools to capture the imaginations of kids of all backgrounds and skill levels, while USA Hockey (ice hockey) built a variety of resources around dry land training to help coaches and athletes build the agility, balance and coordination (ABC) skills around their sport. In many ways, NGBs and their coaches are the easiest to reach because of our governance structure. Hardest to reach are the actual coaches and administrators in the field that are part of individual sports clubs or youth leagues that operate independently. An additional challenge is a full understanding of the concept of physical literacy by the public, which includes many volunteer coaches. Often, even if volunteer coaches have heard the term physical literacy, they will first look for sport-specific resources before thinking about overall athlete development or understanding the concept of physical literacy. Although several of the NGBs have been supportive of physical literacy, they have limited resources to reach every local chapter of their sport. The physical literacy community could work with the state or regional chapters of the NGBs in the same states where they have targeted governors, and offer to work together to help train and inform local sports leagues, as well as coaches, directly about the benefits of physical literacy and to their sport and athletes. In addition, from a grass-roots perspective, we could highlight some existing regional or local programmes in different areas of the country by highlighting their successes. This is where multi-sport and fitness organisations can play a significant role in the promotion and implementation of physical literacy activities and programmes. With that in mind, below are some current programmes that can serve as great examples.

National multi-sport/fitness organisations

One example of a multi-sport organisation, with a significant national reach, that is concerned about overall athlete development and has embraced the concept of physical literacy is the Boys & Girls Clubs of America (BGCA). This national organisation, which is headquartered in Atlanta, Georgia, provides programming for youth through more than 1,100 independently and locally governed organisations and 4,300 club facilities throughout the country, as well as BGCA-affiliated youth centres on US military installations worldwide. The BGCA is focused on after-school programmes with the goal of enabling all young people, especially those who need it most, to reach their full potential as productive, caring, responsible citizens. Their Triple Play programme, which is based on comprehensive health and wellness, strives to improve the overall health of club members ages 6–18 by increasing their daily physical activity, teaching good nutrition and helping develop healthy relationships. Utilising their expertise in youth development, the BGCA combined the existing Triple Play programme with the concept of physical literacy in 2015. Seeing a need to address the lack of available information and resources for coaches, teachers, mentors and parents to assist 'non-competitive teenagers' to develop into 'active for life' adults, they developed a new physical literacy framework. After evaluating multiple 'athletic development models', the BGCA created a model of physical literacy development focused on best practices for staff as well as keeping teens engaged (currently in draft form; see Figure 14.3). Wayne B. Moss, BGCA Senior Director, Sports, Fitness & Recreation, believes that:

> Although this is a good base for expanding the concept of physical literacy throughout the youth development sector, much work remains to be done. The next steps for the lifetime physical activity model include: refining the foci of each stage; expanding the framework to include specific staff practices and competencies for optimal development at each stage of age, ability, confidence, and desire; and developing tools to assess the physical literacy of youth.

With the inclusion of nutrition, the different components form a physical health pathway. All components of the physical health pathway must support the ability, confidence, and desire of young people to be physically active and eat a balanced diet daily. According to Moss:

> This support across programmes and through a diverse set of age and culturally specific and inclusive practices will lead to physical and nutritional literacy. This higher level of literacy will then in turn manifest in more regular health practices and a lifelong commitment and expression of physical health.

Another organisation with a major national impact is the American Council on Exercise (ACE). The ACE is a global non-profit fitness certification, education and training organisation, is committed to getting people of all ages to adopt healthy lifestyle behaviours, and consequently has supported the promotion of physical literacy with the intent of helping set the stage for a healthier, more active and more productive generation of young people. The ACE offers several resources (e.g. youth fitness curriculum, youth and family activity, focused articles and videos, blogs and tips) aimed at educating and empowering parents, schools, health and fitness professionals, and community leaders to help children and adolescents get started on a lifelong journey of physical literacy and movement. In addition, the ACE has provided sponsorship funding for a number of physical literacy-focused projects, including the Aspen Institute's Project Play and Physical Literacy Working Group initiatives, the BOKS before-school physical activity programme with integrated physical literacy concepts (www.bokskids.org), and the U.S. Report Card on Physical Activity for Children & Adolescents (www.physicalactivityplan.org/reportcard/NationalReportCard_longform_final%20for%20web.pdf). According to Cedric X. Bryant, Ph.D., FACSM (ACE Chief Science Officer and member of the Aspen Institute's Physical Literacy Working Group):

> Because the concept of physical literacy is so perfectly compatible with, and complementary to, the ACE mission, it's been a virtual no-brainer to support. That said, the fact that American children received a very low grade

in 'overall physical activity' and 'sedentary behaviours' illustrated the great need to continue to work collaboratively to expand the level of awareness and adoption of physical literacy concepts and principles – in many respects, the health of our future depends on it.

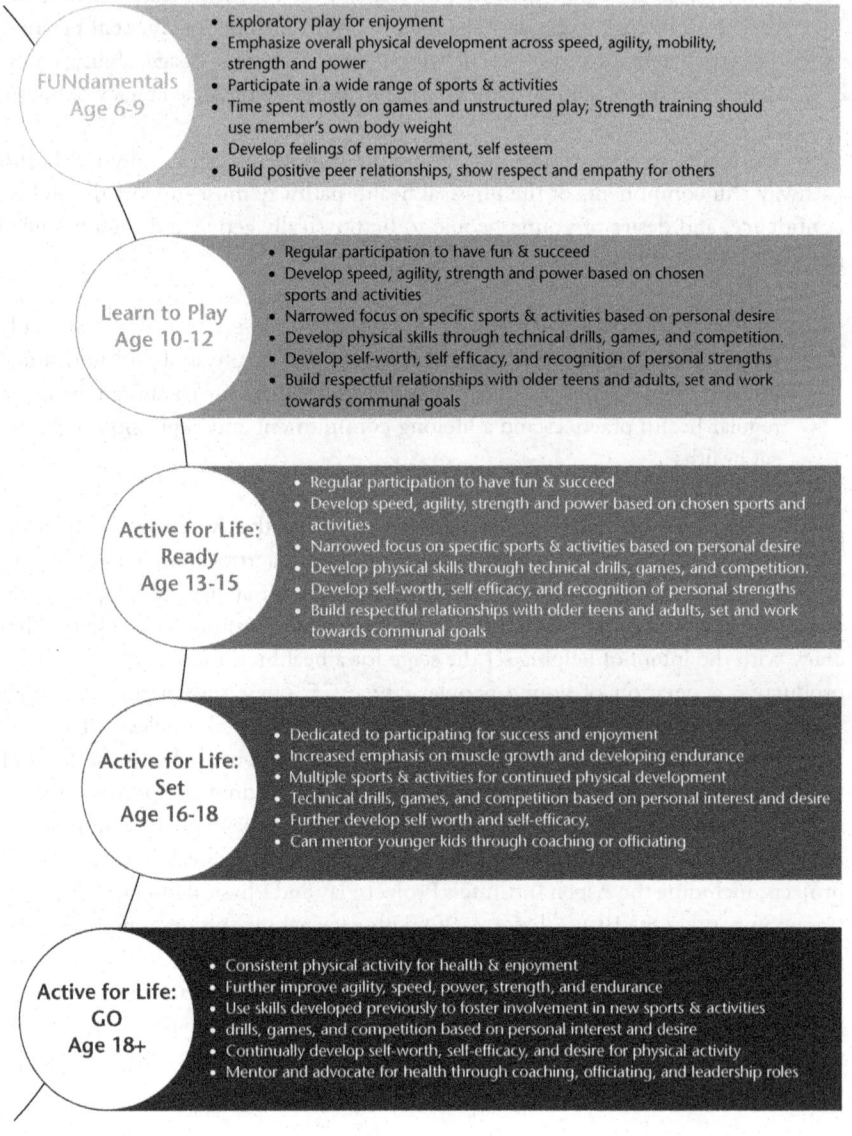

FIGURE 14.3 'A life of movement': the BGCA's lifetime physical activity model

Source: Reprinted with permission of the Boys & Girls Clubs of America

Progress at the regional/local level

One organisation that has fully embraced physical literacy is 2-4-1 Sports (http://241sports.com/), headquartered in the state of Connecticut, which has expanded in other states such as Colorado. Their philosophy is that 'life's 2 short 4 just 1 sport', which is emphasised throughout their trainings, camps and a wide variety of sports clinics. Working primarily in the education sector, their approach to lifelong wellness recognises the mind/body connection and the value of nutrition and mindfulness as they relate to physical literacy. In addition, there is a significant focus on 'sport sampling' (experiencing a range of physical activities) and participating in multiple sports. The overall goal of this holistic approach for the participants is that they become better athletes, better students, and more engaged members of society. According to Founder and Director, Steve Boyle, 'As kids, parents, teachers, and administrators work through our P.L.U.S. (Physical Literacy United States) programming, they will learn how to move, what fuels the body for optimal growth, and how to feel good about themselves while having fun'. For the purpose of highlighting their holistic approach, they have modified the definition of physical literacy to state that it is the 'ability, balance, confidence, desire and explorative nature to be active for life'. In addition, they use a working definition illuminating the name of the organisation ('the ability, confidence, and desire 2 be active 4 – 1 extraordinary life'). Another component that sets their programme apart is that they encourage getting kids to be active with video-based 'BrainErgizers' in the classroom throughout the school. The premise is that kids will not only enjoy the physical activity, but being active will also stimulate their brain and allow them to focus better. Through a partnership with a university, success of the programme continues to be monitored. Although well received at the school and community level, there continue to be some challenges, primarily in reaching and educating parents, as well as obtaining funding to provide these programmes on a larger scale.

Another programme that has achieved community success is Gators in Motion (GIM), an after-school sports-based programme that is the outcome of a partnership between the University of Florida's (UF) Department of Tourism, Recreation and Sport Management and the United States Tennis Association (USTA) Foundation's local National Junior Tennis and Learning programme, Aces in Motion (AIM) (www.acesinmotion.org/gatorsinmotion). The programme focuses on local underserved youth, with a focus on the inclusion of those living in the marginalised communities of East Gainesville. The overall goal to positively change lives is achieved through a combination of academic support, mentoring and sport. Utilising a multifaceted approach to facilitate the holistic development of their participants, GIM provides an after-school component emphasising academic achievement, character development and physical activity. To this end, participants are provided: (1) a space on UF's campus in which they are introduced to college life, exposed to various career pathways from talks with guest speakers and facility tours, as well as access to one-on-one tutoring from college students; (2) a mentoring curriculum emphasising life skills and character enhancement through nine principles of personal development; (3) both a tennis-based curriculum as well as a sport sampling model stressing physical literacy and activity; (4) educational resources regarding a healthy and active lifestyle; and (5) a 'coaches in training' programme highlighting goal-setting skills, community service, and leadership development for previous students wishing to contribute to the future of their community's youth. Together, these components allow for the programme to offer a unique blend of sport, life lessons, and academic tutoring aimed at facilitating personal and life skills development, enhancing academic skills, fostering a desire for education, as well as increasing an understanding of physical literacy and activity. In October 2018, this programme was highlighted in the 'Bright Ideas' section of the *British Journal of Sports Medicine* (Bopp and Roetert, 2018).

Summary comments

Progress related to the understanding, adoption and implementation of the construct of physical literacy in the United States has been steady over the past decade. As is evidenced by the activities of both national and regional organisations, a top-down as well as bottom-up approach is likely going to provide the greatest continued progress towards success of physical literacy-related programs in the United States. Organisations, such as the ones highlighted in this chapter, continue to provide guidance through planning meetings, publications, presentations and social media outlets. Having said that, much work is still left to be done. Unlike many other countries, federal funding for formal physical education and sport-related programmes is not considered a major priority. Sport-related programmes rely on professional and private organisations to support activities, while physical education programmes tend to be a low priority within school budgets, which are a combination of state and federal funding. As such, neither formal system has demonstrated motivation to invest in these areas. Similar to other countries, sedentary behaviour and overall physical inactivity continue to be a problem for all age groups.

Physical literacy can be the solution as it not only focuses on learning the competencies of physical activity, but also addresses the motivation, desire, confidence, enjoyment, and social and ecological benefits of being physically active for the full lifespan. Understanding and teaching the concepts that develop these components of physical literacy can help us address future challenges. These challenges include developing a unified message regarding the construct of physical literacy, the promotion and support of physical literacy-related research, and reaching different sectors of society not currently reached sufficiently, such as public health, business and industry, recreation, transportation/community design, and the older population. Finally, advocacy for the construct at national, regional and local levels, gaining media support and collaboration of each country with key international organisations, such as the International Physical Literacy Association (IPLA), will help in highlighting and amplifying the importance and relevance of physical literacy-related programmes. This book is a great step towards providing an understanding of the history, as well as the current status and future challenges related to physical literacy in each of the countries highlighted. Together, these components allow for the programme to offer a unique blend of sport, life lessons and academic tutoring. The goals are aimed at facilitating personal and life skills development, enhancing academic skills, and fostering a desire for education. As a cohesive unit, they are designed to increase an understanding of physical literacy and activity.

Contributors

I would like to thank the following people who contributed to the content of this chapter: Trevor Bopp, Steve Boyle, Cedric Bryant, Lynn Couturier MacDonald, Wayne Moss, Cheryl Richardson, Robin Schepper, Chris Snyder and Carly Wright.

References

Aspen Institute (2015) *Physical Literacy in the United States: A Model, Strategic Plan and Call to Action.* Available at: http://plreport.projectplay.us (accessed 1 February 2018).

Bopp, T. and Roetert, E.P. (2018) Gators in Motion: a holistic approach to sport-based youth development. *British Journal of Sports Medicine*, published online first, 12 October 2018, doi: 10.1136/bjsports-2018-099528.

Castelli, D.M., Barcelona, J.M. and Bryant, L. (2015) Contextualizing physical literacy in the school environment: the challenges. *Journal of Sport and Health Science*, 4: 156–163.

Centers for Disease Control and Prevention (CDC) (2017) *Active People, Healthy Nation Initiative.* Atlanta, GA: Centers for Disease Control and Prevention.

Corbin, C.B. (2016) Implications of physical literacy for research and practice: a commentary. *Research Quarterly for Exercise and Sport*, 87: 14–27.

Ennis, C.D. (2015) Knowledge, transfer and innovation in physical literacy curricula. *Journal of Sport and Health Science*, 4: 119–124.

GBD 2015 Obesity Collaborators (2017) Health effects of overweight and obesity in 195 countries over 25 years. *New England Journal of Medicine*, 377: 13–27.

Hastie, P.A. and Wallhead, T.L. (2015) Operationalizing physical literacy through sport education. *Journal of Sport and Health Science*, 4: 132–138.

Lounsbery, M.A.F. and McKenzie, T.L. (2015) Physically literate and physically educated: a rose by any other name? *Journal of Sport and Health Science*, 4: 139–144.

Lundvall, S. (2015) Physical literacy in the field of physical education: a challenge and a possibility. *Journal of Sport and Health Science*, 4: 113–118.

National Coalition for Promoting Physical Activity (NCPPA) (2017) *Let's Get Physical.* Washington, DC: National Coalition for Promoting Physical Activity.

Roetert, E.P. (2016) Physical literacy: more than just a new fad. *Physical Activity Plan Alliance Commentaries on Physical Activity and Health*, 2(1). Available at: www.physicalactivityplan. org/commentaries/Roetert.html (accessed 14 March 2019).

Roetert, E.P. and Couturier MacDonald, L. (2015) Unpacking the physical literacy concept for K–12 physical education: what should we expect the learner to master? *Journal of Sport and Health Science*, 4: 108–112.

Roetert, E.P. and Jefferies, S.C. (2014) Embracing physical literacy. *Journal of Physical Education, Recreation and Dance*, 85(8): 38–40.

Roetert, E.P. and Ortega, C. (2019) Physical literacy for the older adult. *Strength and Conditioning Journal*, 41(2): 89–99.

Roetert, E.P., Kriellaars, D., Ellenbecker, T.S. and Richardson, C. (2017a) Preparing students for a physically literate life. *Journal of Physical Education, Recreation and Dance*, 88(1): 58–62.

Roetert, E.P., Ray, J. and Meserve, B. (2017b) Physical literacy for all. *Olympic Coach*, 28(1): 12–14.

Roetert, E.P., Ellenbecker, T.S. and Kriellaars, D. (2018) Physical literacy for clinicians: why should we embrace this construct? *British Journal of Sports Medicine*, 52(20): 1291–1292.

Society of Health and Physical Educators (SHAPE America) (2014) *National Standards and Grade-Level Outcomes for K–12 Physical Education*. Champaign, IL: Human Kinetics.

Society of Health and Physical Educators (SHAPE America) (2016) *SHAPE of the Nation Report*. Available at: www.shapeamerica.org//advocacy/son/2016/upload/Shape-of-the-Nation-2016_web.pdf (accessed 14 March 2019).

Trust for America's Health and Robert Wood Johnson Foundation (2017) *The State of Obesity: Better Policies for a Healthier America – 2017*.

USOC Youth Sport Working Group (2017) *Final Report to USOC Board of Directors*. Submitted for November 2017 board meeting.

Whitehead, (1990) Physical literacy: meaningful existence, embodiment and physical education. *Journal of Philosophy of Education*, 24(1). Available at: www.physical-literacy.org.uk?jpe-1990.php (accessed 14 March 2019).

Whitehead, M. (2013) *International Physical Literacy Association Definition*. Available at: www.physical-literacy.org.uk/ (accessed 14 March 2019).

Personal communications were conducted with:

Steve Boyle, Founder/Director, 2-4-1 Sports – 18 October 2017.
Cedric Bryant, PhD, Chief Science Officer, American Council on Exercise – 8 December 2017.
Wayne Moss, Senior Director, Sports, Fitness & Recreation, Boys & Girls Clubs of America – 13 November 2017.

15

PHYSICAL LITERACY DEVELOPMENT IN WALES

Helen Hughes

Introduction

The development of physical literacy in Wales has been a progressive journey since 2008, and we still have a long way to go. There has been a lot of learning along the way, much of which has stemmed from giving something a try, being innovative and taking risks. Have we got everything right? Maybe not. More importantly, have we learned from the experiences? Yes. We recognise that the key lies within education to lay down the foundations. If physical literacy is not embedded within curriculum delivery as a platform to build upon, any advocacy or interventions that take place outside the school gates will be a harder task. However, education cannot achieve this alone as physical literacy is a lifelong journey for every individual. Everyone is unique with different life experiences, environments and contributors along the way. The place of Sport Wales as an organisation is to help bring the right people together to make a real difference across all communities in Wales. How much or how little our part is, the big picture is still being determined, but at the very least we have been the catalyst in the agenda and encouraged partners to experiment with their thinking, programmes and delivery.

Sport Wales

Sport Wales is the national organisation responsible for developing and promoting sport and physical activity in Wales. We are the main adviser on sporting matters to the Welsh Government, with a responsibility for distributing National Lottery funds to both elite and grass-roots sport across the country. As an organisation, we are committed to developing an active, healthy and successful Wales, where every citizen, from every community, can participate in sport and physical recreation and reach their potential, irrespective of background and circumstance. Since 2000,

Sport Wales has been commissioned to support the development and delivery of sport and physical activity programmes within schools across Wales. The organisation has a proven track record in coordinating the delivery of sport and physical activity within school settings and in the community, and the capability to unite a network of experts across organisations and institutions to work in collaboration. Therefore, Sport Wales are a well-positioned central body to lead on the physical literacy agenda in Wales.

Over the past 17 years, there have been several programmes and initiatives that delivered many successes, but with this came a tremendous amount of learning. In 2000, we introduced the Dragon Sport programme, which aimed to enhance extracurricular provision for 7- to 11-year-olds (Key Stage 2). The year 2002 saw the introduction of the PE and School Sport (PESS) programme, which supported curriculum physical education (PE) through targeted professional development opportunities (Sport Wales, 2001). The success achieved within Dragon Sport and PESS highlighted a gap in provision for secondary schools. This led to the introduction of the 5x60 programme in 2006 targeting secondary schools' extracurricular provision (Sport Wales, 2006).

Finding physical literacy

Sport Wales initially stumbled across the concept of physical literacy a decade ago. In 2008, Sport Wales was given the opportunity to work within the foundation phase (Welsh Government, 2008). In Wales, this phase covers 3- to 7-year-olds. Our remit was to provide guidance and training to support practitioners in their curriculum provision for physical development and creative movement. In retrospect, this was a significant breakthrough for us due to our original remit not starting until Key Stage 2. We were given a blank canvas and a new phase in which to work. This began with seven months of research and consultation, engaging with early years practitioners to ensure that whatever we created was fit for purpose. It was during the research phase that the concept of physical literacy came to our attention.

It was apparent that physical literacy had a lot of synergy with our thinking in terms of the need for a holistic, child-centred approach to teaching and learning, which needed to be at the heart of what we created to support the foundation phase. After nearly three years in development, we produced a resource and training package entitled Play to Learn (Sport Wales, 2010). As a 'People and Programme Development Team' within the organisation, the fundamental shift stemmed from our learning in creating Play to Learn. It provided much more than just a PE resource that would sit alongside a maths or literacy equivalent. Up until this point, we had been activity- or sports-specific in our approaches. Our awareness of the physical literacy concept was not there in those early days of PESS. We would traditionally create specific genres of resources and training such as dance, gymnastics and team games. In Play to Learn, we created something very different, something that was much more holistic in the way it could be delivered, linking across other curricular areas. It took a thematic approach to teaching and learning, which signalled a significant shift from what we had done traditionally. Furthermore, in 2012, we launched the Play to Learn website (Sport Wales, 2012b) to encourage and support parents/carers and family members to play a part.

Adoption of physical literacy

Since 2010, Sport Wales has adopted the concept of physical literacy as a key strand of its core business. Sport Wales introduced the sector's Vision for Sport in Wales in 2011 (Sport Wales, 2011) with an aspiration of getting 'every child hooked on sport for life'. Our definition of 'hooked' was 'participating in physical activity three times or more per week'. A strategic priority within the Vision was 'skills for a life in sport', where every child and young person is helped to acquire the skills and confidence from an early age to foster physical literacy through high-quality, engaging sporting experiences. At an organisation level, this signified a change in approach to both strategic design and delivery, away from siloed, age-specific programmes, to a broader continuum of learning or a 'journey' of experiences. The learning from Play to Learn then resulted in trying to make sense of all the other initiatives in which we had been involved.

The year 2010 saw the tenth anniversary of Dragon Sport, which led to a programme review. It was clear that the programme needed reinventing to ensure we had a continuum leading on from Play to Learn. This led to the introduction of the Dragon Multi-Skills and Sport programme (Sport Wales, 2012a), which replaced the more traditional Dragon Sport. We needed to make sure that all the key players were on the same page, whether that is in a curriculum, extracurricular activities or community programme, adding value and making sense of it in terms of messaging for the end user – the child.

Furthermore, in 2015, Sport Wales conducted its biennial School Sport Survey, which returned 110,000 responses from children across Wales. The survey results identified that young people are more likely to be 'hooked on sport for life' if they develop the skills and confidence both to take part in and enjoy activities. These are critical components of physical literacy, and with the most recent statistics indicating that only 48% are 'hooked' (Sport Wales, 2015b), there is much work to do. With the clear link between pupil voice and its alignment with physical literacy, this provided further traction and merit to commit to exploring physical literacy further.

Following on from the PESS programme, in 2014 we introduced the Physical Literacy Programme for Schools (PLPS) (Sport Wales, 2014b), acknowledging the recommendations of the Welsh Government Physical Activity Report (Welsh Government, 2013). The most recent outcome of this investment was to embed physical literacy at the heart of 'physical literacy beacon schools' for pupils to become 'healthy and confident young people' who regularly build physical activity into their lives. The PLPS funding enhanced teachers' and teaching assistants' knowledge and understanding of the delivery of PE and the physical literacy journey of their pupils across 12 beacon clusters of schools. This enabled the beacon schools to have a better understanding of physical literacy, the types of pedagogical approaches and model-based practices that develop physical literacy, and the holistic relationship between physical literacy and the broader health and well-being of their pupils. The Sport, Physical Education and Activity Research (SPEAR), Canterbury Christ Church University *Impact Evaluation Report* (SPEAR, 2016) of the PLPS programme and the Physical Literacy Framework (now known as the Physical Literacy Journey, or PLJ) highlighted the impact of PLPS interventions on young people. It reported improvements in young people's physical, social and emotional development, as well as young people's engagement, attendance and behaviour. It also demonstrated the effective pedagogy utilised within these interventions.

Moving beyond education

During the final twelve months of PLPS, Sport Wales created a tripartite partnership between higher education institutes, education consortia and schools to support the development of physical literacy across the four regions of Wales. An important feature of this work was the establishment of a collaborative research group. The group included University of Wales Trinity St David's, Cardiff Metropolitan University, University of South Wales, Bangor University and Glyndwr University, and involved using action research in each region to explore the development of physical literacy in schools. The main aim of this research group, chaired by the Director of the Welsh Institute of Physical Literacy, was to gain a deeper understanding of the issues of implementing sustainable change in relation to physical literacy, and as such health and well-being as an aspect of curriculum development.

When we first started talking of 'physical literacy' within the sport sector and across wider partners within education and health, we were faced with a lot of confusion and subsequent questions. At that point in time, we were using the 2012 definition of physical literacy: 'A disposition acquired by human individuals encompassing the motivation, confidence, physical competence, knowledge and understanding that establishes purposeful physical pursuits as an integral part of their lifestyle' (www.physical-literacy.org.uk). We quickly realised that across the sector, there was a need to translate the concept to help people in Wales understand its importance and the role they can play. To aid understanding, we simplified the definition and drew up the following translation or 'equation':

physical skills + confidence + motivation + lots of opportunities = physical literacy

We wanted everyone, including children, parents, grandparents, teachers, coaches and young leaders, to connect with the concept. By breaking down the terminology and explaining the definition and philosophy in simple terms, it was evident that people who then understood physical literacy were excited and engaged in the potential. To get the physical literacy message out there simply and encourage people to engage, we created a suite of communication tools. Our aim was to explain the concept, advocate the importance and suggest that everyone has a part to play in the agenda. Given that we had the remit from the Welsh Government to specifically target education in the first instance, the communication was channelled through the PESS and PLPS projects.

However, initially steps were taken within Sport Wales to ensure that our own staff within the community sport, communication and insight teams had a secure and consistent understanding of physical literacy. This was achieved through staff briefings and inviting key staff to physical literacy events. Some of the communication tools we created satisfied both internal and external messaging. However, while we made inroads, we recognised there was still a significant amount of upskilling to undertake.

Communicating the message

Our first 'tool' was our physical literacy video clip (see Figure 15.1). The video uses a 4-year-old child to deliver a strong message to all, making physical literacy everyone's business. The idea was taken from a Thomson in-flight health and safety message delivered by a child on screen, which seemed to be a very effective approach to grabbing people's attention. We felt we could take the same approach, as people are much more likely to sit up and take notice of a message delivered by a child than by an adult.

This 90-second clip sparked people's thinking as to what physical literacy is. However, the video could only do so much, which was to convey what physical literacy is and its importance. It far exceeded our initial expectations, and did in fact have an international reach, becoming one of our physical literacy success stories.

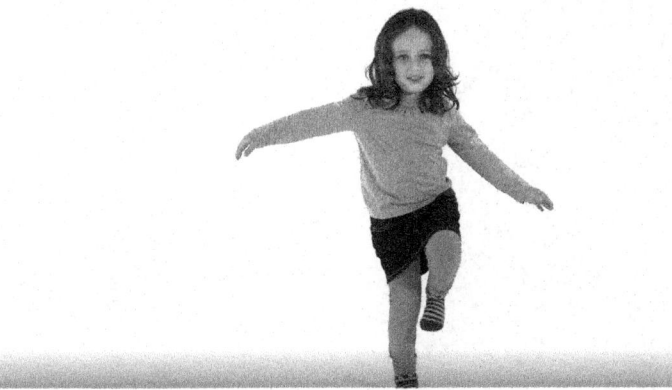

FIGURE 15.1 Amelia from our first 'tool' – physical literacy video clip

Source: Reproduced courtesy of Sport Wales (2013)

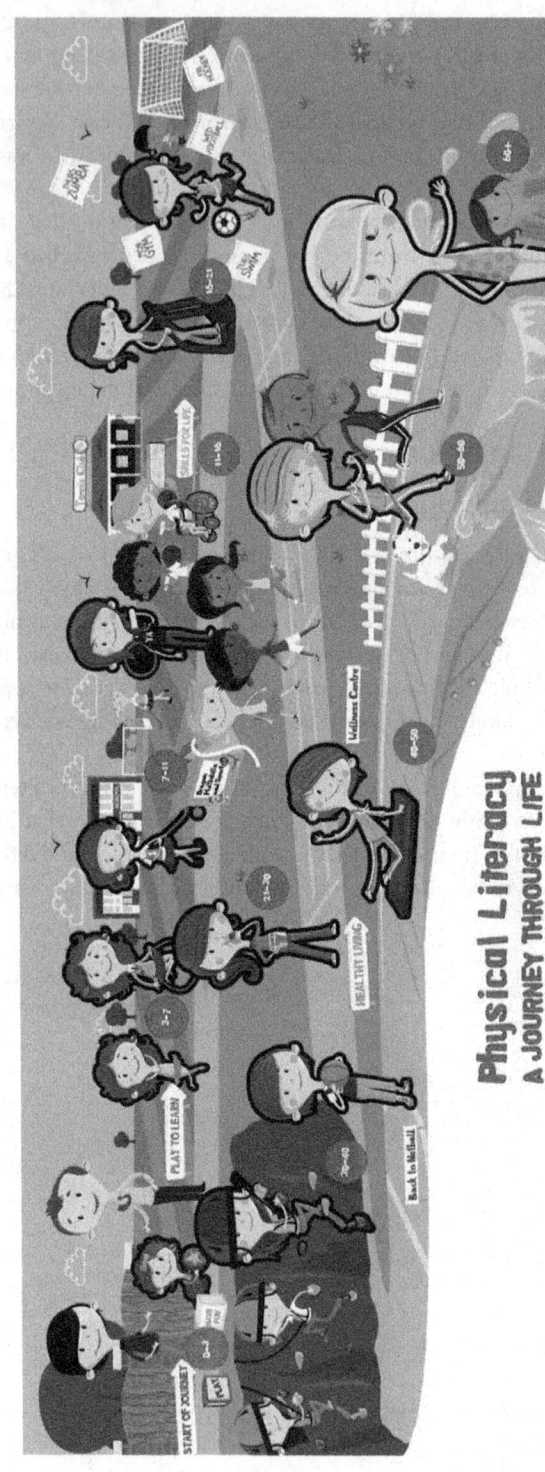

FIGURE 15.2 Sport Wales physical literacy journey poster

Source: Reproduced courtesy of Sport Wales (2014a)

On the flip side, it did make people query whether the video was more weighted towards the physical competency strand of the concept, but the intention was for the 4-year-old to convey all strands. This was a difficult task, which led us to the second phase of our communication tools – the physical literacy journey poster (see Figure 15.2).

Our physical literacy poster allowed us to deliver more layers of messaging beyond that which the video could achieve. This poster was our next chapter, another visual featuring 4-year-old Amelia, but in an illustrated journey concept, or lifecourse from birth through her school years, adulthood and into later life. We could portray what is important as a recipient in the early years (exploring and having fun with parents/carers) through to being a role model in the senior years by passing on lessons learnt and key aspects of knowledge to the next generation. It importantly showcased the phases of the lifecourse, what is important at each stage, and how this changes. It also highlighted key players and influencers along the way, as well as the importance of various environments, all of which are significant in the journey.

We often use the poster as a 'talking tool' when we try to explain the concept. We also provide people with a blank journey template to map out their journey to date, considering the layers of 'where', 'who' and 'why'. This often results in what we call the 'light bulb moment' – realising the layers within their own personal journeys, and recognising that one change, opportunity or key player can significantly alter the course ahead and lead to a different path. The poster to date is still one of the best resources we have that sparks and scaffolds the initial thinking and supports the understanding of the concept. Since developing the video and poster, we created additional materials to add further understanding of the concept:

- a physical literacy section on the Sport Wales website (Sport Wales, 2014c);
- a physical literacy community programme; and
- a suite of hard copy materials supported by training.

Furthermore, feedback we received over time in relation to the Amelia video also raised the question whether we were suggesting physical literacy is just about young children. This was obviously not the intention, so as a result we created version 2 of the video to better reflect our message, which was particularly important when engaging with the health sector (Sport Wales, 2015a). Some of the renewed internal understanding has subsequently shone through via meetings with potential partners. This includes stakeholders such as the Older People's Commissioner, who recognises the potential of physical literacy to impact on older people's agenda and the need to upskill practitioners. Sport Wales colleagues have subsequently presented the importance of physical literacy and raised awareness at health sector events for specific attention to be given to groups such as those with dementia. As a result of this range of dialogue and working with the newly formed International Physical Literacy Association (IPLA), Sport Wales has adopted the IPLA definition due to its simplicity compared to our 2012 definition: 'Physical literacy can be described as the motivation, confidence, physical competence, knowledge and understanding to value and take responsibility for engagement in physical activities for life'. This definition also allows us to address some key messages that could be lost through our simple 'equation', such as knowledge and understanding and valuing the importance of physical literacy.

Developments in education

The year 2015 saw the introduction of two significant policies in Wales. The first was *A Curriculum for Wales: A Curriculum for Life* (2015) (Welsh Government, 2015a). This sets out a new approach to delivery of schools' curricula in Wales from 2022. Sport Wales was commissioned by the Welsh Government to create a physical literacy framework to support the development of the new curriculum. As a result, the Physical Literacy Journey (PLJ) was created as a draft curriculum planning tool to inform the curriculum reform team (Sport Wales, 2016b). The PLJ was used by pioneer leaders (practitioners selected to develop the curriculum) to secure both the understanding of the physical literacy concept and the operationalisation of the concept across the learning continuum. A collaborative approach towards physical literacy will build upon existing and future Sport Wales partnerships, supporting a creative and relevant curriculum. In addition, this will provide an enriched *Pupil Offer* (Welsh Government, 2014), which extends physical literacy beyond the school day into community settings.

The second was *The Well-Being of Future Generations (Wales) Act 2015* (Welsh Government, 2015b). This is an exciting and ambitious piece of legislation to improve the social, economic, environmental and cultural well-being of Wales. Sport Wales are committed to playing our part, and an important element of this is the development of a suite of well-being objectives that are embedded into our governance structure and form the basis for our impact measurement (Sport Wales, 2016a). At Sport Wales, we believe that this piece of legislation provides an exciting opportunity to work more collaboratively across the public sector to create a more active and more successful Wales.

Exploring partnerships

When we began immersing ourselves in learning more about physical literacy, we were still very much at the exploration stage with sectors outside education. As an organisation, we recognised that physical literacy could be seen as the canopy of an umbrella, with the spokes supporting the sectors with which we needed to engage and collaborate. Those sectors include education, sport and health, as well as wider community organisations and groups. Our aim within education was to influence future curriculum planning and strengthen links with higher education and further education in relation to the future workforce. Within health, we saw opportunities to encourage collaborative cross-sector practices, an advocacy role we could play with the potential for upskilling the various interventionists who provide levels of support to families. Within the community sector there are the traditional sporting clubs and organisations that involve a coaching and volunteering workforce. But there are the non-sporting organisations and other national, regional and local organisations that overlap the physical literacy agenda, including housing associations, youth groups such as Girlguiding Cymru and the Urdd – our Welsh-language national organisation.

We have sport development teams within the communities across Wales who have embraced the importance of physical literacy and who are linking with wide-ranging partners to deliver the agenda. As the suite of school-based programmes delivered by local authority partners evolved (Dragon Sport, 5x60 and PESS), they were given the overarching name of 'active young people programmes'. This now offers a more multi-skill-based provision to enable children and young people to explore wider opportunities across various environments. The sport development teams collaborate with partners within health, the early years sector and family groups, and this has resulted in several projects taking place to engage wider audiences, and ultimately increase physical activity levels. The teams utilised our communication tools in their strategies to connect with partners and to help bring physical literacy to life. In addition, they created further materials based on local feedback and need, such as parent/carer packs, to promote home engagement beyond the sessions attended.

Some of the innovations over the last few years included the 'Calls 4 Action' programme (Sport Wales, 2016c), which aims to tackle inequality in sports participation. Its overarching objectives were positive action, changing lives, encouraging new approaches, and increasing regular and frequent sporting activity. These themes and the positive outreach by Sport Wales successfully attracted new partners, including non-sporting organisations. Successful applicants include Girlguiding Cymru, Trevallis Housing Association and Brecon Beacons National Park. Girlguiding Cymru introduced a physical activity programme to their provision, delivering multi-skills and sport-specific and leadership opportunities throughout the Girlguiding network in Wales. Brecon Beacons National Park Authority focused attention on engaging young people living in poverty and with low participation by using the natural environment through the medium of geocaching. Trevallis Housing Association adopted a peer-led approach to foster the principles of physical literacy among parents/carers and their children aged between 3 and 8 years in disengaged communities.

Working with the IPLA

An opportunity arose in 2016 to go to the International Physical Literacy Association (IPLA) inaugural forum, in which we were asked to present our ideas and the intention of Sport Wales. We had 'dipped our toes' into the philosophy at that stage and were trying to make sense of it. The communication tools we had created were simplified translations of the philosophy, recognising that the people of Wales needed to understand and connect with the nature of physical literacy. We were finding ourselves in the middle of these developments in Wales, often acting as a translator. At the IPLA forum, we threw ourselves 'into the lion's den' and presented our intention, where we were at, and our findings to date. The feeling was that there was merit in sharing this with the IPLA, so they could learn from us as much as we could learn from them. Our message was well received and embraced, and provided an opportunity to link with the group and develop a wider network of people who could help shape our thinking going forward. The two-way relationship helped to cement our thinking around physical literacy. In addition, we could share examples of physical literacy in practice, and in so doing discuss challenges faced, quick wins and breakthroughs. We also have a strong link with an IPLA trustee who is based in our education system in Wales, and this strengthens our network and knowledge base on home ground.

Funding issues

Unfortunately, in March 2017, the PLPS funding ceased, resulting in redundancies in staff across the regions in Wales. While Sport Wales actively sought to maintain future funding in this area to secure momentum, we have been unsuccessful due to a fundamental review and step change in the education system being undertaken. Funding to continue supporting this agenda now forms part of the amalgamated funding that has been allocated to the education consortia across Wales. While direct support of funded interventions via Sport Wales can no longer be delivered in schools, a significant number of resources developed by Sport Wales and endorsed by the Welsh Government remain available to schools, including the physical literacy journey (Sport Wales, 2016b). Sport Wales is striving to continue the success of all the aforementioned programmes over the past 17 years and to capitalise on this learning to support school and community understanding of a 'Physical Literacy Journey' through life. A video reel was created in early 2017 to showcase our journey of learning and development to date (Sport Wales, 2017).

There are many layers to consider from the perspective of the individual. This will need to recognise experiences at home, at school and in the community. All these layers interact as they wrap round the individual. Surrounding that is policy development in Wales, which in recent years is aligning itself completely to our physical literacy mission. A multi-level approach of influence has been taken to date – at the Welsh Government level, the CEO and leadership level, and the operational level across our key sectors. There have been successes and a great deal of learning, and this continues to evolve with changes across policy. Future developments predominantly rely on future investment to make the practices widespread across Wales. Sport Wales believes that there is strength in numbers, and that, in going forward, working in partnership with other groups and pooling resources will be the best strategy.

Current status of physical literacy in Wales

We are at the cusp of what could be some fundamental changes ahead. To date, we have made huge strides on many levels. Internally, as an organisation, we have strategic buy-in to physical literacy, which is impacting directly on two of the organisation's well-being objectives. Within our schools, physical literacy has influenced pedagogical approaches to delivering the curriculum. Through PLPS, elements of the great work undertaken are ongoing and leaving a legacy. The new curriculum, currently under construction, will be physical literacy-informed. Developed by the teaching profession for the teaching profession, with support from experts in their respected fields, the Health and Well-being Area of Learning and Experience, when completed, will be a world-leading example of how physical literacy can be operationalised within education, providing a foundation for a continuum of learning from 3 to 16 years of age.

From a community angle, physical literacy has encouraged collaborative approaches across sectors. PLPS also encouraged collaborative practices, with pockets of great cross-sector work taking place within health, libraries and early years settings. There is a lot of good work taking place across Wales, but it is not yet countrywide.

Challenges ahead

While many of the projects to date have seen successes, many barriers or elements of resistance have started to emerge. One resistance to engagement is the perceptions of parents. It became apparent that some parents did not understand and/or see the value in bringing their children along to thematic, multi-skills-type sessions as opposed to sport-specific sessions, which was their comfort zone and therefore perceived preference. To prevent disengagement, some community partners changed their marketing approach from 'multi-skills clubs' to clubs with blended titles to make the sport more visible within the title (i.e. 'Netball Tots' or 'Rugby Tots'). This is also the case when working with national governing bodies (NGBs) of sport as the culture and practices within their club environments are strong in their particular sport. However, the multi-skills approach is encouraging a change in delivery from predominantly group teaching to the use of a much more participant-centred approach. The approach is also resulting in broader skill development, embracing a wider range of activity contexts. Some NGBs have welcomed the opportunity to explore physical literacy further and compare what this could look like in practice.

National governing bodies

Conversations within the Welsh national governing bodies of sport are often challenging in this area. In a nutshell, we are asking them to put the participant first and their sport second. This is difficult as for NGBs, their sport is their business and the reason behind all their work. What we are asking is to ensure all children have every opportunity to become all-round athletes and are involved in experiences that enable them to 'flourish' in life. These issues stimulate a great deal of discussion in terms of the place of physical literacy within their sport and their programmes. It is challenging NGBs' culture and questioning whose place it is to do what. Some sports feel they are promoting physical literacy, so we are looking to work with NGBs to reflect on their thinking, their intention and their programmes. However, we need to work with the sports in a bespoke fashion to see the situation from their point of view, as they are all unique. It is certainly not a catch-all situation, nor a case of us 'telling' them what to do. We need to come up with a collective understanding and see if there is something that can be achieved by working together on this agenda. The direction of travel can only be a good one to challenge thinking and address learning from a range of different perspectives. We have a group of NGBs looking to explore the concept with us further, which links to the new sporting landscape and operating model currently under development in which physical literacy features strongly.

Education sector

Within the education sector, we are now facing a significant step change in approach. It is taking time at the strategic level to interpret the new curriculum going forward and the place of the Health and Well-being Area of Learning and Experience alongside other 'competing' areas of learning and experience. Traditionally, performance in the academic domain has the spotlight and the perceived preference. In addition, there is an acknowledgement that PE and the existing menu of provision is not working as effectively as it could and can disengage some pupils. There has been significant work undertaken with the Welsh Government to develop a common understanding of physical literacy and its relationship to physical activity and well-being. This is evident in the positivity emerging from conversations within the curriculum reform team around physical literacy and the part it should play within the new curriculum, and more broadly within wider community provision.

Health sector

The challenge to overcome within the health sector is the myriad of issues that need tackling and what takes priority. For us, it is recognising the importance of physical activity and its potential impact on the 'prevention over cure' agenda. Sport Wales continues to showcase the benefits of physical activity on the wider health and well-being agenda, in particular the potential to reduce the health consequences of leading sedentary lifestyles and rates of obesity, and increase activity levels. However, the introduction of a new joint action plan between Sport Wales and Public Health Wales (in conjunction with Natural Resources Wales) will seek to address this by working in collaboration and setting out the parameters of who does what. The physical literacy concept provides the perfect opportunity to be the enabler to such a collaboration at a country-level cross-sector. We believe that physical literacy has the capacity to do this.

A cross-sector approach

Our physical literacy community projects, which sit outside the traditional sporting offer, began at a time when significant focus in terms of Sport Wales senior officer time and resource was given to education. On reflection, we quickly recognised that as physical literacy is cross-sector and involves everyone, our resources were proving too limited. It has been effective to a degree, but the learning for us was that there is so much scope to make a difference, which required a breadth of collaboration, the acceptance and reality of overstretching ourselves was surfacing. If we are really going to make a difference with some of these organisations, we need to work with them more closely and target resources effectively. Our aim is not a quick fix; for some, it will be a cultural shift. Embedding physical literacy will require mentoring along the journey to really bring it to life, creating champions to ensure long-term sustainability. They need to come on the journey with us and truly understand the concept and what it means to them. The fundamental shift for us is that it is not a resource, a training package or a product that is imposed on them. Physical literacy is a very valuable concept, and Sport Wales must do all it can to get to the core of what it means to organisations, challenge their thinking, and ensure their understanding is secure as they devise future programmes. There is a lot of merit in what has been done to date, but the learning so far has taught us that more targeted resources to support the development are needed.

Targeted approach

We have taken a similar approach with every organisation to date, a liaison officer being attached to each project or organisation, but this is one of the lessons learned in terms of aligning the right people to the right organisations/projects. We need the right people with the right skills and knowledge to make this a reality. We realised in Sport Wales that we cannot achieve our goals alone and that we needed to collaborate with others. To ensure the right people with the right skills are paired more appropriately with organisations, a team of physical literacy consultants have been recruited. The consultants' skills and expertise are matched with organisations and governing bodies, thus maximising the opportunities for partnership working towards common goals. We are often faced with varying political pressures and change, but physical literacy is not a short-term agenda, and we are in this for the long haul.

Spreading understanding

It is safe to say that when we get past the understanding of physical literacy with partners in Wales, the concept is broadly accepted because when you explain it in terms of human flourishing, it cannot be argued with. When the light bulb goes on and they 'get it', no one can question its importance. How can anyone doubt that we are advocating anything other than a valid goal, when it is ultimately aimed at enabling everyone to be the best they can be in life? But the challenge we have is translating physical literacy into practice collaboratively. What does this look like? How is this any different to what I do in school now, in my coaching sessions, in the messages health practitioners are already delivering? It may not be a case of changing practice significantly; it could be a recognition that what they are doing is already supporting and underpinning physical literacy. For some people, it could mean a small change in focus, while for others it could be a significant shift, that is if they believe it is the right thing for them.

Therefore, the approach that we are looking to take needs to be bespoke, as all partners and organisations will come at it differently. Importantly, we need to make sure it is reciprocated and bought into by them. This comes back to the definition of physical literacy; everyone needs to value and take responsibility for this if we are going to truly see some impact. At the very core of all the work will be the ability to transform the workforce, so everyone is working together, building and enhancing the experiences for young people to allow them to succeed, reach their potential, and set them up to continue valuing their physical pursuits throughout life.

Going forward

Fundamentally, going forward we will have a new vision (Sport Wales, 2018) and strategy that will align to *The Well-Being of Future Generations (Wales) Act (2015)* (Welsh Government, 2015b) and, more recently, Prosperity for All (Welsh Government, 2017). Setting out our stall across policies will help us to develop our future direction and devise strategies that aim to operationalise physical literacy with wide-ranging partners. It will be a challenge, but this next stage of the journey will be an exciting one. We will need to be able to answer the million-dollar question: 'What does physical literacy look like?' Furthermore, we will need to ensure we can demonstrate the impact we are having on the levels of physical activity across the nation. We are not in this alone; we are one piece of a bigger puzzle, but we are keen to collaborate to get it right and make a significant difference. It is certainly a case of 'watch this space' in Wales. Our journey continues.

Special thank you to Gethin Mon Thomas and Marc Gregson for their support in editing this chapter.

References

Sport, Physical Education and Activity Research (SPEAR), Canterbury Christ Church University (2016) *Evaluation Report of the PLPS and PL Framework*. Available at: http://physicalliteracy.sportwales.org.uk/media/40469/spear-cccu-plps_plf-final-report_client-draft.pdf (accessed 28 February 2018).

Sport Wales (2001) *PE and School Sport Programme (PESS)*. Available at: http://sport.wales/community-sport/education/pe--school-sport/about-pess.aspx (accessed 28 February 2018).

Sport Wales (2006) *5x60 Programme*. Available at: http://sport.wales/community-sport/education/5x60.aspx (accessed 28 February 2018).

Sport Wales (2010) *Play to Learn Resources*. Available at: http://sport.wales/community-sport/online-shop/play-to-learn-products.aspx (accessed 12 April 2018).

Sport Wales (2011) *A Vision for Sport in Wales*. Available at: http://sport.wales/media/506916/sport_wales_english_vision_doc_reprint_all_v3.pdf (accessed 28 February 2018).

Sport Wales (2012a) *Dragon Multi-Skills and Sport Programme*. Available at: http://sport.wales/community-sport/education/dragon-multi-skills--sport.aspx (accessed 28 February 2018).

Sport Wales (2012b) *Play to Learn*. Available at: http://sport.wales/community-sport/education/play-to-learn.aspx (accessed 28 February 2018).

Sport Wales (2013) *Physical Literacy Video*. Available at: www.youtube.com/watch?v=R8PIXqp3JpA (accessed 28 February 2018).

Sport Wales (2014a) *Physical Literacy Journey Poster Landscape*. Available at: http://physicalliteracy.sportwales.org.uk/en/ (accessed 28 February 2018).

Sport Wales (2014b) *Physical Literacy Programme for Schools (PLPS)*. Available at: http://sport.wales/community-sport/education/physical-literacy-programme-for-schools-(plps).aspx (accessed 28 February 2018).

Sport Wales (2014c) *Physical Literacy Section*. Available at: http://physicalliteracy.sportwales.org.uk/en/ (accessed 28 February 2018).

Sport Wales (2015a) *Physical Literacy Video Version 2*. Available at: www.youtube.com/watch?v=fyCm6ZLRCbQ (accessed 28 February 2018).

Sport Wales (2015b) *School Sport Survey Results*. Available at: http://sport.wales/research--policy/surveys-and-statistics/school-sport-survey/school-sport-survey-2015-results.aspx (accessed 28 February 2018).

Sport Wales (2016a) *Wellbeing Statement*. Available at: http://sportwales.org.uk/about-us/how-we-work/well-being-statement.aspx (accessed 28 February 2018).

Sport Wales (2016b) *Physical Literacy Journey Website Draft*. Available at: www.physicalliteracyjourney.wales/ (accessed 28 February 2018).

Sport Wales (2016c) *Evaluation of the Impact of Phase 2 of Calls 4 Action*. Available at: http://sport.wales/media/1922957/c4a_p2i_evaluation_first_interim_report.pdf (accessed 28 February 2018).

Sport Wales (2017) *15 Year Physical Literacy Story*. Available at: www.youtube.com/watch?v=zULjFSA3zH8 (accessed 28 February 2018).

Sport Wales (2018) *Vision for Sport*. Available at https://visionforsport.wales/ (accessed 29 October 2018).

Welsh Government (2008) *Foundation Phase*. Available at: http://gov.wales/topics/educationandskills/foundation-phase/?lang=en (accessed 12 April 2018).

Welsh Government (2013) *Schools and Physical Activity Review Report*. Available at: http://gov.wales/docs/dcells/publications/130621-sports-and-physical-activity-review-en.pdf (accessed 28 February 2018).

Welsh Government (2014) *Schools Challenge Cymru: The Pupil Offer* Available at: http://dera.ioe.ac.uk/21783/1/141212-pupil-offer-en.pdf (accessed 28 February 2018).

Welsh Government (2015a) *A Curriculum for Wales: A Curriculum for Life*. Available at: http://gov.wales/docs/dcells/publications/151021-a-curriculum-for-wales-a-curriculum-for-life-en.pdf (accessed 28 February 2018).

Welsh Government (2015b) *The Well-Being of Future Generations (Wales) Act 2015*. Available at: http://gov.wales/topics/people-and-communities/people/future-generations-act/?lang=en (accessed 28 February 2018).

Welsh Government (2017) *Prosperity for All: The National Strategy*. Available at: http://gov.wales/docs/strategies/170919-prosperity-for-all-en.pdf (accessed 28 February 2018).

16

REFLECTION ON INTERNATIONAL PERSPECTIVES

Margaret Whitehead

Introduction

This chapter follows the pattern of Chapter 7 and picks up common themes considered among the chapters written by colleagues from the eight different countries. Strategies to inform and engage with a wide range of personnel have included the running of training courses and the production of general and targeted resources. Colleagues in a number of countries have used research and scholarly writing to investigate and advocate the concept of physical literacy. Many colleagues have been successful in influencing policies and programmes, while all have met and addressed a range of challenges. All have ambitious plans regarding future development. It is seen as valuable to learn as much as possible from the experiences spelled out in the chapters and use these to support those others new to the field.

Training and resources

It is very encouraging to report that a wide range of training events, from large conferences to half-day training sessions and small seminar discussions, have been held to further the work of disseminating physical literacy. CS4L has run a biennial International Physical Literacy Conference, while personnel in other countries such as the United States, Austria and Brazil have included consideration of physical literacy within a range of multi-topic conferences. New Zealand set up a series of workshops, nationally, to introduce the concept of physical literacy. In Dumfries and Galloway, Scotland, seminars were run for teachers and head teachers, for local authority staff and for parents. In addition, colleagues in New Zealand and Dumfries and Galloway have followed the IPLA Foundation Course.

The production of resources to introduce, explain, promote and illustrate aspects of physical literacy has been impressive. Some of these are referred to in the separate chapters. Wales created two videos and a poster. These were produced over a number of years and were developed sequentially to respond to constructive evaluation of previous material. CS4L and New Zealand created a range of booklets and handouts. The Czech Republic drew together a small book, while Dumfries and Galloway wrote a range of bespoke leaflets addressed to different constituencies. Most countries have felt it helpful to produce models or info-grams to clarify the interrelationships between the different aspects of physical literacy. Some of these, regrettably not in colour in this text, have been shown in the chapters.

Research and scholarly writing

A range of research has been carried out. Delphi polls in Australia, Canada and Wales have investigated the understanding of the concept. There have also been research enquiries into teacher and student perceptions of physical literacy and the effect of PETE courses on knowledge related to physical literacy. This last approach has been used in Scotland, Wales and Canada. However, the main focus of the research on both a formal and informal basis has addressed charting progress on individuals' physical literacy journeys. Canada has been particularly proactive in this area; however, Australia, the United States, New Zealand, the Czech Republic and Wales have also carried out investigations and produced schemes (for further details, see Chapter 5).

Not surprisingly, scholarly writing around the topic of physical literacy has principally featured in countries where universities have been central to promoting the concept. Colleagues in Canada have been very proactive, producing over 20 refereed papers, most of which have been written by groups of authors (for these papers, see IPLA, 2019). Topics addressed include conceptual issues, the history of the concept of physical literacy, charting progress, the value of physical literacy, and the relationship of physical literacy to participation in physical activity and to health. Colleagues in Europe, particularly the Netherlands and Norway, have written papers concerning the fidelity of physical literacy to claimed philosophical roots, issues in the field of skill development, and the nature of fundamental movement skills. Academics in Australia have written on psychological areas, as well as conceptual issues inherent in the definition. There have been some papers from colleagues in the United States, mainly clarifying the concept and promoting the spread of physical literacy across different sectors. In addition, IPLA colleagues were invited to draw up an ICSSPE Bulletin (No 65. 2013) and to compile a special physical literacy issue of the US-based *Journal of Teaching in Physical Education* in 2018. In some instances, academics from different countries, such as Australia and Canada, contributed to these publications.

Policies and programmes

It is pleasing to note that those working to promote physical literacy have played a part in the design of relevant policies and strategies at national, state or local level. Colleagues advocating physical literacy have been invited to discussion groups and planning meetings, and have been successful in influencing the outcomes of many of these debates. For example, physical literacy is referred to in *The Well-Being of Future Generations (Wales) Act 2015* (Welsh Government, 2015), the Australian Sports Commission's Organisational Strategic Plan (Australian Sports Commission, 2016), the SHAPE America National Standards (SHAPE America, 2014), and in Scotland *A Healthier Future: Scotland's Diet and Healthy Weight Delivery Plan* (Scottish Government, 2018). In addition, programmes and curricula have been adjusted or refocused such that new school curricula reflect the philosophy of physical literacy, as do schemes of work for those with special needs, adults, the elderly and minority populations. For example, there is recognition of aspects of physical literacy in the New South Wales physical literacy continuum, the New Zealand health and physical education curriculum, and two programmes in the United States, the Connecticut 2-4-1 initiative and the Florida Gators in Motion scheme.

Challenges

With respect to the accounts given in the foregoing chapters, there are a number of challenges that colleagues have had to address. First, they themselves were confronted with the need to read, understand and navigate their way through some philosophical principles, and then be able to stand back to reflect objectively on both the huge potential of fostering physical literacy for all, and the reasons why, in many circumstances, current practices were not seeming to open the door to these benefits. This clear understanding was essential if they were to 'sell' the concept to others. Colleagues in Wales write that this was a demanding process, and colleagues in Canada and New Zealand reflect that they might still need a deeper understanding. Even with this understanding and belief, colleagues need to solve the problem of seeing the situation from the perspective of other groups/constituencies and to present the case in a way that connects with others' perceptions. Persuading practitioners to reconsider aspects of their practice was not an easy task. Those in Dumfries and Galloway took time to rewrite a basic flier, a number of times, into language that would facilitate understanding and appreciation by each audience. Colleagues in Wales describe the value of their poster as a talking point to be explained as appropriate.

Particularly challenging groups included parents, who had their own perceptions of the role of physical education, physical activity coaches, and instructors, who jealously guarded their responsibilities to specific sports and individuals in government who held somewhat entrenched views regarding the purpose of physical activity. These views often included the perception of physical education and physical activity as only of value in promoting physical fitness alongside the identification and nurturing potential talent. Two particular areas are the subject of considerable debate. A common question posed by physical activity practitioners was, 'What does physical literacy look like?' Countries have begun to provide guidance in this area. Colleagues in New Zealand have worked on this and have drawn up quality guidelines for practitioners. The Coaching Association of Canada has created a HIGH5 physical literacy instructor programme. Another way that this is being addressed in both Wales and India is via the establishment of lead schools that exemplify good practice to trial and then disseminate programmes. In India these are known as centres of excellence, while in Wales these were referred to as Beacon Schools and latterly as Pioneer schools. In addition, practitioners have been charged by their managers to provide evidence of the beneficial effects of adopting a physical literacy approach. This has required the creation of instruments to chart progress. Canada has done significant work here, and the United States, New Zealand, Wales, and Dumfries and Galloway, as well as some countries in continental Europe, are trialling a variety of systems.

Other areas of challenge include the need for better physical education training for primary teachers and the finance to carry through significant changes. For example, funding in Wales was cut, and now other ways to finance further developments are having to be investigated. Colleagues in India had significant problems in securing finance from central government, and they have now established a charitable organisation to provide support. Some challenges are specific to a country. For example, in the United States, there is no federal oversight of sport. This responsibility has been handed over to the United States Olympic Committee. In India, an immediate issue is the shortage of trained physical education teachers.

Another way to address challenges is the development of partnerships. Where other practitioners could see the benefit of physical literacy in their own area, this added support in advocating the value of physical literacy. Advocates have set up numerous meetings across constituencies and found ways to be represented on national or local working parties. In addition, they have been alert to opportunities in which physical literacy could become part of a wider strategic planning. Overcoming these challenges and creating opportunities for advocacy has required patience and persistence.

Priorities for the future

Most chapters indicate priorities for the immediate future. A number focus on developing partnerships within and beyond the country in question to aid the spread of the concept. Colleagues in New Zealand and Wales are keen to secure a place for physical literacy in newly nationally identified foci concerned with well-being. Advocates of physical literacy in Canada feel it is important to demystify the philosophy underlying the concept as a precursor to wider adoption. Colleagues in Scotland feel that they need to work on a culture change to provide a receptive context for further development. Colleagues in India are concerned to embrace native content. Those working in Australia feel they need to foster cross-constituency debate to clarify the nature of physical literacy, and those in the United States feel it important to have one unified message to share with a wide range of constituencies. Colleagues in continental Europe want to develop collaboration between the different parties who have influence in respect of developing national educational policies, and those advocating physical literacy in the United States and India identify working at national, regional and local levels as a priority.

Building on from current experience

In sum, there is much to be learnt from the experiences set out in the chapters above. It would seem essential that the IPLA uses these experiences to support, aid and empower those who are at the start of their physical literacy advocacy journey. Significant here is to work with colleagues to deliberate how physical literacy can be aligned with the particular culture of a country. To this effect, it would be very valuable for the IPLA to set up an international advisory board to support colleagues in countries new to the concept. This may involve guidance in understanding aspects of the concept and the production of a resource on recognising and addressing challenges. As each country is unique, initiatives might include a more targeted strategy – possibly the partnering of a country that has established physical literacy with one that is just starting along this road. It is also hoped that the content of this text can provide valuable information.

Overview

The chapters in Part II paint a picture of commitment, vision and hard work. The achievements made to promote physical literacy are impressive and the plans for the future perceptive, challenging and ambitious.

The wide variety of perspectives taken in the preceding chapters is indicative of the depth and breadth of physical literacy. The depth relates to the philosophical roots of concepts as they resonate with cultures and established practices, while the breadth covers relevance in preschool settings, schooling, and physical activity and health for all throughout the lifecourse. Physical literacy has generated debate on a challenging intellectual level, as well as being viewed as directly applicable to solving problems in the day-to-day work of, for example, teachers, coaches and local government personnel.

Such is the range of the backgrounds of colleagues who initially championed the concept of physical literacy that the current state of play varies from country to country. While this can be viewed as indicative of the range of values inherent in physical literacy, these different scenarios present different challenges. For example, those working in the academic field have the challenge to engage with practitioners, and practitioners have the challenge to become familiar with the knowledge base of the concept. It is clear that a key focus of the endeavours of the IPLA and all physical literacy advocates is now to establish a close theory/practice partnership. The development of communication between parties is essential. In this dialogue, perceptive reasoning and analysis from those working in universities can convince and empower practitioners in the field. Alongside this, committed and inspirational practitioners can generate and deliver practices that enrich the philosophical deliberations of academics. Genuine collaboration of this nature is now needed for physical literacy to be securely established in more countries across the world.

While colleagues writing Chapters 8–15 share different scenarios of the development of physical literacy in their country, all respect physical literacy as a valuable concept worthy of serious consideration. Underlying this belief is the view that physical literacy can play a part in enhancing the quality of life. The notion of physical literacy as contributing to well-being and human flourishing is alluded to by all, with colleagues in New Zealand, Canada, Wales, continental Europe, Scotland and India specifically identifying this view. The claim that physical literacy can contribute to human flourishing is the subject of Chapters 18 and 19.

References

Australian Sports Commission (2016) *Organisational Strategic Plan.* Available at: www.sportaus.gov.au/__data/assets/pdf_file/0004/678883/35063_SportAUS_Corporate_Plan_WEB.pdf (accessed 25 March 2019).

Bulletin on Physical Literacy (2013) ICSSPE Bulletin No. 65 (2013).

International Physical Literacy Association (IPLA) (2019) *Physical Literacy across the World: Resources and References.* Available at: www.physical-literacy.org.uk/plaw-resources-and-references/ (accessed 14 March 2019).

Journal of Teaching in Physical Education (2018) Special issue, Operationalising Physical Literacy, 37(3), https://doi.org/10.1123/jtpe.2018-0136.

Scottish Government (2018) *A Healthier Future: Scotland's Diet and Healthy Weight Delivery Plan.* Available at: www.gov.scot/publications/healthier-future-scotlands-diet-healthy-weight-delivery-plan/ (accessed 25 March 2019).

Society of Health and Physical Educators (SHAPE America) (2014) *National Standards and Grade-Level Outcomes for K–12 Physical Education.* Champaign, IL: Human Kinetics.

Welsh Government (2015) *The Well-Being of Future Generations (Wales) Act 2015.* Available at: http://gov.wales/topics/people-and-communities/people/future-generations-act/?lang=en (accessed 28 February 2018).

PART III

Physical literacy

Establishing significance and looking ahead

17

PHYSICAL LITERACY AS A JOURNEY

Liz Taplin

Introduction

This chapter proposes that physical literacy is best described as a journey, and that the journey metaphor helps to clarify the nature of physical literacy. The notion of physical literacy as a journey will be examined in the context of relevant philosophical positions, and consideration will be given to the usefulness of the journey metaphor as an entrée into life history. To this end, the value of seeing the physical literacy journey as a life history, using the wealth of life history theory to underpin description, examination and research into physical literacy, will be explored. Four 'physical literacy as a journey' life histories will then be shared and discussed with respect to aspects of physical literacy.

The 'physical literacy as a journey' metaphor

A metaphor is a figure of speech that is used to help explain one idea by setting it alongside another (Lakoff and Johnson, 1980). The value of using metaphor is that it clarifies meaning, and this is certainly the case with physical literacy, as there remains some confusion regarding aspects of its nature (e.g. the misconception that physical literacy is something only relevant to young children).

The identification of the journey metaphor for the fostering of physical literacy has proved helpful and valuable in underwriting the notion that the concept is not a state acquired and retained thereafter. On the contrary, it is a disposition concerned with the fostering of a positive attitude to physical activity that, ideally, becomes progressively secure as life is lived. The idea of physical literacy as a journey, whereby the individual is heading in a particular direction, with a choice of routes and potential diversions along the way, appears particularly apt.

Accepting the use of metaphor, and appreciating the particular usefulness of the 'physical literacy as a journey' metaphor in both explaining the concept and helping make it reality, is endorsed by Whitehead (2010), who uses the metaphor when explaining that 'each individual will be on their own personal physical literacy journey', and that the important issue is whether or why 'individuals are making progress' (p. 38). She continues to refer to the 'physical literacy as a journey' metaphor when she writes that 'physically literate individuals will be on a journey through which they are interacting effectively with features in an increasing range of environments' (p. 49).

Taplin (2011) reinforces this by further considering the unique nature of an individual's journey, and states:

> No two journeys will be identical because, just like fingerprints differ, so too will genetic make-up, environmental factors, opportunity and a whole host of other factors … each individual will be travelling in different contexts, at different speeds and often in different directions … the journey is unlikely to be smooth and uncomplicated; individuals are unlikely to travel along a constant forward and upward path.
>
> *(pp. 28–30)*

It is the where, when, why, what and how behind life events, and the individual's responses, that create the framework for the physical literacy journey. Furthermore, the physical literacy journey should not be seen as having a fixed destination as it is an ongoing interrelated chain, or sequence, of events comprised of experiences that affect attitudes towards physical activity. The challenge is to make progress on the journey, and to maintain that progress, while also enjoying the present moment.

Links between the journey metaphor and the philosophy underpinning physical literacy

Appreciating the nature of physical literacy journeys can be facilitated by referencing the three underlying philosophies that provide the fundamental rationale behind the concept. Existentialism, monism and phenomenology each in their different way can legitimise the significance of the journey metaphor. Fundamental to existentialism is the notion that humans create themselves as they interact with the world. In these terms, life itself is a journey, a journey through which experiences shape the individual, a journey that is all the richer where experiences are varied and challenging. Physical literacy journeys share this characteristic – being the outcome of experiences that highlight human embodied capability.

The notion of monism – viewing the human as a whole rather than composed of separate parts – is valuable in the context of interpreting journeys. The holistic nature of the human means that any experience will affect all aspects of being (e.g. the affective, the physical and the cognitive). In this context, every experience has an influence on the individual. Physical literacy journeys clearly exemplify this. While the significance and impact of an experience, in which the embodied capability is the focus, will more obviously shape physical competence, the experience will, at the same time, have an effect on the affective and cognitive capabilities. An experience within the field of physical activity is very likely to affect the attitude the individual has towards participation and add to the understanding of the nature of the activity. Examples of these influences can be found in the journeys set out below.

Phenomenology builds on from these two philosophies by proposing that as a consequence of the individual being shaped by holistic interaction with the world, each individual will develop a particular viewpoint from which experiences are perceived. In this sense, any journey essentially builds from previous experiences. This is very evident in respect of physical literacy journeys, as participants will approach any situation or challenge from the perspective of past experiences. This explains the uniqueness of each journey and is exemplified in the journeys set out below.

Journeys, stories and the life history research method

Whitehead (2013) wrote that physical literacy is 'best seen as a journey; a journey unique to each individual' (p. 30). With this is mind, Taplin (2013) has developed life story and life history methodology as a way of exploring the concept of a physical literacy journey. The starting point for this is that the notion of a journey and that of a story are closely related. Macartney (2007) states: 'Journeys and stories sit well together. With all that is magical and wondrous in this world, journeys that become stories and stories that become journeys are among the most precious' (p. 22). Stories can be seen as central in what it means to be human. Sykes (cited in Clough, 2002) supports this claim, suggesting that it is natural for humans to use story 'to understand our lives and the lives of others' (p. xii).

Since the beginning of time, stories have been used in a myriad of formats to educate, inform and entertain, and consequently storytelling, in its various forms, is recognised as an authentic qualitative research method under the broad genre of (auto)biography. Some commenters (e.g. Schwandt, 2001) refer to biography as simply a way to record an individual's life events. Ellis (2004) agrees, and puts forward the view that stories are 'essential to human understanding' (p. 32).

The life story method is often compared, or confused, with the life history method, and while both methods are branches of the (auto)biography genre, there are distinct differences. Atkinson (1998) writes that life story is 'the story a person chooses to tell about the life he or she has lived' (p. 8), and essentially is the participant's own words not altered, or interpreted, by the researcher. Roberts (2002) investigated life story theory as an appropriate method for understanding the lived experience, and reaffirms that life story comprises of the exact words spoken by the individual, unedited and uncut.

Contrary to this, a life history is an account that is edited by the researcher, who may also consider additional material, such as input from significant others, as well as information from written records. Goodson and Sikes (2007) support this view, stating that 'the rendering of lived experience into "life story" is one interpretive layer, but the move to "life history" adds a second layer and a further interpretation' (p. 17).

In the context of exploring physical literacy journeys, the position taken here is that the life story is the account given by an individual recalling and reflecting on their experiences. This account can become a data set for the researcher to interpret and investigate in order to construct the life history.

The life history method is used in the context of this chapter to maximise the impact of the journey metaphor as applicable to physical literacy. In particular, it allows the pattern of individual physical literacy journeys to be captured, facilitating a better understanding of the concept. Physical literacy life histories enable us to map an individual's physical literacy journey and allow us to attempt to reveal the nature of the individual's lived experience. In addition, the life history method allows the researcher to reveal the uniqueness of each person's journey and provides a lens through which key themes, such as significant others and significant events, can be examined.

Using the life history method

The life history method is used here to facilitate reflection and analysis of four physical literacy journeys. As is characteristic of the method, the life histories shared in this chapter were initially collected by way of a face-to-face interview. The interviewer spoke only to encourage the interviewee and kept questioning to a minimum; the interviewees were simply encouraged to tell their story. The word-for-word transcript that resulted from each interview became the life story; the researcher then used the life story to draw up an account of the journey in chronological order and, where appropriate, included direct quotations from the original transcript, which, alongside the perceptions and commentary added by the researcher, created the life histories.

Physical literacy stories (the life story method in practice)

The following four stories focus on individuals from Chile, The Gambia, the Netherlands and England. They are shared not for direct comparison, but to demonstrate how the use of the life history method can illustrate and clarify key principles of physical literacy.

Lucia's story

Lucia (an alias) is a 49-year-old teacher from Chile. Playing for hours on end with her three brothers in the quiet street outside her home was central to Lucia enjoying a happy and secure childhood. With children from the neighbouring houses, they made up games, played football and climbed trees. Everyone joined in, and Lucia was well equipped to compete with and against them all. The never-ending games and the battles she enjoyed with her brothers nurtured her competitive spirit. Lucia recalls, 'I wanted to chase balls; I wanted to climb trees; I wanted to win. I was born wanting to chase my brothers and to beat them'.

When she was not playing, Lucia was on her bicycle, back and forth to the shops, doing laps of the crescent outside her house, and practising how to ride hands-free. If she was not on her bicycle, she was one of the few girls who rode skateboards, as it was a good excuse to be with the boys.

Despite the sibling rivalry, sport was not recognised as a particularly valuable pursuit within her middle-/upper-class family environment. Academic success was the driving factor, and the expectations were high at the private all-girls Catholic school that Lucia attended from the age of 4 until the age of 18. However, physical education was included in the curriculum and participation in sport was encouraged. The range of activities on offer were limited, but Lucia thrived. In particular, she excelled in athletics, and by the age of 12 Lucia was competing for the school at events across Chile. This required her to attend training after school on Tuesdays and Thursdays, as well as on Saturday mornings. Lucia's ability across events meant she was competing in at least six disciplines at every track and field meeting. She knew it was too much, and wanted to do less but better, yet her teachers and coaches would not listen. Lucia felt under pressure and any sense of enjoyment slowly drained away. She began to resent her increasingly muscular body, and detested the public sharing of measurements during the school's annual height and weight monitoring process.

As Lucia entered her teens, she wanted to look like the feminine young woman she was becoming, and recognised her physical body was developing in a way she did not want. She began to feel angry. Lucia wanted to say 'no'. The solution turned out to be easy. As Lucia entered the senior part of the school, physical education was taught by a different teacher, who also coached the school volleyball team. Here was someone who treated the girls as individuals and at the same time created a tremendous team ethos. She gave the girls agency, respected their opinions, and made training enjoyable. Lucia recalls, ' I loved her. She was very inspirational'.

By the age of 15, Lucia had quit athletics. The athletics coaches were cross, but Lucia was happy. She immersed herself in the world of volleyball and loved every minute – training sessions and matches were joyful, life revolved around volleyball. Lucia felt valued.

Life changed when Lucia went to university. There was no volleyball. Instead, there was studying and there were boys! However, the need to be active remained strong, so Lucia joined a gym and dabbled with aerobics. But she was not inspired, which meant participation was minimal, and before she knew it she was in England. With her degree completed and a scholarship to improve her English in hand, she joined a gym, made friends, met her first husband and married. Before long, the first baby arrived and exhaustion set in, with sleep triumphing over the need to exercise. It was a struggle to maintain the active lifestyle of her teens.

Eventually, Lucia, her English husband and her growing family (three boys at this point) returned to Chile, and she was dismayed to find she could not keep up with friends when they went hiking in the mountains. Lucia knew that she needed to exercise, and having heard colleagues talking excitedly about Bikram yoga decided to try a class. She immediately felt a sense of excitement and engagement – yoga allowed her to disconnect from the busyness of life and enabled her to become more comfortable in her body than she had ever been. For eight years, Lucia hardly missed a session. During that time, she divorced, felt herself healing, remarried, had another baby, watched her children grow up, and devoted her life to her family and her teaching.

Some years later, Lucia enthusiastically accepted a promotion at work when it was offered, but the sacrifice was stepping away from her yoga classes because of scheduling clashes. Physical activity had become such a central part of her life that she immediately looked for something else that would fit into her busy lifestyle, and consequently she joined a Pilates class where she felt challenged and pushed to her limit.

As Lucia heads towards 50 years of age, she has a new love alongside Pilates – extreme gardening! Lucia spends up to eight hours a day, whenever she can, constructing, digging and planting. She feels connected to the earth – it makes her feel alive. Lucia is proud of her fitness and health, and wants it to be forever thus – she cannot imagine life any other way.

Buba's story

Buba (who wishes his real name to be used) is 33 years old from The Gambia, where home is a village on the outskirts of the capital city, Banjul, where he lives with his extended family. As a very young child, Buba would accompany his mother to the community garden each day and would sit under the shade of a mango tree while she tended to her work. On one occasion, Buba began exploring, and a few minutes later his mother found him inside a well, close to drowning. He was taken to hospital, given a thorough medical check and put on a drip. The 2-year-old tugged at the tube up his nose, which prevented the fluids from taking effect, so to overcome this Buba's hands were tied to the bedstead by the medic. The restraint was too tight, the blood flow was restricted, and by the time the doctors realised there was a problem it was too late. To save Buba's life, both of his hands were amputated just above the wrist.

The consensus was that Buba's disability meant he had no potential to write, and therefore no potential to succeed in school. Consequently, Buba stayed at home throughout his childhood, watching his peers going off to school while he undertook simple household chores. He played with children from his village and occasionally went with his father to the quarry. As the years passed, he realised he was destined to become a beggar on the streets, and that school was his only hope. Buba knew he had to prove himself, so he persuaded his friend to teach him how to write letters and numbers – initially using a stick (gripped between his two stubs) in the sand, and eventually through mastering the ability to manipulate a pencil on paper. His determination paid dividends, and at the age of 12 Buba was allowed to enrol at school.

Buba recalls starting to play football with a friend in his compound around the age of 5, usually with a ball made of cloth and rope, and occasionally with a plastic ball bought from the market by his father. He surprised everyone by learning to ride a bicycle by the age of 8, applying a light touch to the handlebars with his stubs in order to steer. He enjoyed the sport-focused physical education lessons at school, and participated in rounders and athletics, but football was his passion. Soon after starting school, he was chosen for the school team – his speed, agility and skill stood out, and while there was reluctance to select him for the team because of his disability, his ability made him impossible to ignore. Buba soon caught the eye of local club coach, and thus Buba's competitive football career began, during which time he became a local celebrity. He played junior and senior football, and people came to watch the player with no hands. Buba was usually a substitute who made an immediate impact when he came on. In one memorable cup final, his team was one-nil down with 17 minutes to go. Buba came on from the bench and scored the equaliser, with his team eventually winning on penalties. He felt proud about the role he had played and enjoyed being the 'point of observation'.

Buba's ambition was to play in The Gambian professional league, but friends and advisors said the officials would never allow it as there was concern about how he would fare in the more physical aspects of the game. He reluctantly took the advice of his elders, and decided that if he could not play as a professional he would teach. The decision to set up his own academy seemed a natural one, but football is expensive to run and he was not financially strong. He handwrote application forms, bought material to make bibs, and managed to buy a football, which enabled him to launch his academy. His efforts caught the attention of several foreign visitors, with Football Gambia (a UK-based charity) and Plymouth University, in particular, helping him to attend coaching clinics and providing regular donations in the form of equipment. Currently, the academy has approximately 90 players on its register, spread equally across his three squads (U9, U10 and U14). Buba oversees all the training sessions, arranges matches, and ensures the boys lead healthy, responsible lives.

It is through the academy that Buba looks after his own fitness. He trains with the players each day, runs at least 3 km every day, and regularly plays in a friendly small-sided game. Buba is happiest when he is active and playing football, although he cites coaching his players as being very special as well. He enjoys the way the players copy him and how they listen so carefully to his words. He smiles as he adds that scoring the equaliser in the cup final was also very special.

Hardly a day goes by when Buba does not play, coach or watch football, and he recognises that it is important to keep exercising, explaining, 'it makes you strong and helps prevent sickness'. Furthermore, he promises that 'as long as my legs allow me, I will go and do some exercise ... because physical activity makes me happy and gives me energy'.

Nienke's story

Nienke (an alias) is the middle child of three children who resides in a town in the centre of the Netherlands. Nienke thrived when she started kindergarten at the age of 4 because the focus was on play, music and being outside. By the time she started primary school at the age of 6, Nienke already knew she was good at being physical, and consequently she enjoyed her physical education lessons, which were mainly focused on gymnastics, ball games and swimming.

Throughout Nienke's childhood years, there were always lots of children to play with in the street. Their games were made-up, fun, and required ever-increasing levels of skill. Football was a firm favourite, as was riding their bicycles, and the children would play unsupervised in the street. She and her brother were always outside because they wanted to be. They played all day long – if they were not playing football, they would be cycling in the nearby forest where they followed trails and created adventures. Nienke thrived on being as good as the boys at football and on being accepted by them. She progressed from street football to lessons at school, and then onto playing for the school team.

Nienke's parents both played tennis, and, as an eager 7-year-old, Nienke jumped at the chance to have tennis lessons at a club near to her home when her mother suggested it. She loved the game, and by the time she was 11 she was playing at a good level, competing against children from other clubs and enjoying a good social life. Around the same time that she started playing tennis, Nienke also began going to a local gymnastics club with her brother and her best friend. Her tennis coach, a soft-hearted and gentle man, generated a good spirit and lightness during lessons; her gymnastics coach was strict, and took time to compliment Nienke if she did well. The praise, whomever it came from, motivated Nienke to do better.

She enjoyed the opportunity to challenge herself in gymnastics, but she always seemed to know that it would not be a long-term pursuit. She loved being physical and using her body, but it was not long before she left gymnastics to focus on her tennis. As Nienke developed as a tennis player, she joined a bigger club, and her new coach encouraged her to aim for the national level, but by the age of 14 Nienke's motivation was diminishing.

At secondary school, Nienke found the physical education lessons were not as focused as they had been in primary school, but nonetheless she continued to stand out as one of the physically more able pupils and she accessed a wide range of experiences in different sports. As she entered her teens, Nienke became aware that a lot of the girls either were not good at physical education or did not like it, and an increasing number told her it 'wasn't cool' to play sport. To begin with, she was not particularly affected by peer pressure because she still loved playing football with the boys, but looking back she realises she began toning down her enthusiasm as the peer pressure took effect.

Her parents divorced when she was 13, and although Nienke's mother and father shared the parenting responsibilities, and it worked as well as could be expected for the family, money was scarce. Nienke's involvement in sport began to trail off, although 90 minutes per day of cycling to and from school meant she retained a very good level of fitness. By 14, Nienke was immersed in a new circle of friends. Beer, smoking, motorbikes and music became central to her group, and tennis was replaced with going to music concerts and dancing.

Leaving school at 19 was the start of a painful and difficult few years. Nienke broke up with her best friend, she travelled during a gap year, started and left a university course, and became ill with pneumonia. During this time, there was no participation in organised sport or physical activity, but at some point in her early twenties Nienke realised she needed to exercise – she felt her body was aching and calling out for help. She began trying different activities such as tai chi, running and yoga – all part of her search to fulfil her innate desire to be active. She particularly enjoyed yoga and attended classes several times a week. Yoga felt good for her body and for her soul.

A stress-related illness in her thirties meant a lengthy period away from work, during which time she developed a love of walking, and this became an essential part of the healing process. In her early forties, routines were interrupted once again because of a house move, which resulted in cycling becoming her primary exercise regime once more. Now aged 45, cycling and walking remain central to Nienke's schedule (walking through choice, cycling as a means of transport). These days, trips such as her forthcoming walking holiday to Spain provide her with the adrenaline buzz she needs from her exercise. Looking to the future, she feels sure that she will return to tai chi, and pictures herself participating from a chair when she becomes elderly. But for now, she wants to do more, and claims emphatically that yoga, walking and cycling will feature heavily in her life over the next few years.

Joanna's story

Joanna (an alias) lives in England. She is 41 years old and combines supply teaching alongside an emerging writing career. Joanna describes herself as being 'at the top end of the scales' – she is 5 feet 2 inches tall and weighs approximately 15 stone. Joanna realises she is very overweight, and knows committing to some kind of physical activity is important, but she is finding it hard to find that commitment.

A principal feature of Joanna's life is her passion for music, which she has had from an early age. She attended her first gig at the age of 11, discovered boy bands at 14, and has had a fascination with country music for as long as she can remember. At every opportunity, Joanna goes to concerts, following her favourite singers around England and beyond. Her spare time is filled with listening to music, which forms an ever-present backdrop to her writing. The feeling of elation she describes when attending a concert underpins how she feels about music. This passion is a far cry from her relationship with physical activity.

Joanna had a challenging childhood. She, her younger sister and single mother were a happy family unit, but they had to move frequently, which meant that between the ages of 3 and 8, Joanna never stayed in the same house, the same school, or the same area for more than six months at a time. Added to this, Joanna was in and out of hospital during early childhood, having operations on her ears, nose and throat. Problems with hearing, and later with eyesight, caused difficulties for Joanna throughout her childhood, and continue to do so in adulthood. The family's nomadic existence meant Joanna moved from school to school, and consequently she recalls virtually no participation in physical education lessons until the family eventually settled in one place, a small town in the north of England.

As a child, Joanna would spend time outdoors, but never played rough-and-tumble games like her sister. She never climbed a tree, stamped in a puddle or learned to ride a bike – not because she was not allowed to, but because she had no inclination to play such games. Instead, Joanna enjoyed sitting on the sofa at home, reading or listening to adult conversations. Her mother, who was herself averse to being physically active, was happy for Joanna to do so.

At the age of 11, Joanna started secondary school, and remembers her physical education teacher distinctly. She claims the teacher never liked her and never encouraged her, and with none of the basic skills or confidence usually developed in primary school, Joanna felt excluded. She became adept at excusing herself from lessons, and as a result she rarely participated in any form of physical activity within school.

Despite this, Joanna does have a few positive memories, such as when she was given a pair of pink roller skates for a birthday present, which she enjoyed using. She also felt reasonably comfortable when school physical education lessons focused on dance. Outside of school, Joanna enjoyed occasional outings with her aunt, who would take her hiking on the moorlands nearby.

As a young adult, the only physical activity Joanna engaged in was an occasional visit to an aerobics class and some rollerblading, both of which came out of a pact with a friend to do something crazy. Her university experience was not a positive one, but she persevered and eventually found herself doing a one-year teaching qualification. She shared a flat with a group of young professionals, among whom Joanna felt comfortable. These friends encouraged Joanna to try a few new activities, and she would take up the challenge, trying something once or twice but then leaving it alone. These challenges included abseiling, which she recalls gave her an amazing adrenaline rush, skiing on an artificial slope, running for charity dressed as Santa Claus, and a gruelling commando challenge course. After university, Joanna spent two years teaching English in China, where she joined in a dance class, tried tai chi and went hiking in the mountains. Back in England, she eventually settled into a long-term job as an international advisor in higher education, where she became more and more sedentary, with walking her only exercise.

Joanna was 34 when her daughter, Chloe, was born. Joanna's joy was tempered with feeling physically broken as a result of giving birth. She felt drained physically and emotionally, and it took her months to feel she could face the world again. As her confidence returned, she began to walk to lose weight. Chloe is now an energetic 6-year-old and Joanna finds it hard to keep up, especially as the walking habit has stopped and the weight has increased. Joanna wants to change but is finding it hard. She dismisses joining a gym, is horrified at the thought of joining a sports club of some kind, and has only fleeting interest in the idea of learning to swim.

She dances at music concerts, but beyond this the only form of exercise she will consider is to start walking again. Yet she is afraid to go walking by herself and will not commit to a regular schedule, apart from a recent decision to start walking around the house and up and down stairs while listening to music. The future looks uncertain; Joanna wants to be active but lacks the motivation to put her intention into action.

Commentary

Each of the above narratives has the potential to entertain the reader, but the true value of the life history method is the reader developing their understanding and appreciation of physical literacy. Intriguingly, each reader will take something different from the stories as they come to the stories having had different experiences themselves. It is, however, the role of the life historian to draw out common themes to use as evidence to support a particular enquiry and to investigate variances to test particular hypotheses. For the purposes of this chapter, the stories will be used to consider the lifelong nature of physical literacy, the impact that significant others and significant events have on those journeys, and how the subjects view their participation. It is anticipated that this exploration will help the reader to appreciate the degree to which each individual takes responsibility for their involvement in physical activity and the value they put on that involvement. Finally, aspects of each person's journey, which have the potential for further examination, will be signposted.

Common to all four stories is the clear demonstration that the physical literacy journey is ongoing. Lucia, Buba and Nienke are 49, 33 and 45 years old, respectively, and all have a lifelong appreciation of, and commitment to, physical activity, which has been a part of their lives for as long as they can remember. Regardless of their culture or personal/economic circumstances, their childhoods were full of playful activity with family and friends. They all identify experiences that are positive, such as Lucia's switch to volleyball, and all consider experiences that have had a negative impact, such as the moment Buba realised he would not be able to play professional football. They all value and have a commitment to lifelong physical activity, such as Nienke's determination to develop her yoga practice in the future. At 41 years old, Joanna claims to appreciate the need to be active, but her story indicates a lifelong struggle to commit to a physically active lifestyle. Positive experiences throughout her life have been few and far between, which, combined with scarce encouragement, a fragmented physical education, and very few successes of any note in respect of physical activity, begin to explain her lack of motivation and sedentary life. Joanna views physical activity as a chore and as something that she is not suited too.

In every case, the journeys are influenced by situations that resonate with the affective, the physical and the cognitive. For example, Nienke's love of playing with the boys underpinned her passion for football, Lucia's strength and speed led to her becoming a key member of the school athletic team, and Buba's realisation that he needed to get an education lead to him playing competitive football.

Likewise, for Joanna, it seems her love of music has provided her with some fleeting moments where she enjoys being physical, as she happily states, 'I don't sit still [at concerts] … I will dance'.

Significant others

Whitehead (2010) identified that other people can have a positive or negative effect on an individual's physical literacy journey. The term 'significant others' emerged from Mead's theory of self (Mead and Morris, 1937), and refers to a person who has influence over the individual in terms of self-esteem and behaviour. Significant others are important to an individual's well-being, and they can certainly affect the progress an individual makes on a physical literacy journey. In particular, the affective domain is very much influenced by interface with others. Lucia's engagement with volleyball, Buba's commitment to his football team, Nienke's passion for football, and Joanna's occasional one-off challenges are all traceable back to a significant other encouraging the individual in question.

Not all significant others are positive role models, nor do they necessarily have the individual's best interests at heart, in which case the individual's physical literacy journey can be adversely affected. In some cases, this could be to such an extent that the individual may decide to withdraw from a physically active lifestyle. Tragically, Joanna's physical education teacher in secondary school failed to show the empathy or respect that the fragile young person deserved. Instead, the humiliation Joanna experienced, particularly on the netball court, cemented her decision that physical activity was not for her. Another case in point is Nienke's friendship group in her teens, which drew her into a more sedentary way of being.

Significant others are most commonly parents, other family members, teachers, coaches and peers, but may also include a range of other close acquaintances. As the individual moves into adulthood, significant others may include partners and employers. What these people have in common is that they are important in the individual's life.

In Lucia's case, her siblings were significant others – her playful battles with her brothers during childhood created a platform for her fiercely competitive nature. Her brothers challenged her constantly and ensured the competitive element was ever-present. Similarly, throughout Nienke's early years, her younger brother and local friends were always there to play with, whether it was in the street, the park or the school field. Significant in Buba's life was his childhood friend who was attending school while Buba remained at home. Buba persuaded his friend to teach him how to write, the fundamental skill he required to enable him to enrol at school, which paved the way to his realising his ambition to play competitive football. While Joanna's sister was both active and adventurous, her mother had no inclination towards physical activity and was complicit in supporting Joanna to miss physical education lessons. The lack of encouragement during her early years and the lack of positive role models during adolescence must surely have compounded Joanna's negative views.

Teachers and coaches feature strongly in all four stories. For example Lucia's experiences clearly show both the positive and negative influences these adults can have on their pupils. She gave up athletics because she did not feel valued, whereas she thrived in volleyball because the teacher/coach treated her as an individual and was genuinely interested in her progress. Her friends were also significant. Lucia's words are very powerful when she says of her volleyball friends, 'Everyone was trusted and everyone relied upon each other'.

Significant events

Bourdieu's (1986) theory of habitus suggests that our life experiences, or significant events, influence our habits and dispositions. In the case of the physical literacy journey, life histories highlight the individual's key experiences. The individual might not always have positive experiences, but these significant events are nearly always tipping points that have a considerable effect on the future direction of their physical literacy journey. Sometimes referred to as milestones, which is particularly apt given the journey metaphor, there are a number of significant events, or achievements, that are fairly commonplace in a given culture. In the case of three of our subjects, learning to ride a bicycle was a significant achievement. This milestone gave each person a sense of achievement, gave them a degree of independence, and provided another outlet for them to develop their love of physical activity. Contrary to this, Joanna has never attempted to ride a bicycle and has no desire to do so.

For Buba, undoubtedly the most significant event of his physical literacy journey, and indeed his life, was the incident that resulted in the loss of his hands. This remarkable boy determined that people would know him for his footballing skills rather than pass him on the street as a beggar. For Lucia, the moment she rejected athletics and opted for volleyball marks the time when this 14-year-old took responsibility for her own physical literacy journey. Nienke responded to an innate desire to become active after a considerable time leading a sedentary lifestyle. She felt a need to move, and found yoga to be a vehicle for responding to that need, and this initiated her beginning to find her place in the world. Despite a very negative attitude towards physical activity, Joanna has experienced fleeting moments of exhilaration such as the adrenaline rush she felt while undertaking her one and only abseil. And while being interviewed, Joanna also suddenly remembers going to nightclubs at university purely to dance, which she then links to the joy she feels while dancing at music concerts and the weekly dance classes she attended while living in China. This insight suggests that Joanna may, one day, find an activity – dance perhaps – to which she will feel connected.

Other significant events in the stories play their part – illness, parents divorcing, transitioning from school to school or club to club. Every significant incident has the potential to be a hindrance or to be liberating, but it will usually be life-changing.

General observations

Over the course of their journeys, three of the subjects are mostly motivated and confident. At various times, and in varying degrees, all three show remarkable determination, perseverance and commitment in respect of their continued participation. They are all physically competent and able to take part in physical activity settings that are available to them. They are all knowledgeable about physical activity and are capable of intelligent reflection concerning their participation. They have all persisted as they have aged, which in all cases meant either looking at different activities as they got older or adapting the way they engaged. In contrast, Joanna was unable to build a foundation of positive experiences in childhood and adolescence. The early stages of her journey were such that she was unable to find the compass with which to navigate the challenges and opportunities that presented themselves as the years went by. In respect of physical literacy, motivation, confidence and physical competence are lacking. Now in adulthood, she understands the benefit of physical activity, not least to lose weight, and knows she should be more active. However, something prevents her from prioritising time for exercise above her many other interests.

The life histories also reveal potential threats that might stop even our highly motivated subjects from making progress. Once identified, the individual or a significant other can help manage that threat. Lucia's workload is likely to always have a tendency to derail her planned schedule of activity; she recognises this and schedules her Pilates sessions in her diary in advance. Buba's scarred lower arms have a tendency to become infected, causing him to withdraw from his football academy for periods of time. As he learns how to manage the potential for infection and accesses medication, these periods of withdrawal will hopefully become less frequent. In the past, Nienke's physical activity has petered out when she experienced stress, but she has come to appreciate that exercise, particularly walking in nature, is an antidote to stress.

An interesting process to consider is how Lucia's, Buba's, Nienke's and Joanna's journeys would play out if situated in a different culture. For example, the attitude to those with a disability in The Gambia is different to, say, that in Europe or North America. Buba would most likely have been nurtured as a sporting talent, with opportunities to become a Paralympian, had he been born in, say, England or the United States. Perhaps Joanna's progress would have been more fruitful had she spent her early years in a consistent and supportive school environment.

Culture can also be considered on a local (family) level. For Nienke, physical activity was a family affair, with the parents and three children all playing tennis, whereas in Lucia's family success in academia was seen as the priority. In stark contrast, in Buba's family the daily routine of working to feed the family was the only real consideration, and if playing football in the street kept the children occupied, then so be it.

Whether it was the experiences themselves or the reflection on the experiences afforded by telling their stories, Lucia, Buba and Nienke all came to realise that their physical activity was helpful to overcome stress, recover from illness, or counteract disability. They each saw the value of physical activity, and therefore engaged wholeheartedly. Even Joanna appreciates that there is a link between what she calls 'energy' and physical activity.

The stories illustrate the level of importance that physical activity plays in the lives of our subjects, albeit they live in different countries. Lucia, Buba and Nienke all indicate that their lives would not be as fulfilling were it not for their involvement in physical activity. Their accounts also suggest that their lives are built on an innate desire to be active, as if they have no option but to find an appropriate outlet. Joanna knows that she should be physically active but has yet to discover the positive effects that come from participation on a regular consistent basis.

Lucia talks about wanting to chase balls and climb trees, and she declares her life revolved around volleyball. She refers to a strong need to be active, and recounts how excited and engaged she became when she found a form of exercise that met her needs. She reflects that physical activity is a central part of her life.

Buba realises that his work with the football academy provides the opportunity for him to look after his own fitness. It allows him to play the game he loves, to run and to train. He cannot imagine a life without football, or a life without physical activity – for him, participation means happiness.

Nienke talks about thriving when playing football, and tells us that she eagerly seized the opportunity to play tennis. She explains that she enjoyed opportunities to challenge herself, refers to loving being physical, and says yoga felt good for her body and for her soul. And when ill health befell her, she turned to physical activity for the solution, thereby developing a love of walking in nature.

Joanna acknowledges that being physically active would bring significant benefits – weight loss and increased energy, for example – but she has not as yet appreciated that the 'feel-good' factor she gets from dancing at music concerts is something she could experience on a much more regular basis.

There seems ample evidence within these life histories that involvement in physical activity has the potential to enrich lives and contribute positively to wellbeing and human flourishing.

Conclusion

The physical literacy as a journey metaphor helps us to appreciate the individual nature of our engagement with physical activity. The unique experiences we encounter and our appreciation of how these experiences build, layer upon layer, becomes a process through which we find out about ourselves. The snowballing of experiences and the rich mix of interactions change people, with the resultant transformations leading to a greater sense of self. We are who we are because of the accumulated interactions that we experience.

The use of the physical literacy as a journey metaphor alongside the life history method can be used effectively to bring clarity to the physical literacy concept. The metaphor can be valuable to interrogate and learn more about lifelong physical literacy. As discussed in earlier chapters, all too often physical literacy is mistakenly seen as mainly relevant to the early years. Considering an individual's life history and appreciating that every individual is on their unique physical literacy journey leads to a better understanding of this being a concept that applies throughout our life.

In addition, much can be learnt from reflecting on the journeys described, alerting teachers and significant others to the part they play in fostering physical literacy. Empathy, creating opportunities and giving encouragement can be very powerful influences in respect of promoting participation. Lack of support, insensitivity and negative attitudes can have long-term consequences, even a lifelong avoidance of active participation.

Life histories chart an individual's journey and demonstrate the principles underpinning physical literacy. In addition, the process of being interviewed can have a significant effect on the subject, as space is created for the individual to reflect on the past and think to the future, thus serving to raise self-awareness. Stories about physical literacy journeys illustrate that the concept is about individuals achieving their potential and highlight the fact that it is an ongoing feature of life. Further research using the life history method could well make a very valuable contribution to the understanding of key determinants of fostering physical literacy. In time, this type of research might also bring out characteristics of physical literacy journeys that are unique to life in a particular culture or country.

References

Atkinson, R. (1998) *The Life Story Interview*. London: Sage.

Bourdieu, P. (1986) The forms of capital. In J. Richardson (ed.), *Handbook of Theory and Research for the Sociology of Education*. New York: Greenwood, pp. 241–258.

Clough, P. (2002) *Narratives and Fictions in Educational Research*. Buckingham, UK: Open University Press.

Ellis, C. (2004) *The Ethnographic I: A Methodological Novel about Autoethnography*. Walnut Creek, CA: Rowman AltaMira.

Goodson, I. and Sikes, P. (2001) *Life History Research in Educational Settings*. Buckingham, UK: Open University Press.

Lakoff, G. and Johnson, M. (1980) *Metaphors We Live By*. Chicago, IL: University of Chicago Press.

Macartney, T. (2007) *Finding Earth, Finding Soul: The Invisible Path to Authentic Leadership*. Embercombe: Mona Books.

Mead, G.H. and Morris, C.M. (1962) *Mind, Self, and Society from the Standpoint of a Social Behaviorist*. Chicago, IL: University of Chicago Press.

Roberts, B. (2002) *An Introduction to Biographical Research*. London: Open University Press.

Schwandt, T. (2001) *Dictionary of Qualitative Inquiry*. London: Sage.

Taplin, L. (2011) Physical literacy: an introduction to the concept. *Physical Education Matters*, 6(1): 28–30.

Taplin, L. (2013) Physical literacy as a journey. *ICSSPE Bulletin*, 65: 57–62.

Whitehead, M. (2010) *Physical Literacy throughout the Lifecourse*. London: Routledge.

Whitehead, M. (2013) Definition of physical literacy and clarification of related issues. *ICSSPE Bulletin*, 65: 29–34.

18

HUMAN FLOURISHING AND PHYSICAL LITERACY

Elizabeth Durden-Myers and Margaret Whitehead

Introduction

Part I of this book focused on clarification of the definition of physical literacy, and the development of the thinking concerned with value, implications for practice and charting the physical literacy journey. Part II shared with readers how physical literacy has spread and is being interpreted across the world. Part III opened with the developing work on the notion of physical literacy as a journey, and how this metaphor can illuminate areas of personal experience and add to the understanding of individual journeys. This chapter extends the consideration of value as presented in Part I. This earlier discussion was concerned with the legitimacy of physical literacy, first as securely grounded in philosophy and second from a social justice perspective. This chapter aims to look more widely and to make a case for the value of physical literacy as having the potential to make a significant contribution to life as a whole, as a component of human flourishing.

There are four sections to this chapter. The first addresses the nature of human flourishing, while the second looks at whether the notion of human flourishing is in tune with the philosophical roots of physical literacy. The third section considers how far physical literacy shares the characteristics of human flourishing, and the fourth considers how far the constituent traits of human flourishing are comparable with those in physical literacy. It will be suggested that on account of the congruence of physical literacy with a range of aspects of human flourishing, fostering physical literacy has the potential to make a positive contribution to human flourishing.

What is human flourishing?

Human flourishing is a term used to describe a disposition whereby individuals are thriving or living optimally (De Ruyter, 2004). This would also encompass the notions of wellness and living a good life. Each of these descriptions judge the quality of life from a slightly different perspective; however, VanderWeele (2017) argues that regardless of the different interpretations of well-being or human flourishing, most would concur that, ideally, this would include a positive experience in respect of five broad areas of human life: (1) happiness and life satisfaction; (2) health, both mental and physical; (3) meaning and purpose; (4) character and virtue; and (5) close social relationships. All these are arguably at least a part of what is meant by flourishing. Each of these areas also satisfies two important criteria in the context of physical literacy: each is generally viewed as an end in itself, and each is, in most circumstances, universally desired. The nature of human flourishing or quality of life is complex, and relates both to the individual and the cultural context. However, to judge that someone has a good quality of life, it would be expected that most of the five areas of human flourishing cited above would be in evidence, with no overemphasis on, or omission of, a specific area that might threaten flourishing as a whole.

Rasmussen (1999) describes human flourishing as the ultimate end of human conduct. However, human flourishing is not purely focused on the end goal, but also includes an awareness of the value of the means to achieve these ends. A flourishing life is something that is seldom achieved at a stroke. Therefore, the means to foster, for example, happiness, health, meaning and purpose, and close social relationships (VanderWeele, 2017), should not be viewed only as stepping stones to human flourishing, but also as partial realisations or expressions of this human disposition (Rasmussen, 1999). Human flourishing therefore values equally the means and the ends of striving towards, and attaining, a life that thrives and flourishes. To flourish as humans is a desirable endeavour. It can be considered as the ultimate aim of life, which is not just simply to exist, but instead to flourish in existence. The notion of human flourishing encompasses many different aspects of human life, each of which can contribute towards flourishing. The question is, 'What contribution can physical literacy play in promoting human flourishing?'

Shared philosophical basis of human flourishing and physical literacy

Before looking in detail at the relationship between human flourishing and physical literacy, it is useful to consider how far, from a philosophical point of view, the two concepts share common ground. Physical literacy has roots in monism, existentialism and phenomenology (Whitehead, 2010), and it is suggested that these philosophical concepts also align with human flourishing.

The central tenet of monism is that a human is not comprised of separate aspects of being, such as the body and the mind, but is one intricately intra-dependant whole. It is evident in all discussions of human flourishing that this view is endorsed. As mentioned above, human flourishing is described as a disposition or a way of living. Wolbert et al. (2015) refer to human flourishing as a dynamic state, with no particular aspect of human nature singled out. Physical literacy is also described as a disposition that essentially draws on all areas of human nature.

Existentialists argue that human beings create themselves in interaction with the world of animate and inanimate features. Human flourishing embraces this view by including reference to areas such as environmental mastery and positive relationships with others (Ryff and Keyes, 1995). Wilson-Strydom and Walker (2015) describe interaction as the seedbed of human flourishing and advocate involvement in a range of interaction avenues. This view is supported by Wolbert et al. (2015), who argue for the value of experiencing life in all spheres. In a similar way, effective fostering of physical literacy is best realised in involvement in wide and varied contexts, both in respect of the physical environment and interaction with other people.

Finally, there is congruence between human flourishing and physical literacy in the context of phenomenology. This philosophical position is concerned with highlighting the notion that each individual interprets and acts in the world from a unique standpoint. Past experiences are carried forward and frame future perceptions. On account of this situation, every individual is unique and should be respected as such. This position is integral to human flourishing as it is stressed that each individual should take responsibility for their particular preferences and lifestyle. Wolbert et al. (2015) propose that 'Striving for a flourishing life is a life-long journey in which one keeps asking what might bring out the best of oneself' (p. 127). Agency, autonomy and having a purpose in life all feature in human flourishing, and this would seem to endorse a phenomenological view of the individual at the centre of the enterprise. Within physical literacy, there is also the clear indication that each person is a unique individual who should take responsibility for participation in physical activity.

It would seem that there is no dissonance between human flourishing and physical literacy in respect of philosophical foundations, and this augurs well for underwriting physical literacy as an acceptable component of, and contributor to, human flourishing.

Characteristics of human flourishing

In order to articulate how physical literacy can contribute to human flourishing, it is useful to consider Rasmussen's (1999) interrelated characteristics of human flourishing. These are identified as being objectively good, inclusive, individualised, agent-dependent, self-directed, and socially constructed. Each of these characteristics is explained briefly and then related to physical literacy.

Objectively good

Objectively good as a characteristic of human flourishing is derived from the Greek word *eudemonia*, which translated into English means happiness (Annett, 2016). However, human beings are inclined to seek a deeper sense of happiness than mere attainment of pleasure and avoidance of pain. Ryan and Deci (2001) and VanderWeele

(2017) give particular attention to aspects of human flourishing that could promote flourishing on account of their being objectively 'good' and contributing to 'the good life'. In addition, human beings are inclined to seek not only the good life for themselves, but the good life for and with others. This sense of mutual flourishing is embedded in the notion of the common good (Etzioni, 2015). In short, happiness should be sought after by working from 'good' motives and intentions rather than selfish and unethical intentions.

Physical literacy similarly incorporates the notions of being 'objectively good'. The physical activities promoted in nurturing physical literacy are generally viewed as enhancing the good life, being intrinsically worthwhile and maximising potential. It would be seen as unacceptable if participation in a physical activity was entered into knowing that this could possibly cause distress to others or put them in any danger. In most cases, in respect of physical activity, the participation of an individual in physical activity offers the opportunity for others to be involved in and benefit from this engagement. In this way, participation is very much in the common good (Ryan and Deci, 2001; VanderWeele, 2017). Physical literacy and engagement in physical activity would seem to play a significant role in human flourishing in being intrinsically 'good' and providing opportunities for meaningful activity.

Inclusive

Human flourishing is inclusive in that it is accessible and obtainable for all, regardless of endowment or personal circumstances. Individuals can flourish by striving to live optimally and by maximising their personal human potential (Durden-Myers et al., 2018). Inclusion, more broadly, can be fostered in environments in which individuals with a whole host of unique (often marginalised or minoritised) identities can find opportunities to succeed and belong. Such an inclusive environment can contribute to the establishment of close social relationships.

Physical literacy embraces this foundational notion of inclusivity in the sense that all individuals, irrespective of their knowledge, skills and endowment, are encouraged to explore and develop a broad movement repertoire. When experiences are offered in a wide variety of environments, this maximises engagement in physical activity, and thus can capitalise on particular human potential.

Individualised

Human flourishing is individualised because it is dependent on who and what constitutes that person (Rasmussen, 1999). This means that individuals will flourish in different ways and involve different means, which will be specific and unique to that person.

Physical literacy also shares this individualised view, and values the distinctive and unique nature of perception, development and aspirations as exhibited by each human being. Physical literacy aims to embrace this by suggesting that each individual is on a personalised and unique journey, with no two journeys being the same.

Therefore, it is not appropriate to compare individuals with one another as this approach threatens the individualised nature of human flourishing, and indeed physical literacy. Instead, the creation of personal goals and aspirations that relate to the individual is recommended. This approach encourages individuals to find personal authentic meaning and purpose in life, which can promote both physical literacy and human flourishing.

Agent-dependent

Human flourishing is agent-dependent. Flourishing does not merely happen or occur independently of the individual. In order for flourishing to be nurtured and expressed, it falls to the individual to be proactive in attributing meaning or value to particular circumstances. A person needs to have a hand in creating the conditions by which to flourish. There must be a synergy between these conditions and the individual.

In relation to physical literacy, the provision of physical activity experiences and environments are provided in ways that individuals can grow to value and find meaning in these activities. Individuals are provided with authentic opportunities to pursue movement and physical activities that are personally meaningful (see explanatory glossary), thus establishing a relationship between the individual, the activity and the environment.

Self-directed

Human flourishing is self-directed. This means that human flourishing must be attained through the individual's own actions and efforts, and cannot be purely achieved in responding to external factors that are beyond an individual's control (Rasmussen, 1999). Each individual is on their own path to a flourishing life, and this path must be travelled as a result of that person's own volition following self-selected goals (Durden-Myers et al., 2018).

Within the definition of physical literacy, the notion of individuals taking responsibility for their own engagement in physical activity alludes to the self-directed nature of lifelong physical activity. Individuals are encouraged to exercise independent decision-making and to take action in the interests of participation in physical activity. Providing individuals with the opportunity to be self-directed allows them to engage in movement tasks that are meaningful and purposeful. Thus, to foster physical literacy as a lifelong journey, an appropriate range of opportunities for physical activity should be provided for all age groups. The provision of choice encourages self-direction in decision-making, which not only recognises differences, but can help to nurture physical literacy in all.

Socially constructed

Rasmussen (1999) also describes human flourishing as a socially constructed concept. Human beings are naturally social animals. Human flourishing therefore embraces this aspect of human nature, and incorporates the relationship between the individual, the environment and others. Flourishing in this context is realised through interaction with a wide range of cultural and/or context-specific factors, including the individual's social world. Understanding the interconnected nature between an individual and their environment is key in creating circumstances that support and further human flourishing. Flourishing is likely to be evident in communities that recognise the role they play in nurturing their population. Communities should appreciate that personal values, aims and effectiveness are both unique to the individual and developed in concert with the social milieu. Annett (2016) explains that this is a win–win situation as the flourishing of the individual is interlinked with the flourishing of the community.

Similarly, physical literacy is socially constructed and situated within social community, whether this is a school, a local community or a state/country. Engagement in physical activities that are established within a community should feature in programmes that foster physical literacy. These experiences in recognised forms of activity are likely to be more readily meaningful to an individual. This promotion of physical activity and physical literacy not only creates opportunities for individual development, but also helps to foster and establish communities that value physical activity. This is again a win–win situation.

The characteristics of human flourishing identified above provide an outline of the nature of flourishing. These refer to being objectively good, inclusive, individualised, agent-dependent, self-directed and socially constructed. It is argued that all these features readily align with characteristics of physical literacy, and this synergy would suggest that the promotion of physical literacy has the potential to enhance human flourishing.

Constituent traits of human flourishing

A second area of congruence that needs to be considered is the alignment of the constituent traits associated with human flourishing with those of physical literacy. This section sets out some of these traits, which have been proposed by writers such as Ryff and Keyes (1995), Kekes (2002) and Seligman (2011). There is considerable common ground covered by these analyses; however, the description drawn up by Ryff and Keyes (1995) is seen as representing the major aspects of human flourishing. They list human traits of autonomy, personal growth, self-acceptance, a purpose in life, environmental mastery, and positive relationship with others. Ryff and Keyes (1995) also identify vitality and optimism in their writing, but do not include them specifically among their constituents; however, as these are very apposite to physical literacy, they have been included in the following discussion.

It is suggested that to describe an individual as flourishing, there should be evidence of each of these constituent traits. In brief, it might be expected that an individual evidences:

- *autonomy* in exercising independence, self-determination and agency, taking responsibility for shaping their life;

- *personal growth* in a proactive interest in learning, accomplishment, and a wide-ranging and enquiring attitude to new opportunities;
- *self-acceptance* in realistic self-perception, positive self-esteem and acceptance of personal potential;
- *a purpose in life* in having a clear sense of direction, commitment and perseverance regarding the task at hand, and a sound vision of the future (i.e. personal clarity relating to values by which to live);
- *environmental mastery* in the ability to effect productive relationships with a wide range of environments (this is achieved though perceptive understanding and imaginative, apposite response);
- *positive relationships* with others in showing good interpersonal skills of listening, understanding and empathizing, as well as advising with sensitivity;
- *optimism* in being positive about the future, displaying a robust confidence and showing resilience in the face of challenges; and
- *vitality* in having energy, drive, commitment and enthusiasm.

Table 18.1 sets out the ways in which physical literacy can foster each of these constituent traits. The table is created with reference to the definition and the attributes of physical literacy, which can be found in Chapter 2. It is useful to refer to these earlier sections in reading the table. For example, the 'autonomy' listed among the constituent traits of human flourishing can be furthered by those aspects of physical literacy that indicate the individual should take responsibility for participation in physical activity. The 'personal growth' constituent of human flourishing can be supported in the development of physical competence and effective interaction with the environment. The motivation and confidence identified in the definition of physical literacy can be seen as having the potential to contribute to the traits of human flourishing relating to 'self-acceptance', 'optimism' and 'vitality'.

There seems little doubt from the discussion above that physical literacy can contribute to human flourishing in respect of contributing to constituent traits as set out above. These are identified as autonomy, personal growth, self-acceptance, a purpose in life, environmental mastery, positive relationships, optimism and vitality. This congruence supports the claim that physical literacy has the potential to make a wide-ranging and significant contribution to human flourishing.

Conclusion

This chapter has set out a case for physical literacy to be acknowledged as making a valuable contribution to human flourishing. The two dispositions share some common philosophical roots and are closely aligned in respect of characteristics and constituent traits. The next chapter will discuss the relationship between human nature and human flourishing, as well as considering physical literacy as a key aspect of human nature, and thus an essential part of human flourishing.

TABLE 18.1 Constituent traits of human flourishing and their exemplification/place in physical literacy

	Nature of the constituent trait	*Inclusion of the constituent in physical literacy*
Autonomy	Independence, self-determination, agency, responsibility, freedom and liberty.	Physical literacy aims to encourage individuals to be responsible for adopting a physically active lifestyle. Participants are encouraged to take ownership of their involvement in physical activities. Promoting individual *autonomy* is an aspiration embedded within physical literacy.
Personal growth	Proactive interest in learning and accomplishment. Wide-ranging and enquiring attitude to new opportunities. Ambitious and forward-thinking.	Physical literacy aims to develop confidence through progressive achievement appropriate to age and endowment. Growth and accomplishment are realised in effective interaction in physical activity in a wide variety of environments. This depends on individual perception and imagination, as well as application of movement patterns. *Personal growth* is a very significance aspect of all work to foster physical literacy.
Self-acceptance	Realistic and positive self-perception. Acceptance of, and contentment with, personal potential. Awareness of strengths and weaknesses. Sound self-esteem and self-concept.	Those advocating physical literacy strongly support showing respect for each person as unique with individual potential. Realistic self-perception is fostered through developing motivation and self-confidence. Assessment of physical literacy is ipsative (i.e. based on previous performance). Encouraging feedback on effort, progress and achievement is recommended. *Self-acceptance* permeates the work in physical literacy not least in celebrating steps individuals take in realising their individual potential and developing a positive sense of self.
Purpose in life	Clear sense of direction, commitment and perseverance. A sound vision of the future. Personal clarity relating to values by which to live.	Proponents of physical literacy see involvement in physical activity as opening the door to a rich range of opportunities that can play a part in defining life. Physical activity offers new horizons and can feature in mapping life experiences for the future. It can change lives. Engagement in physical activity in the context of physical literacy can add meaning and *purpose to life*. The valuing of physical activity in its own right is a priority.

Environmental mastery	Productive relationships within a wide range of environments. Astute perception, understanding, imagination and apposite responses. Productive use of previous experiences.	Physical literacy is grounded in existentialism, and thus meaningful involvement in a range of situations and environments is central to the concept. Effective interaction involves alert perception, imagination and creative ways to apply movement patterns. *Mastery of the environment* lies at the heart of physical literacy.
Positive relationships with others	Good interpersonal skills of listening, understanding and empathising. Establishment of mutual trust. Caring and responsive attitude. Adds positively to group enterprises.	Much engagement in physical activity takes place alongside others, and indeed relies on the actions of others. To achieve effective participation, individuals are guided to develop mutual respect, empathy and responsiveness in relation to others. The fostering of physical literacy includes the realisation of *positive relationships with others* so that experiences for all are meaningful and rewarding.
Optimism	Positive attitude towards the future. Robust confidence and resilience in the face of challenges.	The fostering of physical literacy depends on developing the motivation and confidence to look ahead to rewarding experiences in the field of physical activity. Realistic self-acceptance alongside support from others engenders resilient application in the expectation of progress. Physical literacy is imbued with *optimism* in the confidence and excitement of further meaningful experiences in the context of physical activity.
Vitality	Energy, drive, commitment, zest for life, enthusiasm, and sound embodied health and well-being.	Founded on the intricate complexities and extensive abilities of human embodied life, physical literacy has the capacity to energise and enhance life (Almond, 2015). The effort required for participation, and the quality of subsequent experiences, engenders a thirst for more active involvement. The *vitality* that is realised in involvement in physical activity is a distinguishing characteristic of physical literacy.

Source: Adapted from Ryff and Keyes (1995)

References

Almond, L. (2015) *Characteristics of Physical Literacy*. Unpublished paper.

Annett, A. (2016) Human flourishing, the common good, and Catholic social teaching. In J. Sachs, L. Becchetti and A. Annett (eds), *World Happiness Report 2016: Volume II*. Available at: http://worldhappiness.report/wp-content/uploads/sites/2/2016/03/HR-V2_web.pdf (accessed 18 March 2019).

De Ruyter, D.J. (2004) Pottering in the garden? On human flourishing and education. *British Journal of Educational Studies*, 52: 377–389.

Durden-Myers, E., Whitehead, M.E. and Pot, N. (2018) Physical Literacy and Human Flourishing. *Journal of Teaching in Physical Education*, 37: 308–311.

Etzioni, A. (2015) *The Common Good*. Cambridge: Polity Press.

Kekes, C.L.M. (2002) The mental health continuum: from langishing to flourishing in life. *Journal of Health and Social Research*, 43: 207–222.

Rasmussen, D.B. (1999) Human flourishing and the appeal to human nature. *Social Philosophy and Policy*, 16: 1–43.

Ryan, R. and Deci, E. (2001) On happiness and human potentials: a review of research on hedonic and eudaimonic well-being. *Annual Review of Psychology*, 52: 141–166.

Ryff, C.D. and Keyes, C.L. (1995) The sructure of psychological well-being revisited. *Journal of Personality and Social Psychology*, 69(4): 719–727.

Seligman, M.E.P. (2011) *Flourish: A New Understanding of Happiness and Wellbeing – and How to Achieve Them*. London: Nicholas Brealey.

VanderWeele, T.J. (2017) On the promotion of human flourishing. *Proceedings of the National Academy of Sciences of the United States of America*, 114(31): 8148–8156.

Whitehead, M.E. (ed.) (2010) *Physical Literacy throughout the Lifecourse*. London: Routledge.

Wilson-Strydom, M. and Walker M. (2015) A capabilities-friendly conceptualisation of flourishing in and through education. *Journal of Moral Education*, http://dx.doi.org/10.1080/03057240.2015.1043878.

Wolbert, L.S., De Ruyter, D.J. and Schinkel, A. (2015) Formal criteria for the concept of human flourishing as an ideal: the first step in defending flourishing as an ideal in education. *Ethics and Education*, 10(1): 118–129.

19

HUMAN FLOURISHING, HUMAN NATURE AND PHYSICAL LITERACY

Elizabeth Durden-Myers and Margaret Whitehead

Introduction

The previous chapter sought to establish the relationship between human flourishing and physical literacy. It was argued that there is a clear synergy between human flourishing and physical literacy in respect to philosophical roots, characteristics and constituent human traits. The congruence between these two human dispositions would seem to provide a sound context to articulate support for the value of physical literacy. To consider further this source of endorsement, this chapter considers how physical literacy can gain further credibility via being a significant aspect of human nature. This possibility arises on account of the close relationship between human flourishing and human nature. The chapter also explores the relationship between physical literacy and human needs, the nature of human resources, and the primacy of movement.

Human flourishing and human nature

The nature of human flourishing has been outlined broadly as living a rich and rewarding life with the opportunity and freedom to develop chosen aspects of human potential. In other words, fostering human flourishing could be seen as realising all those aspects of being that together constitute human nature. Thus, there is a sense in which humans will flourish if their nature as humans is respected, nurtured and celebrated.

Two important aspects of human nature are human needs and human potentials. The close relationship between human flourishing and human nature, as comprised of needs and potentials, has been underwritten by a number of writers, such as Kekes (2000), Nussbaum (2000), Younkins (2010) and Wilson-Strydom and Walker (2015). Younkins (2010) writes that 'there is an inextricable relationship between human flourishing and human nature' (p. 1). Wilson-Strydom and Walker (2015) and Nussbaum (2000) elaborate on this view, identifying value as the essential link. For example, Wilson-Strydom and Walker (2015) write that 'flourishing from a capabilities approach point of view is thus understood as the extent to which a person is able to be and to do what they have reason to value being and doing' (p. 4), while Nussbaum (2000) expresses the view that human flourishing is 'a striving to achieve a life that includes all the activities to which [on reflection] they [a person] decided to attach intrinsic value' (cited in Wilson-Strydom and Walker, 2015: 3).

The notion of human nature and human needs will be touched on from a psychological perspective, while the issue of human nature and human resources will relate to social justice. In both cases, a link to physical literacy will be made. These are both areas that would benefit from further study and research.

Human nature, human needs and physical literacy

Writers such as Maslow (1970), Manfred et al. (1989), Doyal and Gough (1991) and Ramsay (1992) characterise human nature as a form of life that revolves round the fulfilment of particular needs. From the variety of suggestions (see Alkire, 2002), two clusters of needs are set out in Tables 19.1 and 19.2. Maslow (1970) identifies five human needs that he argues have to be satisfied in a hierarchical order, from the physiological perspective upwards. In his view, self-actualisation is the paramount need to which humans are drawn (see Table 19.1). Manfred et al. (1989) identify nine needs that stem from the condition of being human and are to be understood as interactive, with only subsistence and survival as essential fundamental needs (see Table 19.2).

Looking through these two lists, it seems there is no problem in identifying how physical literacy could contribute to satisfying many of these. The concern for the affective domain in respect of physical literacy will feed into the realisation of self-esteem and identity. Attention to the physical domain will contribute to physiological needs and needs in respect of participation and leisure. Cognitive aspects of physical literacy will play a part in satisfying needs for understanding and creativity. In addition, the aspiration of empowering individuals to take responsibility for decision-making will feed into the needs for self-actualisation and freedom. Physical literacy can play a role in the fulfilment of human needs, and thus is in alignment to human flourishing in this respect.

TABLE 19.1 Maslow's (1970) hierarchy of needs

Hierarchy of needs	Brief description
Self-actualisation (highest order need)	Achieving one's full potential, including creative activities
Esteem	Prestige and feelings of accomplishment
Belonging and love	Intimate relationships and love
Safety	Security
Physiological (most basic need)	Food, water, warmth, rest

TABLE 19.2 Manfred et al.'s (1989) fundamental human needs

Human needs	Brief description
Subsistence/survival	Have physical and mental health
Protection	Receive care and consideration
Affection	Be shown respect and generosity
Understanding	Have opportunities to exercise capacities such as curiosity and intuition
Participation	Be valued as a participant
Leisure	Have opportunities to experience tranquillity and spontaneity
Creativity	Have opportunities to exercise imagination, curiosity and inventiveness
Identity	Experience a sense of belonging and self-esteem
Freedom	Have opportunities to express autonomy and open-mindedness

Human nature, human potential and human resources

The second approach to describing human nature is the identification of what could be seen as human potential. Again, there are a range of views. For example, Younkins (2010) proposes that the principal areas of potential are:

  i. an intent to thrive and live to maturity;
 ii. an ability to think rationally and formulate personal views and perspectives;
iii. an insatiable curiosity to make sense of the world;
 iv. a determination to achieve self-improvement;
  v. an ability to consider implications of actions and plan ahead;
 vi. an ability to take account of others and the environment in decision-making; and
vii. an ability to attribute value to particular features and actions.

Human potential has also been described as relating to that which we are able to accomplish. These are often referred to as human resources. The list above can be interpreted as embracing human resources. For example (ii) infers the ability to reason, (iv) infers the potential to self-reflect and make decisions, and (vi) infers an ability to be sensitive towards others. However, a frequently used way to look at human resources is from the perspective of capabilities. Capabilities have been developed by two authors, Sen (1993) and Nussbaum (2000), and have been discussed fully both in Whitehead (2010) and earlier in this text. As explained in Chapter 4, capabilities can be described as 'functionings' or what humans are capable of being and doing. Nussbaum's (2000) list includes, inter alia, the senses, emotions, practical reason, and control over one's environment. As explained in the earlier chapter, Nussbaum is working from a social justice perspective, and argues that all humans have the right to develop and use their potentials or capabilities throughout life. From this perspective, the link between human flourishing and human potential might be expressed as a situation in which individuals have the opportunity to draw on and enhance their individual potential. It was argued earlier in this text that there is a strong case for physical literacy to be seen as a human capability in its own right, in addition to playing a part in many other capabilities. On these grounds, as a unique and significant mode of human functioning, physical literacy can be recognised as a valid aspect of human nature. If human flourishing is to some extent tied to optimising human potential, the fostering of physical literacy as a capability would seem to gain both credibility and value.

The aforementioned broad description of human flourishing could be developed to read as 'living a rich and rewarding life with the opportunity and freedom to address and develop those human needs and potentials to which an individual attributes the most value'. In other words, human flourishing is most likely to be achieved in situations perceived as valuable on account of personal needs being satisfied and personal potentials being fostered. While humans share common needs and potentials, each person is a unique being, and in this context the specific nature of human flourishing will be particular to the individual.

Human nature and the nature of humans as essentially embodied

A final area in which to consider the relationship of physical literacy to human nature, and thus to human flourishing, returns to the philosophical roots of the concept, now substantiated by cognitive scientists. This was referred to briefly in Chapter 4. While this perspective builds from the notion of the human embodied nature being a significant resource – among other resources, a further important perspective is the notion that movement capability contributes to human nature by being the ground of wider holistic development.

This will be exemplified in looking briefly at the role of the embodied dimension in interacting with the world, the centrality of movement in early development, and the way that our embodied nature infiltrates life as we grow from early childhood to adulthood and into older adulthood.

The role of the human embodied dimension in interaction with the world, and the influence this has on the realisation of becoming fully human, has been covered both in Whitehead (2010) and in Chapter 4 in this text. To reiterate the position set out earlier, it was explained that humans perceive and act on the world from the perspective of an embodied being. All perception, and much understanding, is imbued with human bodily nature. This would seem to signal that human nature and human embodiment are inseparable. The importance of interaction with the world springs from the view put forward by existentialists, who propose that humans create themselves as they interact with the world. It follows that all those avenues through which contact is made with the environment are significant in life. Gill (2000) describes the significance of human motility or embodied capability as the very vehicle through which individuals observe, interact with and respond to the world around them. In this interrelationship, the individual develops an embodied sense of self alongside enhanced perception, observation and fluent response. In addition, individuals come to know the world they inhabit. With reference to understanding the environment, Gibson (1979) refers to an appreciation of possibilities for action as presented by the world. He calls these affordances. Affordances describe the way that humans perceive how the world can be acted upon. Perception of affordances and the response to these are not readily appreciated as they function below the level of consciousness (see explanatory glossary). Gill (2000) refers to this situation via the work of Polanyi (1964), who describes embodiment as the axis of all tacit knowing and explains that we know much more than we can tell.

The role of movement in relation to human development and human functioning has in the past been predominantly approached from the dualistic perspective, with movement seen as of value particularly to facilitate other ends such as cognitive, emotional and social development. However, recently, psychologists have come to adopt a less dualistic position advocating that acting and knowing are inseparable (Carlson, 1997; Rosenbaum, 2005). As a result, more monist perspectives of our embodied nature have emerged, one of these being the notion of the primacy of movement. In this respect, humans are judged as innately moving beings, and from the earliest stages of life have an insatiable curiosity that stimulates a desire to move. There seems an inbuilt urge to interact and engage with the immediate environment to make sense of the world (Almond and Myers, 2017). This is true throughout life, but during early years movement is especially important as infants and children are drawn to explore the world around them. In this interaction, they come to know themselves and gain confidence as they gradually become aware of the nature of the environment. The child's urge to move provides the very source of their capacity for optimal development. It is argued that the importance of the very early movement experiences cannot be underestimated. As Sheets-Johnstone (2000) explains, in the early months of life, 'we were all apprentices of our own bodies: we learn our bodies and learn to move ourselves' (p. 344). Similarly, Goddard-Blythe (2004) talks about movement being the essential stimulus to human development, including the cognitive and the affective as well as the physical domain. This incidence of embodied activity contributes significantly to fulfilling the needs to explore and be creative and at the same time realise potential in unlocking innate human resources. The physiological thinking behind this claim makes for a fascinating read (Haggard et al., 2002; Gibbs, 2006; Barton, 2012). It is remarkable that this desire to move, through which children learn so much, does not require instruction or intervention. All that is needed is an environment rich in variation, stimulation, and importantly contexts in which they are free to move. The early development of the child who is stimulated by exploring the world through movement can be seen as the very first step in developing a platform whereby physical literacy can be nurtured, and subsequently contribute to human flourishing.

A reliance on movement does not fade after early childhood. In fact, it is claimed that the human embodiment underpins and permeates many aspects of human nature throughout life. For example, Lakoff and Johnson (1999) discuss the role of movement in the formation of concepts and in language development, while Leder

(1990) refers to Merleau-Ponty's view that 'abstract cognition itself may sublimate but never fully escapes its inherence in a perceiving, acting body' (p. 7).

Much of the recent work on the holistic nature of the human condition does not single out embodied potential, but sees it as intimately involved in most other human characteristics. For those interested in this line of enquiry, there are numerous leads to follow. The work of Gibson (1979) signals this perspective in claiming that perception and action operate in concert. Terms in neuroscience that describe this view are 'embodied cognition', 'enactivism' and 'essentially embodied existence'. Embodied cognition is championed by Gibbs (2006) and Adams (2010). Central to this view is the assertion that embodied activities shape human cognition (Gibbs, 2006: 10). Enactivism, which is discussed by Varela et al. (1993) and Hutto and Myin (2013), echoes existentialism in being a philosophy in which cognition is described as arising through a dynamic interaction between an acting organism and its environment. The notion of an 'essentially embodied existence' is proposed by Maiese (2016). She writes that the 'self is nothing more and nothing less than a dynamic, minded, living, essentially embodied process – in effect a life form or a form of life' (p. xiii). This is a useful quotation as it draws together many of the ideas encompassed in the new thinking. These developments are thought-provoking, very valuable and warrant examination. Above all, they signal a radical change in the way human embodiment is conceived by many of those working in this field.

These perceptions of human nature as being rooted in the human embodied presence in the world would seem to underwrite the proposal that physical activity, action and embodiment constitute an essential aspect of human nature. Human embodied potential is deeply embedded in most aspects of human nature, and this signals a central role for human embodiment, and thus for physical literacy within human flourishing.

Conclusion

In this chapter, the notion that human flourishing has a close relationship with human nature raised the question as to how far human embodied potential could be seen as integral to human nature.

The relationship between human nature and human needs, potentials and resources was outlined, and the contribution of physical literacy to both these areas was noted. Next, the view of the human as essentially embodied was discussed. From the wealth of debate around this area, three perspectives were taken. These were the contribution of embodiment to the essential ongoing interaction between the individual and the world, the role of the human embodiment in early development, and finally the place of embodiment in the new thinking about the 'essentially embodied existence'. In all these respects, there was evidence that human embodiment is an integral feature of human nature and human life. This gave further legitimacy to the claim that physical literacy can make a valuable, and perhaps essential, contribution to realising human nature, and thus human flourishing.

References

Adams, F. (2010) Embodied cognition. *Phenomenology and the Cognitive Sciences*, 9(4): 619–628.

Alkire, S. (2002) Dimensions of human development. *World Development*, 30(2): 181–205.

Almond, L. and Myers, L. (2017) Physical literacy and the primacy of movement. *Physical Education Matters*, 12(1): 19–21.

Barton R.A. (2012) Embodied cognitive evolution and the cerebellum. *Philosophical Transactions of the Royal Society*, 367: 2097–2107.

Carlson, R.A. (1997) *Experienced Cognition*. Mahwah, NJ: Lawrence Erlbaum Associates.

Doyal, L. and Gough, I. (1991) *A Theory of Human Need*. Basingstoke, UK: Macmillan.

Gibbs, R.W. (2006) *Embodiment and Cognitive Science*. Cambridge: Cambridge University Press.

Gibson, J. (1979) *The Ecological Approach to Visual Perception*. Boston, MA: Houghton Mifflin.

Gill, J. (2000) *The Tacit Mode: Michael Polanyi's Postmodern Philosophy*. Albany, NY: State University of New York Press.

Goddard-Blythe, S. (2004) *The Well Balanced Child*. Glocestershire, UK: Hawthorn Press.

Haggard, P., Clark, S. and Kalogeras, J. (2002) Voluntary action and conscious awareness. *Nature Neuroscience*, 5: 382–385.

Hutto, D.D. and Myin, E. (2013) *Radicalizing Enactivism*. Cambridge, MA: MIT Press.

Kekes, J. (2000) The meaning of life. In P. French and H. Wettstein (eds), *Midwest Studies in Philosophy, Volume 24: Life and Death – Metaphysics and Ethics*. Malden, MA: Blackwell, pp. 17–34.

Lakoff, G. and Johnson, M. (1999) *Philosophy in the Flesh*. New York: Basic Books.

Leder, D. (1990) *The Absent Body*. Chicago, IL: University of Chicago Press.

Maiese, M. (2016) *Embodied Selves and Divided Minds*. Oxford: Oxford University Press.

Manfred, A., Max-Neef, M., Elizalde, A. and Hopenhayn, M. (1989) *Human Scale Development: Conception, Application and Further Reflections*. New York: Apex.

Maslow, A.H. (1970) *Motivation and Personality*, 2nd edn. New York: Harper & Row.

Nussbaum, M.C. (2000) *Women and Human Development: The Capability Approach*. Cambridge: Cambridge University Press.

Polanyi, M. (1964) *Personal Knowledge*. New York: Harper & Row.

Ramsay, M. (1992) *Human Needs and the Market*. Aldershot: Avebury.

Rosenbaum, D.A. (2005) The Cinderella of psychology: the neglect of motor control in the science of mental life and behavior. *American Psychologist*, 60: 308–317.

Sen, A. (1993) Capability and well being. In M. Nussbaum and A. Sen (eds), *The Quality of Life*. New York: Clarendon Press, pp. 30–53.

Sheets-Johnstone, M. (2000) Kinetic tactile-kinesthetic bodies: ontogenetical foundations of apprenticeship learning. *Human Studies*, 23(4): 343–370.

Varela, F.J., Thompson, E. and Rosch, E. (1993) *The Embodied Mind*. Cambridge, MA: MIT Press.

Whitehead, M.E. (ed.) (2010) *Physical Literacy throughout the Lifecourse*. London: Routledge.

Wilson-Strydom, M. and Walker, M. (2015) A Capabilities-friendly conceptualisation of flourishing in and through education. *Journal of Moral Education*, http://dx.doi.org/10.1080/03057240.2015.1043878.

Younkins, E.W. (2010) Human nature, flourishing, and happiness: toward a synthesis of Aristotelianism, Austrian economics, positive psychology, and Ayn Rand's objectivism. *Libertarian Papers*, 2(35): 1–49.

20

THE SIGNIFICANCE OF PHYSICAL LITERACY IN HUMAN LIFE, CONCLUSIONS AND THE WAY AHEAD

Margaret Whitehead

Introduction

As indicated in Chapter 1, the overarching intention of this book was to build from the introductory text *Physical Literacy throughout the Lifecourse* (Whitehead, 2010) to substantiate a case for the importance and value of fostering physical literacy. This intention issued in the consideration of three areas. First, there was a need to clarify certain aspects of physical literacy that were undermining the acceptance of the concept. Second, it was seen as significant and pertinent to share with readers how physical literacy was being adopted and developed across the world. Finally, it was judged legitimate to reflect on the positive messages conveyed in these narratives, and to propose that the concept has significant potential to contribute to the quality of life for all. This proposal of value was backed up by reference to life history research and the congruence of physical literacy with many aspects of human flourishing

Part I

Part I focused on clarification. The role of philosophy has been a barrier to some people accepting the concept. Hence, most chapters in Part I include a reminder for readers of the underlying philosophy and how this provides a rationale for many aspects of practice. As suggested in Chapter 5, it is asserted that 'the philosophical basis of physical literacy, far from being an impenetrable aspect of the concept, actually serves to clarify the nature of the work. There is nothing mystical about the philosophy; rather, it provides clear guiding principles'. The second area of clarification concerned the nature of the definition and the appropriateness of the use of the word 'literacy' alongside 'physical'. This was addressed in Chapter 2. Modifications to the definition were explained, and a case was made that the notion of 'literacy' was very much in line with descriptions of other aspects of human life. In addition, the case made by UNESCO in supporting the concept of literacy as encompassing valuable and productive communication between humans and their world was outlined.

Significant among the areas of clarification in Chapter 3 was the complex and contentious issue of the relationship between fundamental movement skills and physical literacy. A range of alternative views were shared, and these issued in a number of challenges. It is accepted that participants need to acquire a range of movement abilities, but these are only preliminaries to effective participation in a variety of contexts. Research is needed to ascertain certain aspects of movement development, the nature of the movement abilities that can cater for participation in all forms of physical activity, and the best way to foster these abilities so that they are readily drawn on in activity situations. Chapter 4 addressed the value of physical literacy to participants of all ages and endowments. In this chapter, a strong case was made for physical literacy to be accepted as a human capability in its own right. In addition, an argument was presented in which it was proposed that physical literacy can be seen as an end in itself, rather than predominantly a means to other ends.

Chapter 6 was designed to clarify the implications of adopting fostering physical literacy as an aspiration in physical activity. Building from broad principles based on the underpinning philosophy, key recommendations were set out. This overarching guidance was supported by short sections, each relating to different groups of participants. The rationale for including this specific guidance was to remind readers of the fact that physical literacy is not confined to, or only relevant in, the context of education. Chapter 6 addressed the contentious area of charting progress. This is a complex and challenging area. The IPLA principles were set out together with an example of an instrument designed to be used in all settings, with only minor modifications. Examples from Canada, the United States and Australia were included to show the huge amount of work and time that has been devoted to this area. The IPLA welcome all these developments, but would caution that in the interests of fostering physical literacy, the use of any instrument to chart progress should be a positive motivational experience for all participants.

In summary, Part I was designed to provide a sound and carefully thought through basis for arguing for serious consideration of the legitimacy of physical literacy. It is proposed that based on the underlying philosophy and the growing acceptance and adoption of the concept across the world, there are grounds for physical literacy to be respected, investigated and, as appropriate, adopted.

Part II

While Part II was compiled to set out how physical literacy is being developed across the world, it also serves to consider the answer to two questions. These are:

- Is there evidence that physical literacy is being acknowledged as a useful concept in countries across the world? In other words, have these narratives substantiated the claim for the value of the concept worldwide?
- Has the definition of physical literacy maintained its integrity in the context of different cultures?

With reference to physical literacy being acknowledged as a valuable concept across the world, there seems little doubt, in reading Chapters 8 to 15, that this is the case. Overall, physical literacy has been seriously considered and adopted in many sectors in the countries included. Many saw physical literacy as valuable in contributing to fostering physical activity throughout the lifecourse, playing a part in fighting obesity and contributing to overall quality of life for all. The introduction of physical literacy has initiated new thinking, new partnerships and new policies. In addition, governments have been made aware of the need to address problems associated with inactivity and consider a range of solutions. In academic circles, colleagues across the world have been motivated to carry out a wide range of research and write papers on a variety of aspects of physical literacy. Tribute must be paid to all those who have worked immensely hard to introduce the concept in their country, advocate and effect changes in practice, and lobby for support at all levels.

With reference to the adoption of the IPLA definition of physical literacy, there would seem to be evidence that, at root, this has been seen as acceptable and has retained its baseline integrity. As indicated in Chapter 2, looking across the definitions currently in use, all address the key aspirations of promoting participation in physical activity for all throughout life and the need to appreciate the holistic nature of each participant. Alongside these two aspirations most countries embrace a third consideration, being the unique nature of each participant. It is accepted that some differences in wordage will develop, but this can be seen to represent a considered adoption of the concept, under a description that is relevant to a particular context/culture/country, rather than the rejection of the core definition. Where the three guiding aspirations/considerations identified above provide the rationale for practitioners' work, there is every possibility that a lifetime habit of participation can be established.

Part III

Part III builds on the positive messages from the writers in the international perspective section of this text. There were two areas worthy of consideration: first, to reflect on the value of physical literacy to the individual; and second, to locate the experiences surrounding physical literacy in the wider context of enriching human life. The first generated an investigation into the use of life history research methods with individuals across the world, while the second issued in an investigation into human flourishing and how far physical literacy can be seen to play a part in securing this enviable human disposition.

Chapter 17 proposed that using a journey metaphor in respect of physical literacy, and subsequently adopting a life story/life history research method in respect of physical literacy journeys, had the potential to provide a deeper understanding of individuals' experiences. Examples were taken from individuals in Chile, The Gambia, the Netherlands and England. Experiences recounted by the first three individuals clearly demonstrated that involvement in physical activity was a very important aspect of their lives. Only one made physical activity the focus of his occupation, while the other two took part in physical activity in their non-working hours. Both these two people found physical activity rewarding and pleasurable, and while life circumstances changed, they repeatedly took steps to return to physical activity. Notwithstanding the fact that they came from very different cultural settings, for all three physical activity was an important contributor to the quality of their lives. For the fourth individual, physical activity had seldom been a positive experience, and while she occasionally had good intentions to be active, there was insufficient motivation to follow these through.

Examination of each of these life stories is very revealing, not least in the way that significant events and significant others both played a key part in the twists and turns in the journeys shared. From this brief consideration of individuals' physical literacy journeys, it might be suggested that irrespective of culture, physical activity, and hence physical literacy, has the potential to play a key part in enriching lives, thus making a positive contribution to human flourishing.

Chapter 18 considered the repeated claims that physical literacy enhanced the quality of life. Quality of life was interpreted as human flourishing, and the role of this chapter was to consider how far physical literacy can be seen as contributing to this desirable state of being.

It is interesting to note that, as indicated in Chapter 16, the notion of physical literacy as contributing to well-being and human flourishing is alluded to by all writers, with colleagues in New Zealand, Canada, Wales, continental Europe, Scotland and India specifically identifying this view.

It was argued in Chapter 18 that there are three principle areas of alignment between the two concepts: first, the two concepts share similar philosophical roots; and second, characteristics of human flourishing such as inclusivity and individuality were advocated by proponents of physical literacy. In respect of these two areas, there was evidence of a potentially productive interrelationship between human flourishing and physical literacy. In addition, for someone to be said to be flourishing, it is suggested that the individual should show evidence of a number of constituent personal traits, such as autonomy, self-acceptance and optimism. Examination of physical literacy alongside these traits indicated that promoting this disposition can make a valuable contribution to each trait. In this way, fostering physical literacy cannot only enhance life via increasing breadth of opportunity; it can at the same time make a positive contribution to overall human flourishing.

Chapter 19 focused on the notion that human flourishing was, to a considerable extent, tied to aspects of human nature. This posed the question as to the relationship of physical literacy to human nature. The three sections of this chapter relate to: physical literacy and human needs; physical literacy and human potential; and human embodiment as the ground of human existence. It was suggested that in fostering physical literacy, many human needs were being fulfilled, such as developing self-esteem, understanding, creativity and self-actualisation. Furthermore, it was proposed that as a human capability, physical literacy highlighted a human potential or resource. In both these ways, physical literacy was closely related to capitalising on aspects of human nature, and thus contributing to human flourishing. Finally, readers were reminded that from a philosophical point of view, individuals create themselves in interaction with the world. This interaction is significantly realised via human embodied interaction with the world. In fact, interaction plays a key role in early development, and subsequently in many aspects of life. Human nature is essentially expressed from the perspective of an embodied being. In this way, physical activity, and thus physical literacy, is not just an expression of human nature; it is constitutive of human nature.

Conclusion

The series of arguments that have been worked through in this book would seem to indicate that there is growing support for the notion of physical literacy. The spread of the concept across the world evidences broad interest in and acceptance of the concept. The life histories shared are revealing and begin to show potential for this type of research. Much can be learnt from the twists and turns in the journeys and the fulfilment achieved through participation in physical activity. In addition, the close alignment between physical literacy and human flourishing provides the makings of a secure foundation for justifying the value of physical literacy for all, whatever age, whatever endowment and whatever culture in which they live.

It is reassuring to know that, notwithstanding cultural differences, perception of the value of physical literacy is recognised across the world. Given that humans are at root embodied beings, this widespread perception of value is not surprising. The fact that the three key principles of physical literacy, being the commitment to lifelong participation, the perception of individuals as holistic beings, and the acceptance of the uniqueness of each individual, are broadly accepted and enacted would seem to indicate that the concept is both flexible and robust. In sum, with reference to the areas addressed in this text, there would seem to be evidence that physical literacy can be supported as both relevant to all and at the same time can accommodate interpretations that reflect different countries and cultures across the world.

Postscript

That the concept of physical literacy is gaining recognition and respect should not mask the fact that there is still a great deal of work to do. In reviewing the material covered in this text, the following areas warrant attention and action:

1. The creation of an international advisory board to support development in countries across the world (see Chapters 7–16).
2. Continued collaboration with countries across the world, each with their unique culture, to substantiate the value of physical literacy in its contribution to human flourishing (see Chapters 18 and 19).
3. The development of research into physical literacy journeys from across the world, in the form of life histories, to identify key determinants of fostering physical literacy (see Chapter 17).

4. The gathering of models of good practice from across the world in respect of different constituencies such as coaching and working with those with particular needs (see Chapter 5).
5. The establishment of an international working party to progress the development of instruments to chart progress across all age ranges and constituencies (see Chapter 6).
6. The establishment of an international study group to take a lead in securing close and productive links between theory and practice (see Chapter 16).
7. Further study into the nature of the human condition, particularly the central role of, and the relationship between, the lived body and the living body (see Chapter 4).
8. The development of knowledge concerning the relationship between phylogenetic development and ontogenetic development of movement in the young child, and between basic movement techniques and movement patterns apposite to a wide variety of physical activity situations (see Chapter 3).

References

Whitehead, M.E. (ed.) (2010) *Physical Literacy throughout the Lifecourse*. London: Routledge.

EXPLANATORY GLOSSARY

Early years movement development

Ontogenetic development: Development that occurs as a child matures. Genetically programmed. Outcome of nature.

Phylogenetic development: Development that occurs as a result of learning. Environmentally dependant. Outcome of nurture.

In the early years, there is a reciprocal relationship between ontological physical development and learning that supports physical competence. Growth opens up new possibilities for developing phylogenetic physical competence while increasing competence stimulates growth. In this way, at this stage, development and learned competence go hand in hand.

Meaningful experiences

The concept of meaningful movement experiences is frequently referred to as being important in fostering physical literacy. For an experience to be meaningful, it needs to be purposeful, engaging, relevant and rewarding.

A purposeful experience might be described as one that has a clear goal that is perceived as worthwhile by the participant. This goal is likely to be seen to have the potential to feed forward to further opportunities.

An engaging experience is one that attracts the full attention and application of the participant who is absorbed in the challenge.

A relevant experience is one that builds on from previous experiences that are significant to the individual.

A rewarding experience is one that issues in some element of progress, success, pleasure and satisfaction. In this context, it is likely to enhance self-confidence and self-esteem.

In the context of physical literacy, a meaningful experience could be characterised as one that, in fostering motivation, confidence, physical competence, and appropriate knowledge and understanding, issues in a growth of a commitment to sustain physical activity for life.

Physical illiteracy

The question is often asked whether a human being can be physically illiterate.

This is not a straightforward question. There are three perspectives that can be taken: two result in a rejection of the notion of physical illiteracy, and one supports there being a disposition we could call physical illiteracy.

First, it could be seen as a non-question. It was clarified elsewhere (Whitehead, 2010, 2013) that there is no fixed 'state' of being physically literate. It would follow from this that neither is there a fixed 'state' of being physically illiterate. Physical literacy is a disposition to capitalise on human embodied potential. Those who do not exhibit this disposition are simply not involved in this area of life. It is not that they are physically illiterate, but rather that they are not making any progress in respect of developing this human potential. From this perspective, physical illiteracy does not exist.

Second, human embodied beings rely on movement potential to stay alive. For example, humans speak, breathe and blink. In addition, for example, humans walk from room to room, carry out daily tasks concerned with hygiene and nourishment, and drive the car to work. In this sense, humans rely on movement to stay alive. To be alive is to move. Physical illiteracy cannot occur in a living being. From this perspective, physical illiteracy does not exist.

Third, there is the perspective that physical literacy is a term attributed to capitalising on the human potential to move, and in so doing interact with the world, learn more about themselves in the world and refine physical potential. As more is asked of physical potential, a human grows in self-mastery, becomes adept at interacting with the world, and co-creates with the world significant and rewarding experiences. These experiences are often described as meaningful, and have the potential to add to the vitality, excitement and quality of life. In these situations, it can be said that the individual has a positive attitude to physical activity and can be described as making progress on their physical literacy journey. From this perspective, those who avoid any movement beyond the absolute minimum needed to stay alive, and never ask more of their physical potential, could be described as physically illiterate. From this perspective, physical illiteracy could exist as a recognised disposition.

References

Whitehead, M.E. (ed.) (2010) *Physical Literacy throughout the Lifecourse*. London: Routledge.

Whitehead, M.E. (2013) The value of physical literacy. *ICSSPE Bulletin – Journal of Sport Science and Physical Education*, 65. Available at: www.icsspe.org/content/no-65-cd-rom (accessed 14 March 2019).

Embodiment

Embodiment in the context of physical literacy is best used as a description of the nature of the human being as manifest in the world. The term can be used as a noun, viz. human embodiment, or it can be used as an adjective, viz. embodied potential or embodied dimension.

While it is perhaps odd to use a noun to describe a state of being, the notion of human embodiment is a reminder that there is more to the human condition than a pseudo-mechanical object. Merleau-Ponty (1996) develops this idea in putting forward the view that the body should not be understood as a machine to be trained and disciplined. Rather, it should be understood as a preconscious disposition of human existence.

In the context of physical literacy, the term embodiment is used in preference to the term 'body', as 'body' has inescapable connotations with the human body as an object or instrument. This concept of the 'body' is too readily related to dualism, and is therefore to be avoided where possible. The section below sets out ideas concerning modes of the body or modes of embodiment.

References

Merleau-Ponty, M. (1996) *Phenomenology of perception* (translated by C. Smith). New York: Routledge.

Modes of embodiment/modes of the body

One of the key issues in the debate about the nature of human being concerns human embodiment. For many centuries in the developed world, debate centred on how the body and the mind related to each other. However, current philosophical thinking has moved on from this in its description of human being as characterised by an essentially embodied existence. This belief issues from the view that it is impossible to separate the body (or human embodiment) from the human mind.

What is now perplexing thinkers is how what are referred to as the 'two modes' of the body (or the embodiment) relate to each other.

These two modes are named the 'lived body' and the 'living body' (e.g. Maiese, 2016).

The 'lived body' is described as the embodiment as lived, operating below the level of consciousness as a perceptual faculty (see below).

The 'living body' is described as the functional body that we can consciously control. This could be understood as the body as object. Human consciousness allows humans to 'stand back' from their lived embodiment and view this aspect of themselves as an instrument.

This is a key area of research with which proponents of physical literacy need to keep abreast.

The notion of 'different bodies' is not new; Sartre (1957) refered to the body for self and the body for others, while in the Chinese language there are three words that refer to forms of human embodiment: *shen*, animate embodiment-as-lived; *ti*, inanimate embodiment-as-object or instrument; and *shi*, embodiment-as-corpse (Brownell, 1995).

References

Brownell, S. (1995) *Training the body for China: Sports in the Moral Order of the People's Republic.* Chicago, IL: University of Chicago Press.
Maiese, M. (2016) *Embodied Selves and Divided Minds.* Oxford: Oxford University Press.
Sartre, J.-P. (1957) *Being and Nothingness* (translated by H. Barnes). London: Methuen.

Human embodiment as a perceptual faculty

Human embodiment needs to be appreciated as having a perceptual faculty. This perceptual faculty generates meaning. In interacting with a physical aspect of the world, an awareness of a particular characteristic of this aspect is established. The aspect is thus endowed with a specific meaning. This meaning is created in the embodied interaction with an aspect of the world that involves use of the skeleto-muscular system. The way that this embodied system needs to be deployed in an interaction endows that feature of the world with a particular characteristic that is stored in the memory. These characteristics could be understood to describe how this aspect of the world can be related to (e.g. how it can be handled, how it can afford support). This perceptual information is generally held below consciousness. The interrelationship between the 'living body' and the 'lived body' in the context of perception is currently subject to debate.

All incidences of interaction and simultaneous perception are initiated by the human characteristic of intentionality. Intentionality is a term used to describe the innate and insatiable urge humans exhibit to relate to the world (Whitehead, 1990, 2010). One outcome of this urge to develop an embodied relationship with the world is the establishment of affordances (see below).

On account of our embodied nature and of the fact that human embodiment provides the fundamental way of interacting with the world, the world 'known' by humans is imbued with characteristics generated by the human embodied perceptual faculty.

References

Whitehead, M.E. (1990) Meaningful existence, embodiment and physical education. *Journal of Philosophy of Education*, 24(1): 3–13.
Whitehead, M.E. (ed.) (2010) *Physical Literacy throughout the Lifecourse.* London: Routledge.

Affordances

Affordances are generally described as opportunities for action in the environment of an organism. There is a sense in which features in the world 'call for' a particular response.

They invite involvement of an aspect of the human embodied capability. In other words, features/objects present themselves as 'climbable' or 'requiring a certain amount of power or care in their handling' or 'unstable'.

Affordances are endowed on features in the world on account of their having been involved in previous interaction. Once there has been contact with a feature, this experience becomes part of memory and is drawn on in future encounters. Affordances are not self-generated characteristics; they arise from previous interaction.

The concept of affordances was initially proposed by Gibson (1979) but has been picked up and analysed by other writers (e.g. Sanders, 1999), who proposes that individuals only respond to perceived affordances in situations that they choose to be the most desirable. Rietveld and Kiverstein (2014) argue for the need to widen the scope of affordances from a focus principally on features of the world to include all aspects of the sociocultural context.

It is interesting to note that the notion of affordances was an element of Merleau-Ponty's (1968) work. He created the concept of the chiasm to describe the intertwining of the human being with the world. In a sense, this concept brings together the existential notion of interaction between the individual with the world, the embodied perceptual potentialities of the human, the characteristics of the world, and indeed affordances. It is a cycle that cannot be taken apart, as that which is understood about the world has been generated by characteristics of the embodied human being. We are through and through beings in the world and of the world, and the world we inhabit is the world we create.

References

Gibson, J.J. (1979) *The Ecological Approach to Visual Perception*. Boston, MA: Houghton Mifflin.

Merleau-Ponty, M. (1968) *The Visible and the Invisible*. Evanston, IL: Northwestern University Press.

Rietveld, E. and Kiverstein, J. (2014) A rich landscape of affordances. *Ecological Psychology*, 26: 325–352.

Sanders, J. (1999) Affordances: an ecological approach to first philosophy. In G. Weiss and H.F. Harber (eds), *Embodiment: The Intersections of Nature and Culture*. New York: Routledge, pp. 121–141.

AUTHOR INDEX

Almond, L. 10, 30, 45, 57, 65, 154–155, 182, 197, 273–274, 269, 271
Archer, M.S. 33, 44
Arnold, P. 38–39, 44
Ashworth, S. 49, 57

Barnett, L.M. 20–22, 25, 30–31, 106, 108, 114, 119, 120–124, 145, 154, 182, 197
Biggs, J. 116–117, 120

Cairney, J. 90, 94, 106, 120–121, 182, 197
Canadian Fitness and Lifestyle Research Institute 128–129, 130–131, 135, 139–140
Canadian Heritage 140, 127–131, 140–141
Chen, A. 49, 56, 181–182, 197
Clark, A. 33, 44
Claxton, G. 33–34, 44
Corbin, C. 205, 213

Dekkers, W. 144, 154
De Ruyter, D. 255, 264
Dewey, J. 24, 30
Duda, J. 53, 56–57
Dudley, D. 30, 94, 106–107, 116, 120–122, 183, 196–197
Durden-Myers, E. 21, 30, 44–45, 49, 56–57, 123, 186, 189, 258–259, 264

Edwards , L. 118, 121–123, 182, 188, 197

Freire, P. 17–18

Gibbs, R. 169–171, 282
Gibson, I. 189
Gibson, J. 269–271
Gill, J. 34, 44, 268–269, 271
Goddard-Blyth, S. 60, 269–271
Goodson, I. 241, 254
Gordijn, C. 147, 154
Gulbin, J.P. 110, 121

Heritage School India 195, 164

IPLA 4, 7, 18–19, 27, 30, 76–78, 83, 93–94, 101

Johnson, M. 33, 44, 239, 259, 269, 271
Jurbala, P. 26, 30, 139, 141, 148, 154

Keegan, R. 111–112, 114–115, 121–123, 197
Kekes, C. 260, 264–265, 271
Keyes, C. 257, 260, 263, 264
Kiez, T. 14, 19
Kirk, D. 21, 30, 49, 56–57, 108, 121–122, 155
Kriellaars, D. 14, 18, 88–90, 94, 121, 197, 214

Lakoff, G. 239, 254, 269, 271
Leder, D. 269, 271
Lodewyk, K. 87–88
Longmuir, P. 86, 94, 133, 141, 190–192, 198
Lounsbery, M. 107, 122, 205, 213
Lundvall, S. 182, 198, 205, 213

Maiese, M. 33, 44, 270–271, 280–281
Maslow, A. 266, 271
Maude, P. 60, 63, 57
McKenzie, T. 107, 122, 205, 213
Merleau Ponty, M. 31, 144, 270, 280, 283
Morgan, K. 30, 53, 121, 197
Mosston, M. 49, 57

Nussbaum, M. 34–36, 44, 265–267, 271

Oliver, K. 53, 57

ParticipACTION 86, 127, 141–142
Physical and Health Education Canada
    87–88, 126–127, 132, 141–142
Polanyi, M. 34, 44, 269, 271
Pot, N. 20, 22–23, 25, 30, 264

Randall, L. 92–93, 132, 142
Rasmussen, D. 256–259, 264
Robinson, D. 25, 92–93, 108, 123, 132,
    135, 142
Robyens, I. 34, 44
Roetert, E.P. 205, 207, 212–214
Ryff, C. 157, 260, 263–264

Sanders, J. 122–123, 282
Sartre, J-P. 280–281
Saura, S. 24, 31
Sen, A. 34, 44, 267, 271
SHAPE America 90–91, 95, 100–101,
    202–205, 214, 232, 235

Sheets-Johnstone, M. 269, 271
Sport Australia 91–92, 105–106, 110,
    115–118
Sport England 4
Sport New Zealand 100–102, 167–168, 180
Sport Wales 100, 102, 179, 215–219,
    220–224, 226–229
Standal, O. 9, 18, 22, 24, 31, 34, 44
Sykes, P. 241

Taplin, L. 240–241, 254
Telford, R. 106, 108, 120, 122–124
Tremblay, M. 86–87, 94, 190–192

UNESCO 4, 14–18, 106, 109, 124, 272

Valera, F. 33, 44
VanderWeele, T. 256–258, 264
Vasickova, J. 152, 155

Welsh Government 215–217, 219, 222,
    224, 226, 228–229, 232, 235
Whitehead, M.E. (2010) 3–5, 8–9, 13–14,
    19, 75–76, 82, 196, 256, 272, 279
Whitehead, M.E. *see* the reference lists for
    Chapters 1–6, 17–20 and Glossary
Wolbert, L. 257, 264

Younkins, E. 265, 267, 271

Zimmerman A. 24, 31
Zwozdiak-Myers, P. 53–54, 57

SUBJECT INDEX

aboriginal peoples 113, 134–136
achievement goal theory 49; *see also* motivation
active for life *see* lifelong
advocacy 103–107, 114, 162–163, 175–176, 212–215, 222–224; *see also* communication tools
affective domain 9, 11–12, 115, 127; in assessment 89–91; and different participants 61–66; and human flourishing 266–269; in journeys 240–241, 249–250; and monism 20, 52, 75–76; in practice 172, 187–190; in physical and food literacy 194–199
affordances 34, 269, 281–282
all ages *see* lifelong
ambience of sessions 28, 48–49, 52–53, 56, 63, 68, 70–72
Aspen Institute 102, 103, 114, 119, 142, 202, 207, 209, 213
Assessment 74–96: in Australia 91–92, 106, 108, 112; in Canada 86–90, 125, 132–133, 139; in Europe 148; and fundamental movement skills 24; in India 162; instruments 86–92, 132–134; ipsative 25,67; for learning 53, 57, 62, 64, 83; misunderstandings 84–85; operationalization 51, in Scotland 183, 193; in United States 90–91, 203; *see also* charting progress
attributes of physical literacy 5, 11–13, 16, 20, 27, 30, 45–48

Australia 105–125; assessment 91–92, 106, 108, 112, coaching in 112, 115–116; Council for Health in 106, 109; cultural context 105; curriculum in 106–107, 109, 112; defining statements in 115; Delphi procedure 171; health in 106–113, 115–116; lifelong 92, 95, 105–106, 115; partnerships 113; physical education in 106–109, 113, 116; Physical Literacy Standards Framework in 91–92, 114, 116, 118; research in 105–111, 114–115, 119; sport 113, 116–117; strategic planning 105
awareness of physical literacy 87, 99–100, 132, 167, 171–172, 175–176, 206, 210, 216, 221

body: modes of 280–281; lived 33–36, 22, 280–281; living 33, 35, 280–281; *see also* embodiment

Canada 125–143; assessment in 86–90, 132–134; coaching in 128, 131, 135; consensus definition in 125, 127, 130, 139; disabilities in 134, 137; education in 125, 127–134, 138–139; health in 125–137; lifelong 126; multi-sector involvement 131–132; PHE in 125–137; physical education in 127, 129–132, 137, 139; recreation in 125–129, 131, 137–113 research in 127, 129, 132–139; sport in 125–129,131–133; Sport for

All(S4L) in 103, 125–126, 128, 131–138;
Vivo (adults) 129; women and girls
in 134–137; working with minorities
134–138
capabilities 24, 34–37; and life skills 39–41;
and Nussbaum 34–36; and Sen 34, 267
challenges for the participant 11, 24, 27,
35, 39–43, 50–55, 61–64, 71–72
challenges to establish physical literacy:
issues from across the world 99,
230–234; and charting progress 79–81;
meaningful experience 278; in New
Zealand 167,169, 172; in Scotland
190–191; in United States 201–203,
207, 211–213; in Wales 224–225
charting progress 74–95; IPLA draft 78–81;
ipsative assessment 25, 42, 52, 67, 76,
262; instruments 85–95, 132–134;
misunderstandings 85
child development 42, 58–63
clarification of physical literacy 19–31; goal
or process 26
coaching 46, 58, 65–67, 85, 89, 103, 232,
277; see also Australia; Canada; United
States; Wales
cognitive domain 9, 11–13, 20, 29, 91–92;
in Australia 107, 112–116; in Canada
127, 130, coverage in charting progress
75–76, 79–80, 84–85, 89; and human
flourishing 266–269; and journeys
240–241, 249; in New Zealand
172–180; in Scotland 196–198; in
United States 203; working to promote
40–41, 50–52, 61–66
collaboration 102–104, 233–236; in
Australia 105–109; in Canada 128–134;
in Europe 148–154; in New Zealand
171–179; in Scotland 192; in United
States 207, 212; in Wales 216, 226
commitment to physical literacy; benefits
41–42, 62–66, 70; in Canada 126;
clarification 24–30; in definition x, 4–6,
8, 10–12 22–24, 276, 279; in Europe
147; in journeys 249–250, 252; in
Scotland 196; in United States 209
communication tools 219, 221, 223
community 4, 14–15, 17, 103, 126,
129, 131, 134–138, 160–163, 177;
community sport 101, 167–168,
170–171, 175, 178–179
confidence 8, 11–12, 26–30, 35, 37, 39,
41–43; in Australia 115–116; in Canada
127, 129, 133, 136, 138; in charting
progress 74–84, 86–93; in Europe

154, 160; in New Zealand 167–169;
in operationalising 47, 52, 55, 60–68,
71–73; in Scotland 181, 184, 186,
192–195; self-confidence 40, 43, 56, 63,
65, 68, 182; in United States 201–202,
209–214; in Wales 215–218
content of sessions 48–50, 66, 73, 83, 86,
145, 148, 165, 191, 233
context for the adoption of physical literacy
100–101
culture 3, 10, 15–17, 23, 25, 233–234,
273–276; in Australia 105, 109, 112,
116, 118–119; in Canada 125, 136; in
Europe 143, 147, 152, 154; in India
158, 162–165; and journeys 249,
252–254; in Scotland 168, 170, 173,
179; in United States 182, 185, 191,
196; in Wales 222, 225–227

Delphi exercise 114–116, 122, 231
disability see particular needs
dissemination 151, 165, 203
domains 5, 9, 11, 13–14, 20; in Canada
127; in charting progress 78–83; in
Europe 154; in New Zealand 170, 174;
in operationalising 50–51, 62–63; in
United States 184–196; see also affective
domain; cognitive domain; physical
domain
dualism 9, 32, 34, 62, 84

early years: characteristics 27; charting the
journey 83; child development 22, 278;
implications for physical literacy 59–63;
relevance 6, 254; in Scotland 182, 197;
in Wales 221–223
elements of physical literacy 55, 72, 76, 82,
84, 127, 172
embodiment 8–16, 20, 22, 275–276,
279–282; in Australia 106, 118; in
Canada 135, 138; and capabilities
32–38; and charting progress 78–82; in
Europe 145–148; and human flourishing
263, 268–270; and journeys 240–241;
in New Zealand 169; see also body;
embodied dimension
embodied dimension 8, 19, 13–15, 34–37
empathy 43, 68, 112, 250, 254, 263
enactivism 33, 270–271
essentially embodied existence 33, 270, 280
Europe 143–156; adoption of physical
literacy 145–147; assessment 148;
curriculum development 147–150;
Dutch physical education 146–147;

Europe wide variations 151–155; history of physical education in Europe 143–144; lifelong 152–154; philosophical traditions 143–146; research in 144, 149, 151–152, 154; sport in 146–151
evidence based education 114, 145, 197
existentialism 10, 17–18, 28, 32, 48, 76, 138, 240, 163, 270

food literacy 15, 16, 36, 102, 181, 184, 186, 185–195
Foundation-Talent-Elite-Mastery (FTEM) Model (Australia) 110, 121
fundamental movement skills 5, 19–25; across the world 102, 231; in Australia 106–108; in Canada 126–127; in Europe 145–146, 148–149; in New Zealand 156, 171–172; and research 273; in Scotland 182
future plans 119, 139, 154, 165, 179, 212, 228, 276–277

games for understanding 28, 149
girls and women 135–137, 194; journeys of 242–244, 246–249

health and well-being: in attributes 12; in capabilities 35–36; in charting progress 81–86; in health literacy 14–16; and human flourishing 244–245, 253–256, 263; and human needs 267; life skills 41–43; value 62–64, 69, 72; see also Canada, United States, Wales
Heritage School India 159
high quality physical education 29–30
holism see monism
human flourishing 4, 6, 18, 145, 187, 227, 235, 253–271, 274–276; and assessment 262; characteristics of 267–270, 275; constituents of 260–261, 270, 275
human nature 265–271; human needs 266–267

implications of adopting physical literacy 45–73
India 156–166; advocacy 160–161; assessment 162; becoming aware of physical literacy 157–158; cascade method in 160, 162; caste in 159; coaches 161; cultural context/philosophy 158–159, 164; community in 160–163; lifelong 163; National Curriculum 159, 171; physical literacy champions in 16; physical literacy 'days'

in 163; physical literacy teachers in 161–162, 164–165; research in 158–160, 165; resource institute in 162; traditional cultural games in 165; way ahead 165
individual as unique 10, 12–13, 24, 101, 274, 276; and charting journeys 74–76; and human flourishing 262; in journeys 27–29, 240–242; in operationalising physical literacy 48, 52–55, 61, 65–68, 71; in United States 203; value 36, 41–43; in Wales 215, 228
intentionality 281
IPLA 4, 5, 11, 19, 37, 41, 74–76, 93, 101–102, 234, 273; and charting progress 5, 75–85, 193–194, 230, 273; future plans 276–277; video 4; working with others 4, 6; in Europe 153; in India 157–158, 160; in New Zealand 169, 179; in Scotland 192; in United States 212; in Wales 221, 223, 232, 234

journeys 239–254

knowledge and understanding see cognitive domain

learning/teaching approaches 48–50, 58–73
leisure 15–16, 46, 58, 162, 185, 266, 268; personnel 70–71
life histories/life stories see journeys
life skills 39–41
lifelong 9, 85; charting progress 77; clarification 26; in definition 11–17, 4; developing commitment 62, 65; as a goal 9, 85; in human flourishing 259, 267; and journeys 253–254; and value 10, 27, 38, 42–44; see also Australia, Canada, Europe, India, United States
Lifestyles Of Our Kids (LOOK) project (Australia) 106, 108
Literacies 14–17; physical and food literacy 181–199; relations between literacies 102; see also health and well-being
long term athlete development (LTAD) 110, 125–128, 131, 134–138, 146, 151, 202, 206

maori peoples 102, 135, 168, 170, 179
meaningful experiences 15–16, 24–26, 40–41, 278–279; in Canada 137; and human flourishing 259–260; operationalising physical literacy 47, 50, 64; in Scotland 194; value 39
means and ends 5, 38–39, 256, 273

mental health 184, 200, 256, 267; stress 43, 247, 252; *see also* well-being
metaphor 148, 239–242, 251–253, 255, 274
modes of the body *see* body
monism 9–10, 17–18, 28, 32–35, 48, 76, 138, 141, 240, 256
motivation 108, 111–114, 126, 133–134, 146, 152, 176, 186, 212; in affective domain 11–12, 75, 115–116; and assessment 23, 76–92, 193; and health 261–262; in journeys 246, 249, 252; and life-long 167, 182; as means to physical literacy 47, 75; and philosophy 76; in promotion of physical literacy 52–53, 60–73, 218; value of 42–43, 75
movement: capacities 21–23, 61, 112; development 23, 59, 273, 278, forms 50, 55, 61, 64, 75; literacy 9; in definition of physical literacy 15, 17, 20–25, 41–42, 46; in Europe 146; and human flourishing 262–263; in operationalising physical literacy 50, 55, 61; patterns: in charting progress 76–79; and research 277; in Scotland 184
multi-sport organisations 207–208

National Governing Bodies of Sport (NGB) 103, 107, 202, 206–208, 225–227
New Zealand 167–181; coaching in 176; community settings 177–178; cultural context 174–175; educational settings 176–177; health issues 160, 162; 170–172, 175, 177–178; international collaboration 169–170; lifelong 167–187; next steps 175–179; play 176; research in 168–170, 172, 179; Sport New Zealand's approach to physical literacy 172–174; sport sector 171, 173–176 ; teacher training 174–175, 177; working in partnership 172–178, 181
next steps/future/way forward *see* future plans

obesity: in Australia 111; in Canada 86, 132–133 in Europe 154; in India 156; in Scotland 182, 184–185, 196; in United States 200–201; in Wales 226; world wide concern 100, 274
older adult population 27, 43, 46–47, 58, 72, 83, 113, 221, 252, 268
ontogenetic development 22, 268
operationalising physical literacy 45–73; with different age groups/constituencies

58–73; key recommendations 49–53; philosophy underpinning 47–53; planning for 54; ref content/method/ ambience 49–53; regarding programme structure 55
opportunities for considering physical literacy 101

particular needs 47, 103; in different countries 88, 103, 116, 137–138, 169, 207; implications of working with 68–69; in journeys 244–245, 252; value for those with 43
partnerships 102
pedagogical models 28–29
personal responsibility 8–9, 29; in Canada 127; in charting progress 82–83; with different groups 27; and human flourishing 257, 259–262, 266; and journeys 249, 251; and literacies 12, 15–17; in New Zealand 169, 173, 179; in Scotland 186–187; in United States 201; in Wales 222, 228; working to develop 41–44, 49–51, 62–67
phenomenology 10, 12, 28, 32, 48, 75–76, 138, 183, 188, 240–241, 256–257
philosophy: as basis of concept 10, 32, 34, 41, 100, 232, 270, 272–273; and charting journeys 74–83; in Europe 144–147; and human flourishing 255, 270; in India 157–158, 164–165; and journeys 240; in New Zealand 178, operationalising physical literacy 45–48, 50–56 65–67; in Scotland 185; in United States 211; in Wales 218, 223
phylogenetic development 22, 278
physical activity throughout life *see* lifelong
physical domain: physical competence 8, 11, 19–20, 24–30, 42, 101; and human flourishing 261; in Australia 105; in Canada 127, 130, 133; in charting progress 74–96; in journeys 241, 252; in New Zealand 169, in Scotland 186–187, 193–194; in United States 201; in Wales 218, 222; *see also* Fundamental Movement Skills
physical education: current situation 100; in Australia 10; and being physically educated 29, 30, 169; in Canada 130; in Europe 143, 146–147; and high quality 29–30 169; in India 159, 164; in New Zealand 170, 174; and physical literacy 3, 5, 28, 85, 108, 139, 143, 146, 176, 205; referred to in journeys 243,

245–246, 248–250; as related to health 102, 146–147, 204, 232; in United States 201–203; in Wales 216;
physical education teachers and physical literacy 28, 46, 58, 63, 113, 130, 160–164, 233
play 14, 35, 46, 52, 59–60, 71; in Australia 110; in Canada 139; in New Zealand 168, 177; in United States 210; in Wales 226–227
primary school 42, 46, 58, 60; in Australia 108, 113; in Europe 150; and journeys 246–248; in New Zealand 177; in Scotland 183, 185, 194
priorities for the future *see* future plans
policies and programmes to effect physical literacy 231–232
public health 99, 129, 131, 181, 188, 196

quality of life 15–16, 69, 81, 235, 272–275, 279; in Canada 128, 137; in India 159; in Scotland 181, 235, 272, 274–275, 279
quantified self 145

reflection by participants 36, 40–43, 51–52, 61–64, 73, 77–81, 100; in Australia 116–118; in Europe 150; and human flourishing 266–267; on journeys 242, 252–254; in Scotland 183, 189
reflection on physical literacy 6, 11, 14, 30, 91–93; in Australia 105; in Europe 152; in India 156; on journeys 242; in New Zealand 171–172, 178; in Scotland 181, 184; in Wales 226–227
reflection by teachers 53–56, 75, 192, 232, 252–254
relational paradigm 144
relevance throughout life *see* lifelong
research 4, 6, 86–88, 266, 273, 280; fundamental movement skills 21–25; and journeys 239, 241–242, 254, 272–274, 276; *see also* Australia; Canada; Europe; India; New Zealand; Scotland; United States; Wales
resources refer to IPLA website
responsibility *see* personal responsibility

Scotland 181–200; assessment 192–194; carrying out research 182, 188–192, 194; context 181–183; creation of advocacy material 183–185; creation of physical and food literacy 184–188; first steps 183–184; mounting training

courses 183–185, 192, 194; planning ahead 191–194; testing the concept 188–191
secondary school 27, 42, 177, 185, 216, 248, 250
sedentary behaviour 59, 61, 100; in Australia 111–112 in Europe 144, 153–154; reference journeys 248–249, 250–251; in Scotland 196; in United States 210, 212; in Wales 226
self-determination theory 49
self-reflective practice *see* reflection
self-perception 77–78, 100, 112, 261–262
session planning 53–54
significant events 251
significant others 28, 66, 67, 187, 241–242, 249–250, 254, 275
special educational needs/disability *see* particular needs
Sport England 4
sport identity 145
System of Observed Learning Outcomes (SOLO) Taxonomy 116–118

tacit knowledge 34, 269
talented athletes 42
teachers of physical education 28, 46, 58, 63, 113, 130, 160–164, 233
teaching approaches/methods *see* learning/ teaching approaches
traditional cultural games/sports 164–165, 171, 217, 223, 227
training of teachers 230, 233; in Australia 106, 112; in Canada 130, 133, 135–136; in continental Europe 147; in India 160–164; in New Zealand 174–175, 177; in Scotland 183–185, 190–194; in United States 207–209, 212–216; in Wales 216, 221, 227

UNESCO 4, 14–17, 106, 109, 124, 272
unit planning 53–54
United States 200–215; assessment 90–91, 203; coaching 202–203, 206–207, 210, 212; the cultural context 200–201; health 200–212; lifelong 201–215, 249; the military 204–205; multi-sports organisations 208–212; physical education 201–204; research in 200–201, 205, 212; sport 206–208; way ahead 212–213

value of physical literacy 32–44, 231–234, 272–274, 276; in Australia 107, 111;

in Canada 127; in context of human flourishing 255–271; in context of physical literacy journeys 239, 249, 251–252; in Europe 143–148, 152; in New Zealand 169–170, 73–74, 176, 178; in United States 200–203; in Wales 222, 225, 228
videos – Active for Life: IPLA 1; from Wales 219, 221, 224, 231

Wales 215–233; advocacy 227–228; beyond education 218–219; coaching in 223, 228, 232; communication and creation of materials; 219–222; in education 218, 222–227; going forward 228; health in 215–218, 221–228; physical education 216–218; reaching other constituencies 222–224; research in 216, 218, 228, 230–231: spreading the concept 217–218
way ahead *see* future plans
well-being 12, 20, 41, 43, 46, 232, 235, 275; in charting progress 77, 80; and human flourishing 256, 26; in India 159, 163; in journeys 250; in New Zealand 170, 177–179; in Scotland 184–190; in United States 21; in Wales 218, 222, 225–228